The Caregiver's Guide

The Caregiver's Guide

Helping Elderly Relatives Cope with Health and Safety Problems

Caroline Rob, R.N.
with Janet Reynolds, G.N.P.

HOUGHTON MIFFLIN COMPANY / BOSTON

Library of Congress Cataloging-in-Publication Data
Rob, Caroline.
The caregiver's guide : helping elderly relatives cope with
health and safety problems / Caroline Rob, with Janet Reynolds.
p.   cm.
Includes index.
ISBN 0-395-50086-9. — ISBN 0-395-58780-8 (pbk.)
1. Aged — Home care.   I. Reynolds, Janet.   II. Title.
RC954.R63   1991   91-4221
649.8 — dc20   CIP

Printed in the United States of America

Book design by Lisa Diercks

MP 10 9 8 7 6 5 4 3

This book, precisely as its title suggests, is a guide to help you do the best job you can of assisting an older person with medical and safety concerns and living arrangements, including the procurement of help from specialists. Many of the procedures discussed in the book necessitate instruction from a nurse or other health-care professional before they are applied in any individual's case. You should not perform procedures discussed in the book unless they are part of a care plan worked out with the older person's primary care physician. The author and publisher are not liable for adverse consequences arising from use of information presented in this book. Always contact your health-care provider if you have questions about how to provide care for any individual, and as a rule, always stay within the limits of your training and capabilities.

To my husband, Michel Zaleski,
to our children, Katharine and Olivia,
and to my parents, Charles and Mary Rob
— C.R.

Contents

Foreword

THE FASTEST-GROWING SEGMENT of the American population is people over the age of sixty-five. In 1880 this segment numbered less than 2 million, about 2 percent of the total U.S. population. A century later this age group had grown to more than 25 million, or 11.3 percent. By the year 2030, it is anticipated that 20 to 25 percent of our country's people will be over the age of sixty-five. While these numbers are impressive, what is even more interesting is the increase in the number of the "oldest old," those over the age of eighty-five, who often are frail and in need of support and caregiving. In 1980 the oldest old represented 1 percent of the total population, and they are expected to rise to 3 percent in 2030 and to more than 5 percent in 2050!

It is hard to predict what all this means for those who provide care for older relatives and friends. Nonetheless, we can assume that the burden of care will increase and will be borne primarily by family members, as older relatives experience decreases in mobility, visual acuity, hearing, and other bodily functions. Although entire families are often involved, 70 percent of the time the primary caregiver for a frail older American is a woman. It is said that the average American woman spends seventeen years raising children and eighteen years caring for aging parents.

During the child-rearing phase, parents can turn to a wealth of written material, including helpful "hands-on" information. Dr. Spock, Penelope Leach, Drs. Fries and Pantell, and others have written books with advice about when to call the doctor and other details on various health topics concerning children. Unfortunately, when this same parent has questions on care for her parents, no analogous books have been available until now. The caregiving daughter, son, friend, or spouse typically has had to fend alone in gaining accurate information about health topics affecting the older person.

The Caregiver's Guide is a book for families with aging relatives and friends. It provides sensible, basic information about chronic conditions to which the elderly are prone, and helps caregivers distinguish illness from normal aging. Because illness often presents differently in older people, problems too often can be ignored by older people or their families or even misdiagnosed by their doctors. Many of the symptoms of disease may incorrectly be ascribed to old age. Also, a symptom such as falling or confusion may be the result of medication side effects or of several different medical or surgical conditions. The book helps the caregiver learn that pneumonia may occur without fever or that a change in behavior may be the first clue to a heart attack.

The Caregiver's Guide helps readers recognize health problems for what they are and shows how to get them treated according to current standards of geriatric practice. The chapters are organized by conditions common in older people, making it easy to find information about specific problems such as memory loss, lung disorders, bladder problems, visual impairment, or cancer. The focus throughout the book is on providing up-to-date medical information on chronic disease and medication side effects, advice about medical emergencies, and concrete tips on handling both mental and physical conditions at home. Particularly valuable are the practical suggestions for optimizing function and the day-to-day management of geriatric conditions at home. The final chapter is a useful guide to accessing the social service system and network of support in communities around the country.

The book stresses that good communication is essential between doctors, patients, and caregivers. It also notes the importance of identifying a primary care physician who is especially knowledgeable and sensitive to the needs of older patients and who is in charge of the patient's overall care. The knowledge that *The Caregiver's Guide* provides can facilitate meaningful, constructive dialogue among all parties. This book will also help families, floundering through the medical system, to home in on suitable, satisfactory medical help and assist them in identifying appropriate alternatives.

The Caregiver's Guide is written by a medical journalist who is experienced in caring for elderly people, in collaboration with a nurse practitioner who runs a geriatric clinic. While most physician training is directed primarily toward the recognition and cure of disease, a nurse's training is directed toward managing patient care on a day-to-day basis, encouraging the highest possible independent function.

The Caregiver's Guide fills an important need. It is a useful addition to the resources available for older Americans and their families. I recommend it to people working with or caring for older adults. In caring for an older parent, spouse, friend, or patient, the goals and challenges are to help the person lead as normal a life as possible despite physical or mental impairments. *The Caregiver's Guide* will go a long way in supporting and helping caregivers meet this challenging goal.

Carol Hutner Winograd, M.D.
Associate Professor of Medicine
Chief of Clinical Programs in Geriatric Medicine
Stanford University School of Medicine

Director of Clinical Activities
Geriatric Research, Education and Clinical Center
Palo Alto Veterans Affairs Medical Center

Introduction

THIS BOOK HAD its genesis in a New York City hospital when I was taking care of Hap Hatton, a dear old friend who was ill. One night when I was looking for a nurse to do a second shift for me, Janet Reynolds, a supervisor and geriatric nurse practitioner, came to my rescue and helped me find a nurse to do the job.

Over the next year Janet became a mainstay for me and for my friend's extended family. She found solutions to difficult problems and always answered questions about my friend's condition honestly and forthrightly. She told us what to expect and how to prepare for contingencies — figuring out how Hap's case should be handled, where he should go for care, and who should take care of him. She was also helpful in advising us about how much and what kind of help we could provide for him at home.

Several months after Hap's death, Janet called me and suggested that because I was a nurse and a medical writer, I should write a book with some assistance from her about taking care of elderly parents or friends. As a geriatric nurse practitioner, Janet had much experience with families who were taking care of their older relatives. Along with a social worker she had started a caregiver support group at St. Vincent's Hospital in Manhattan, where she heard from the group's attendees that they had no resources to turn to for straightforward, practical information on how to help their parents cope with continuing medical problems and sudden illness. These caregivers were often confused and frightened about all their responsibilities and they wanted a source that would tell them what to do, much as Janet had told me what to do when I was caring for Hap.

It seemed like a great idea. I was aware that our population is aging rapidly and that it simply isn't true that Americans stick their old people into nursing homes or institutions as soon as difficulties become apparent. The truth is that most older people live at home, and when they get sick or debilitated in any way, they're usually cared for by their family — typically by their spouse or a daughter. Only when families have exhausted themselves in caring for the older person do they give in and decide to look for an institution that can provide full-time care. The idea of being able to provide information to family members and friends about how to give care themselves and procure it from others appealed to me enormously.

And so that's how we began. This work is designed for you, a person taking care of someone older who's debilitated in some way and who needs your help. Early on, we found dozens of books that spoke of the guilt, the frustrations, the isolation, the time constraints, the anger, and even the encroaching grief that come from watching someone you love deteriorate physically and sometimes mentally and emotionally. But nowhere did we find a "Dr. Spock" to help take care of an older parent, even though people today are likely to spend many more years caring for dependent older relatives than they put in caring for dependent children.

Here you have the book, we hope, that will fill that gap with the practical information you need. We tell you how to deal with the nitty-gritty questions about the older person's health condition in a way that effectively addresses how to manage it at home — wherever that may be.

We know that it's scary not to know whether you're doing the right thing, and whether doctors, indeed, are providing the best care possible — not just to treat the symptoms of the disease, but to treat the disease itself in a way that allows the older person as much independence, mobility, and pleasure in life as possible.

The chronic conditions and diseases that seem to increase with old age are confusing. We hope that after reading all we have to offer, you will be able to distinguish between an illness that needs quick medical attention and a condition that's normal to old age and can be managed successfully with minimal medical intervention or a change in daily routine, such as a change in diet or exercise.

We hope to clarify many issues you are likely to run into as your parent becomes older and more disabled. We tell you a lot about how older bodies age and how problems present themselves differently in an older person than they do in someone younger. (An older person can have a raging infection without a high fever. Similarly, an older person who has a heart attack may not feel chest pain like a younger person but instead may act mentally confused, ashen pale, and complain of not feeling "right.")

We give you information so that you can distinguish between illness and normal aging. If you have a relatively healthy older parent who has been active and energetic but suddenly begins acting slightly depressed, forgetful, and confused, you may wonder: Is this a sign of dementia? Is Mom or Dad losing it? Getting Alzheimer's? We hope that you'll learn here that if you see these signs you should suspect your parent's medication before anything else. Odds are that if a relatively healthy parent is on medication and suddenly becomes depressed or confused, it's the medication that causes the symptom, even if it's one she's been on for many years. If it's not that medication, you'll learn here which clues to look for, which questions to ask, and which doctor to see to explain this condition or learn what to do about it.

Similarly, we answer other questions that may come up as you care for your parent:

- Should my mother be on thirteen medications? If not, what can I do about it?
- If Grandpa has angina and is popping nitroglycerin pills, should he be? What do I do if I see him clutching his chest?
- If my parent gets a diagnosis of cancer, what's next? How do I know that the diagnosis is right, and how do I help in choosing the best course of treatment?
- What advice or support can I give if my mother whispers to me that my Dad can't hold his urine any more? What do you do in a case like this?

We know that because older people often see a variety of specialists for many conditions, it's hard to get the whole picture on their health. Rarely does any one doctor have the time to relay all the information needed about your parent's overall health and health management. Then too, doctors often don't know about the seemingly small details that are critical to a person's care and comfort at home. Nurses, who live their lives providing patient care, do know about these issues.

Janet and I, as nurses, hope to fill you in on that larger picture of your parent's health care and management. As nurses, we also intend to give you the most up-to-date and effective information that's available. We know that your job isn't easy. Often you are juggling your career, your marriage, and your children as well as caring for an older parent or relative. If the older person cannot be left alone during the day or night, or if you have to get up in the middle of the night, prepare all the meals, change sheets, or help your parent dress, your job is even more stressful. We hope to reduce your stress and make your job easier by providing you with a framework for understanding the older person's condition — a practical guide for making sense out of medical jargon and doing whatever it is you need to do to care for an older person at home in the best way possible. From this guide, you should know how to ask the right questions to translate any health-care professional's directions. You should know too where to go for at-home professional help when your parent or friend is about to return from the hospital after a stroke or an operation. You will learn how to handle emergencies and know when to call an ambulance.

We hope you will read the whole book, but you can also get help each time you need it by turning to the index and zeroing in on a particular problem.

As we investigated specialties — from those involving muscle and joint disorders to heart disease, to problems with lungs, diabetes, cancer, and incontinence — we found many new approaches to caring for older people that really reduce pain and dysfunction and vastly improve conditions that previously inhibited older people's ability to stay mobile and involved in their own care.

In the final chapter, we tell you about services and health agencies that will provide information and support when you need those. Too many people fall into the trap of going on alone, without reaching beyond the doctor's office and whatever the doctor can tell them. You may have heard the myth that aging services don't exist, but that's not true. In every large and medium-sized city and in all rural counties, an Area Agency on Aging has been set up to help families locate services that help older people and their families with all sorts of problems involving health and living arrangements. For every major disease, you will find organizations that will help you understand which treatment is appropriate for the older person and where that treatment can be found. The information these organizations provide is great, and yet they are underutilized. During our interviews with caregivers who finally went to these organizations for help, one of the remarks we heard most was, "Why on earth didn't we do this sooner?" Remember, you *can* get help when you need it. There's a treatment for everything these days if you know where to find it. It may not be a cure, but it can be a help.

We also want you to remember that although we don't directly address your personal stresses here, it's important for you to take care of yourself. You can't do the best job for anyone else if you're overworked and overtired. In the final chapter we delve into all the social services available in your community. Many of these services are for your older parent or friend, but we also list services that will be helpful to you.

— Caroline Rob
New York City
1991

1

What's Normal
When It Comes to Aging?

OUR SOCIETY IS CONFUSED about what it means physically and emotionally to grow old.

If you've ever been around people in their sixties, seventies, eighties, or nineties, you've probably heard some of them say, as a way of explaining:

- "You know how it is when you get this old, you get dizzy when you stand up."
- "My old bones ache all the time."
- "You can't go to the opera or the symphony if you have to go to the bathroom all the time."
- When you get as old as I am, it is difficult breathing on the way up the stairs."
- "It's impossible to be happy at my age; I've given up trying."
- "My skin never stops itching, but I can't do anything about it."
- "At my age, I can't sew any more. I always feel like there's a film of cellophane over my eyes."

Although you may have believed the speaker — and certainly the speaker believes it — *not one of these complaints is a normal part of aging*. Each is a symptom of a disease or condition that could be addressed and corrected, or at least relieved, by medical intervention.

Normal aging does not involve getting dizzy, confused, forgetful, or incontinent. Nor are cataracts on the eyes, skin diseases, other chronic ailments, or depression to be expected as part and parcel of growing old.

It shouldn't surprise any of us that so many older people themselves don't know the difference between being old and being sick. Old age is not a popular subject in our culture. It's taboo at most social gatherings, and young people find the prospect of growing old tedious, if not downright frightening or disgusting. For many years, most of us are able to put the prospect of growing old out of our minds. Thus it is that when we — or our parents — suddenly become old, physical changes can become distressing or confusing simply because we don't understand what those changes mean. We have no idea what to expect.

Far too often, when people think of physical aches, pains, or dizziness as signs of getting old, it doesn't occur to them or to their children that they should have medical attention or adjustments in their way of doing things. This lack of attention can be tragic in affecting the quality of the life an older person leads. It can also be a terrible waste of life when failure to report serious symptoms and get appropriate medical attention leads to permanent damage, incurable illness, or death that could have been avoided.

At the heart of negative attitudes about growing old is a persistent belief that disease is a fundamental part of aging. It's not. Many older people grow old naturally, comfortably, and free from disease. Some ninety-year-olds will tell you they have never used any medication, not even aspirin! They are blessed with strong constitutions brought to them by good genes and healthy lifestyles, and perhaps, simple good luck.

That doesn't mean normal aging is problem-free, however. Normal aging does bring changes in some body functions, depending on the individual, and slowing down of the body's systems. At the least, very old age almost universally involves a dimming of vision, hearing, touch, taste, and smell, but these changes are generally gradual and can be addressed as they happen — beginning with reading glasses in our forties and fifties, and often graduating to hearing aids in our seventies.

Remember that aging is a highly individual process that affects people in unpredictable ways. It's just the opposite of infancy and childhood, when specialists can predict the ages for physical growth and the development of skills with amazing accuracy. In old age, we have no uniform timetable, and chronological age can be a very poor indicator of how old someone is physically. For convenience, people who work with older people divide them into three age categories:

the young old (people sixty-five to seventy-four), the "old old" (seventy-five to eighty-four), and the "very old" (eighty-five and older). But even these categories can be misleading. Because people are living so much longer than ever before, we may soon need a new category for the "very, very old" — people ninety-five and more.

Some people show the signs of aging very young, but others manifest very little deterioration or slowing down until they are in their seventies or even eighties. Even *within* the older person's body, organ systems age at different rates that often are independent of their owner's chronological age. A person in her eighties may have a very "young" heart and yet have very "old" skin, but a sixty-five-year-old may have very "old" kidneys and a relatively young hormonal system and strong bones. But even though the declines are different and unpredictable, most older people do experience them, and find they have to make adjustments. Many see that their kidney function decreases with age, and most report that eventually all their organ systems begin to behave less efficiently.

Gerontologists have theories about why the body ages, but generally it's agreed that the loss of efficiency comes about as some cells wear out or actually die and do not replace themselves. This process is sometimes referred to as the One Percent Rule — meaning that most organ systems seem to lose roughly 1 percent of their functioning each year, starting at about age thirty. This phenomenon is illustrated particularly well by young athletes, who draw upon every iota of their physical strength during competitive performances. When they are teenagers or when they're in the twenties, they're functioning at their maximum efficiency and have enormous reserves to call upon. Once most of these athletes hit their thirties, however, they begin to "go over the hill," no longer able to draw on the full extent of their reserves, and their peak performances become a matter of history. That, of course, is why we see so many more Olympic athletes in their twenties than in their thirties or forties.

The result of the One Percent Rule is that by the time most people reach their seventies, they start to experience more dramatic evidence that they don't have the stamina or quick reflexes of their youth. They can't swim as many laps without getting winded, or they can't draw on endless reserves if they're working or playing tennis. Age becomes most apparent to them if they're under some kind of stress, such as the setback of an illness, or a tragic life change, such as the death of a loved one. Often in these circumstances older people find that they don't have the staying power they used to have, nor do they bounce back as quickly as they might expect.

It's also true that aging seems to make people more susceptible to diseases that were fended off, or more easily endured, during youth. Four of five older persons develop some kind of chronic condition or disease — whether it's high blood pressure, arthritis, heart disease, or difficulty with vision or hearing. Most of these conditions can be managed in a way that allows older people to go about their business and gather plenty of joy from living, despite the need to slow down a bit or plan their schedules more carefully. Taking antihypertensive medications for high blood pressure or choosing a sport that is not hard on arthritic joints, for instance, allows the older person to live an independent and satisfying life that continues on a steady course.

As aging continues, however, problems sometimes amplify and become disabling and distressing. As people become older, they often seem much less bothered by the imminence of death than by the prospect of being dependent on the care of others.

This is where you come in. As a caregiver, you are taking on the job of helping an older parent, a spouse, or a friend who can't manage in some way or in a number of ways. Your goal at any stage in this job is to be supportive and help this person lead as normal a life as possible, despite any physical incapacities. Although your goals and expectations may change as the person becomes more encumbered by illness or physical problems, always try to keep in mind the goal of helping that person to be as independent and self-sufficient as possible. Being able to make choices and determine the course of one's life is basic to everyone's sense of well-being, whether we are young or old. Certainly, the need to be independent is not one of the things that recede with age.

But in your role as supportive friend to an older relative or friend, it may be useful for you to watch for any shifts in that person's health that need addressing. Usually the older person will be able to tell you about any needs, and it's essential that you listen. It matters particularly that you take health complaints seriously. There *are* solutions to almost all health-related problems older people face, so that if you bring a positive attitude to the incident, you can often make a difference in your relative's or friend's ability to manage the problem before it gets out of hand.

Even if your relative is a hypochondriac, this behavior is a symptom of needing attention. Perhaps it's a message to try to help this person get involved in community activities or to do something else to relieve his or her loneliness or depression, like getting on the phone and calling other family members to come over and visit more. It's also possible that the older person's complaints simply express depression that he or she doesn't want to tell you about for fear that you will interpret it as a failure of character. Aches and pains may, in fact, manifest inner turmoil that could be relieved by talking to a counselor or joining a support group.

Indicators of Illness Change with Age

One thing you both should realize is that medications and illnesses can cause shifts in behavior that aren't easily recognized in an older person. Older people are often so different physically from younger people, and from the way they themselves *used to be,* that their symptoms of disease or response to a medication can be baffling. It's especially baffling to anyone who doesn't know that symptoms of illness change with age. It's not at all uncommon for an older person to be ill and not show the classic symptoms such as fever, pain, and nausea that you usually associate with the illness. For instance, a younger person having a heart attack usually has crushing chest pains, pain shooting down the left arm, and a gray, pallid look to the skin. Older people may also have these symptoms, but it's not unusual for them to have a heart attack without any of the classic, dramatic signals. They may simply become extremely restless, confused, and short of breath.

The medications that control chronic conditions may mask symptoms or alter the way in which the disease shows up. Older people are also more sensitive to medicines, and so medication itself is often the source of a new symptom — even with a medicine they have taken for years.

You need to look out for the obvious signs of illness when your parent is not feeling right, but you also need to know that any dramatic change in behavior can signal a medical emergency. Often disorientation, confusion, or a big change in your parent or friend's mental state and ability to function normally will be the only clue that something is wrong. A bad pneumonia, for example, keeps oxygen from passing through the lungs. Then not enough oxygen can get to the brain, which causes confusion. It's common for an older person with pneumonia to simply act "fuzzy" or confused, but not to run a fever or have any chest pain or coughing.

Realize too that a lot of diseases can look alike in older people. Early, subtle signs of Parkinson's disease and arthritis can look the same, and depression can seem the same as a neurological or hormone problem. Don't ignore any of these difficulties. Treat them with the same vigor in an older person as you would in a young one.

Screening Tests Are as Important as Ever

Remember that screening tests are vital at any age as a preventive measure, but they matter especially for older people. As people age, the chances increase that diseases will come to full expression.

To be sure, you can't force your parents or older friends to go to the doctor's office for the annual physical, but you can encourage them. Even if they feel great, such a visit can reassure them that their health is stable. If anything is wrong it can be diagnosed and treated at an early stage. Many diseases commonly affecting older people give little warning of their presence. No one can usually "feel" a dangerously high cholesterol count, glaucoma, early signs of cancer, or high blood pressure.

If your parent, spouse, or friend is homebound and unable to make trips to the doctor's office, clinic, or hospital, you may be able to arrange for testing to be done at home, by either a doctor or a nurse practitioner.

Although the schedule of tests that follows is generally recommended by geriatricians, some tests are not covered by insurance. If price is a deterrent, call your Area Agency on Aging to see where tests are provided free of charge or at a minimal rate. Quite a few communities have free health-screening programs for older people.

Essential Screening Tests and Exams for People Sixty-five and Older

Blood Pressure. Older people should have their blood pressure checked at least once a year. Those who already have high blood pressure should have more frequent testing.

Electrocardiogram (EKG). By age sixty-five, everyone should have a baseline EKG. After that, it should be conducted according to the patient's general health status and the family history of heart disease.

Cholesterol. From age sixty to seventy-five, testing should be done at least every two and a half years. After seventy-five, have this test annually.

Gastrointestinal Tract Cancer Test. According to the American Cancer Society, a test for blood in the stool should be done once a year. A proctosigmoidoscopy or examination of the colon with a scope instrument should be done every three to five years, based on the advice of a physician.

Breast Exam. This test should be given by a health professional at least once a year, and an older woman should give herself a monthly check.

Mammogram. After age fifty, the American Cancer Society recommends that this x-ray of the breast should be given once a year.

Cervical Pap Smear. If three consecutive annual examinations have been normal, a Pap smear may be taken less frequently, at the discretion of the physician who does the annual gynecological checkup.

Testicular Exam. A health professional should conduct this exam once a year, but an older man should give himself a monthly check as instructed by his doctor.

Prostate. A rectal examination for prostate should be done at the annual physical.

Eye Exam. Always tell your spouse, parent, or friend to consult an eye specialist if changes in vision occur. A basic eye exam should be conducted along with the annual physical. The American Academy of Ophthalmology recommends that everyone over sixty-five have an eye exam done by an eye specialist once every two years. It should include screening for glaucoma.

Dental Exam. An older person should see a dentist every six months whether or not she or he has natural teeth. Dentures need fit checks to prevent gum disorders and irregularities of the jaw.

Hearing Exam. A basic hearing test should be done along with the annual physical. Your older parent or friend may be unaware that they are not hearing as well as usual, but if their hearing problem becomes apparent to you, encourage them to consult a specialist.

Immunization. Influenza can be complicated and even life-threatening to an older person if it leads to pneumonia. The government pays for free immunizations for anyone over age sixty-five. Call your Area Agency on Aging or the local chapter of the American Lung Association for information about where in your area flu shots are given. The American Lung Association also recommends that people older than sixty-five have the pneumococcal vaccine, which provides protection against the most prevalent forms of bacteria that cause pneumonia. The pneumococcal vaccine is given once for a lifetime; however, recent research shows that revaccination is a good idea for some individuals, especially those who are frail.

2

Dealing with Losses in Vision and Hearing

NO OLDER PERSON is spared changes in vision, and few older people hit their mid-eighties without becoming at least slightly hard of hearing.

If you looked around the library at a senior citizen's center, everyone in the room would be wearing glasses for reading and some people might have devices with them to help clarify kinds of seeing problems other than reading up close. Besides their glasses, plenty of older people — particularly the oldest — would also be wearing hearing aids tucked in or behind their ears.

Because eyes and ears do give out, it's essential that older people have annual checkups for vision and hearing. Problems that come up because of normal aging can always be helped after they are identified, but more important, diseases — which can come on gradually without any pain — can be found and treated before they lead to permanent damage.

You as a committed family member or friend must make sure that an older person gets proper medical attention and glasses or hearing aids, whenever necessary. Beyond these preliminaries your encouragement and help may be needed at home so that the new devices are worn successfully and not left in a drawer. Also, everyone who spends time with the older person needs to be well aware of disabilities, to avoid any misunderstandings about what the older person can and cannot do. Recognizing their limitations will allow you to organize the house or apartment in a special way so that they can safely carry on basic tasks necessary for independent living.

Checkups Are Essential

Although many older people go for annual medical checkups, including attention for their eyes, large numbers in all walks of life stay away. It is a tragedy for an older person to lose sight or hear only muffled sounds, when simply going for checkups could have prompted appropriate and timely medical or surgical treatment, or special glasses, or a hearing aid. If you know that an older person is not getting eyes and ears examined at least every year, you must do all the persuading you can for a checkup.

Just a look at the number of older people who have severe disabilities in vision and hearing should put all of us on red alert to the unquestionable need for this attention. The National Center for Health Statistics estimates that "self-reported difficulties with vision," even though conventional glasses or contacts are in use, are:

25% for people aged sixty-five to seventy-four
39% for ages seventy-five to eighty-four
52.1% for those over eighty-five

For hearing loss, the numbers are even higher:

33% for people aged sixty-five to seventy-four
45% for ages seventy-five to eighty-four
62.3% for those over eighty-five

Lost among these statistics are millions of older individuals who have great difficulties, only because their vision or hearing problems were neglected. Those who can't see well live in a precarious world of blurred images. The joy of seeing nature, reading, and performing simple tasks is taken away from them. Those who are hard of hearing miss the full tone of the melodious sounds around them, as well as the noises that warn of danger, such as honking cars, screeching tires, and shouts of "Don't do that, please!" Perhaps worse than any of these missed sounds, they can't hear conversation; they can become socially isolated.

The frustration of being misunderstood is another pain-filled aspect of having failure of sight or hearing. Older people who are unable to see and hear properly are often labeled "disinterested," "stupid," "just plain rude," and worse still, "senile."

The Resistance Factor

If you find yourself exasperated in your attempts to get an older relative or friend to go to a vision or hearing specialist, you are up against a common but nonetheless trying barrier. It may help if you recognize some of the usual reasons older people refuse help for failing vision and hearing:

• Vision and hearing losses usually come on gradually and painlessly. Often older people get used to changes and scoff at them as "normal."

• Fear of losing a driver's license is devastating. Most eye doctors feel obliged to tell patient and the family when tests show vision is no longer good enough for safe driving.

• Mentally impaired, confused, or generally frail older people are especially unlikely to complain of blurry vision and poor hearing. Yet, they must get help, for any disturbance in their perception of the world makes disorientation worse.

• Many people resist confirmation that their eyes and ears are failing because they don't want to end up with "badges of old age" — heavy glasses or a hearing aid.

• Cost can be an issue. Special glasses, other optical aids, and hearing aids are prohibitively expensive. Most of the costs of eye and ear exams are not covered by Medicare, nor are glasses, other optical aids, and hearing aids. The one exception is that Medicare will pay for glasses after cataract surgery.

• People who are in their eighties and beyond often imagine that cataract surgery is dangerous and unpleasant. Thirty years ago cataract surgery was a risky operation and could result in blindness. Also, the patient had to lie still for several days with sandbags on either side of the head. All that has changed.

The Double Loss

One loss is bad enough, but many older people suffer the double hardship of difficulty in both sight and hearing. People who lose the effectiveness of one sense always rely heavily on the other, and those with a double loss do not have this ability.

If your parent or friend does have dimmed vision and dulled hearing, you must be especially alert to safety issues, but you must be even more sensitive to the need for companionship and communication with others. Fear of moving around is a big worry, but the very worst trial is their difficulty in communicating.

Those who have a double loss become isolated from the give-and-take of simple chatter and the enjoyment of shared ideas. Even a slight loss of vision combined with impaired hearing can leave one terribly depressed. Not being able to see well can make listening and coming up with appropriate responses exhausting and complicated for someone who is hard of hearing, because they usually watch people's lips for clues to the words they use, and their facial expressions and gestures for the emotional and situational context.

VISION PROBLEMS

Normal Aging Changes in the Eye

As the eyes age they undergo normal changes in structure and function. These changes cause both difficulty in seeing and discomfort within the eye.

We will describe these so-called normal changes that many older people experience and how the changes can be made less burdensome by glasses or common-sense adaptive strategies.

Normal as they are said to be, such changes must be reported to an eye specialist, who can rule them out as symptoms of a serious eye disease. A specialist will also be able to provide the older person with suggestions for managing discomfort and other problems.

Farsightedness
Quite early in life, around our forties and fifties, the eye lens thickens and loses its ability to focus on anything we're looking at up close. As we age, this farsightedness gradually gets worse. In fact, the clinical name for this condition is *presbyopia* or "old" eyes. If she strains and squints to see the phone book, or to thread a needle, it's time for your mother to get new glasses.

Difficulty in Shifting Vision
Many old people keep their ability to see far away, but have trouble zooming their gaze in close. People with this problem need to go slowly about their daily routines so that their eyes can accommodate to different tasks. Attention to safety is crucial, for the risk of accidents from missing a step or bumping into things increases. An older

person who has a dazed and confused expression as you approach may simply be adjusting focus from near to far.

Nearsightedness

Not being able to see faraway objects is known as nearsightedness (myopia). The Center for Health Statistics reports that by age sixty-five, half the people have a visual acuity of 20/70, or less (something that can be seen at 20 feet, a person with perfect vision can see from 70 feet).

People who are nearsighted in younger years inevitably become more farsighted, just as everyone else does as they get older. Without bifocal glasses or contact lenses, such people see everything — up close and far away — as one big blur. Although bifocals are a big help, older people who are near- and farsighted usually have more difficulty than other older people in shifting their vision from near to far.

Reduced Peripheral Vision

Many older people have a restricted range of vision to either side. Their eyes take in less light and therefore fewer images. But also, the eye itself can sink back from surrounding structures. People with poor peripheral vision should *not* drive.

Need for More Light

The aging eye takes in less of the available light, and so to see well older people need a great deal more light than do younger people. A twenty-year-old needs 20 watts of illumination to see properly, but a sixty-year-old needs 40 watts, and an eighty-year-old 60 watts.

Older people also require more time to adjust to changes in light levels, from a darkened room to a lighted one. Consistent and vivid light throughout the house is vital.

Exaggerated Glare

Older eyes need more light, but they also respond poorly to glaring light. An older person — not wearing sunglasses — can be temporarily blinded by bright sunlight, and may also feel sharp pains in the eyes after stepping outdoors. Shiny surfaces such as linoleum floors, polished furniture, and walls painted with glossy paint can also create eye distress.

Many older people give up driving at night because of the glare from oncoming headlights and reflections from wet pavement.

Color Changes
Plenty of very old people have difficulty in seeing the difference between shades of blue, green, and violet. The blue end of the light spectrum is filtered out by the older person's eye lens, which becomes yellowed as part of aging. This washing out of colors can be dangerous, if the older person identifies medications by their color.

Floaters
Many older people see small specks in their field of vision. *Floaters* are frequently visible when looking at a plain background, such as a blank wall or a blue sky, or when reading.

Although floaters appear, annoyingly, to be directly in front of the eye, they actually float deep within the gel of the eye. Eye doctors frequently receive calls from older patients frustrated by the specks. The best way to deal with floaters is to shift the eyes back and forth, up and down so that the floater can swirl out of the way in the fluid within.

Cornea Becomes Less Sensitive
A very old person may not feel something in the eye — a scratch or an irritating infection — even though the usual signs of damage are present, such as redness, watery eyes, or pus. Contact-lens wearers of all ages have similar corneal insensitivity.

Dry Eyes
Often older people notice that their eyes are dry and scratchy, because the water content of tears is decreased. The dryness is there because the tears change to a less viscous consistency and easily fall off the eye. Eyedrops called artificial tears can be bought at any drugstore and applied several times a day to alleviate this annoyance.

Difficulty in Seeing Contrasts
Some older people can't recognize contrast and the depth between surfaces, especially those in the gray tones. Cracks in pavements and steps can go unnoticed, and an entire staircase can look smooth as a slide.

Adaptive Help and Safety Tips for Failing Vision

Proper Lighting Makes a Big Difference

- Use many light sources evenly distributed around the room.
- Minimize shadows with consistent lighting.
- Make sure bulb wattage is high enough.
- Put light switches on the outside of rooms so that the older person never has to fumble around in a dark room.
- Use three-way bulbs and dimmer switches to control light intensity.
- Put nightlights in hallways, the bedroom, the bathroom.
- Put intense light at the top and bottom of staircase and steps.

Cut Out Glare

- Use sheer curtains or blinds in rooms that take in bright sunlight.
- Don't use fluorescent lights; they produce more glare than incandescents.
- Don't use wax on floors, and use low-gloss wax on furniture.
- Cover or get rid of shiny furniture or counter surfaces. Paint walls with matte-finish paint.
- Encourage your parent or friend to wear sunglasses with ultraviolet protection. Plastic lenses can give up to 50 percent more protection than glass lenses.

Create Contrasts and Recognition with Color

- Contrasts should be used in the design of all rooms. The walls should be a different color than the floor, and also the furniture. Staircases should contrast with other flooring.
- Light objects should go on dark surfaces, or vice versa. For instance, plates should contrast with a table surface, a telephone should contrast with the bedside table.
- Mark edges of steps and stairs with light paint or tape.
- Put glow-in-the-dark, brightly colored tape around light switches, doorknobs, and keyholes.
- Use light-colored mugs and cookingware when pouring hot liquids.
- Use colored containers and dishes. Clear glass "disappears."

Three *Common* Eye Diseases

The following diseases need to be looked for during the annual medical checkup and during visits to the eye specialist. Treatment in the first phase of their development can prevent an older person from suffering unnecessary loss of sight.

Cataracts
Look through a piece of crumpled cellophane and you can simulate the blurry, clouded vision of someone who has a severe cataract. You'll see why people with cataracts often say, "I feel like a curtain of film is over my eyes." A cloudy, opaque area in the lens of the eye, the cataract scatters light and generally interferes with vision.

Around half the people over seventy-five show some signs of a cataract in one or both eyes; cataracts are indeed very common, especially in the "very-old" group. It is said that everyone would develop cataracts if they lived long enough, because they are caused by progression of normal age-related changes. So far, research has not been able to find why cataracts form earlier in some people.

Although very safe and effective surgical techniques are available for treating cataracts, they are still the most frequent cause of visual impairment in the elderly and the third leading cause of legal blindness in the United States. Cataracts cause severe damage when they "ripen" and become fluid-filled so that they press against vital eye structures. The eye doctor following an older person will recommend surgery well before a cataract reaches this final stage in development.

Once a doctor has identified a cataract in the eye, the decision has to be made whether or not to remove it. When the cataract causes no visual impairment, and does not greatly limit one's ability to function, it is usually left alone and just watched. Sometimes a cataract can sit in the eye for several years without causing changes in vision. Don't be surprised if the doctor does not recommend surgery. Certainly, though, if you have doubts about any medical recommendations, it is always a good idea to get a second opinion.

Some influences can make cataracts worse in the fragile aging eye, or actually provoke their formation. Ultraviolet (UV) sunlight is now thought of as a culprit in cataract formation and as an accelerant to cataracts once started. The older person who has a cataract should try to wear UV-protective sunglasses and a wide-brimmed hat when spending more than a few minutes in the sun. Chemical injury by household agents such as soap and insect repellent, infections, and even a blow to the eye can also worsen a cataract.

Cataract Surgery. This type of surgery is a great boon. It has a 90 percent success rate without complications and accounts for most operations performed on the elderly. The natural lens of the eye is removed from the eyeball by an ophthalmic surgeon and replaced with a plastic substitute lens. One way to do the operation is for the surgeon to remove the lens intact through a wide incision in the front of the eye. Another operation draws the contents of the lens capsule out of the eye through a large-bore needle.

In 90 percent of cases a clear plastic lens is implanted directly in the eye during surgery; otherwise, thick glasses or contact lenses are prescribed. Today elderly people are almost always given the plastic lenses because they are safe, effective, and trouble-free.

If an older person you know wears cataract glasses prescribed years ago after surgery, recommend talking to an eye specialist about an implanted lens. Cataract glasses are definitely second best because they provide no side vision. The glasses are also extremely thick, heavy, and unattractive.

Cataract surgery sounds frightening, but it is not nearly as bad as it sounds. Usually the patient is given local anesthesia and the surgery is painless and over within less than an hour. If one has cataracts in both eyes, one eye is operated on at a time, for vision can take at least six weeks to recover after surgery. A patient almost always goes home on the same day and normally would feel no discomfort beyond a mild tugging sensation from the stitches.

Postoperative Care. The older person will certainly need special attention in the days after surgery. Here's what to expect during the recovery, so that you can plan for it.

• It takes about six to twelve weeks for the eye to completely heal and adjust to an artificial lens. During the healing, vision may be blurred in the operated-upon eye. Vision should return to where it was before the cataract was removed. Keep your expectations realistic and in line with the older person's general eye health.

• Transportation has to be arranged for a number of routine doctor visits, and for any other purposes. In most cases patients should not drive for several weeks after cataract surgery, especially in the days right after surgery. The surgeon will want to observe the eye more than once in the first week and possibly at other times during recovery.

• After surgery a patient is told to avoid activities that can increase pressure within the eye (intraocular pressure) and disrupt the stitches. Avoid any kind of vigorous exertion and do not bend forward or lift anything heavy.

• Constipation needs to be prevented, because straining on elimination increases intraocular pressure. Provide and encourage a high-fiber diet and plenty of fluids.

• If the older person begins to feel nauseated or is starting a cold call your eye doctor *immediately*. The doctor may want to prescribe medication to avert sneezing or vomiting, for either could put a great deal of pressure on the eye and disrupt stitches.

• Cataract patients wear an eye patch for protection in the first few days and nights after surgery. The patch needs to be worn during sleep with the head lying on the unaffected side if the older person doesn't enjoy sleeping on his or her back all night. Sometimes the doctor will prescribe interim glasses for the few weeks it takes for the recovering eye to settle down to normal.

• The patch should be worn during bathing or showering for two weeks after surgery. Water and soap should never enter the eye during everyday face washing.

• Consider making regular hair-washing appointments at a beauty salon or barbershop during the first six weeks. If your parent wants to have the washing done at home, do the job by bending his or her head gently backward, *not* forward, over a sink.

What Is a Secondary Cataract? Although cataract surgery is considered a very safe and successful sight-saving operation, roughly 40 percent of those who have it experience a "secondary cataract," a clouding of the new lens capsule at the back of the eye that supports the new lens. Cloudy vision from a secondary cataract may take months to several years to form.

To remedy the cloudiness, a painless laser procedure can be performed in just a few minutes in the doctor's office. This procedure usually causes rapid improvement in vision and rarely leaves complications.

Glaucoma
The disease glaucoma is known as the sneak thief of sight because it has few early symptoms, and, when left undiagnosed and untreated,

it can lead to blindness. Although fewer older people develop glaucoma than cataracts, it is considered a much more serious disease because of its ability to cause permanent damage quickly.

Glaucoma starts when the consistency of the eye's fluid content becomes abnormally viscous and therefore unable to drain effectively through the eye's plumbing system. The backup of fluid causes the eyeball to balloon unnaturally but painlessly against the optic nerve. Those with advanced glaucoma have tunnel vision, which means they can see clearly at the center of their field of vision, but dimly around the periphery.

The disease runs in families and is especially prevalent among black people. The simple, painless check for glaucoma should be performed annually on everyone over age thirty-five.

Some cases of glaucoma can be relieved with laser surgery. Usually the disease is easily treated with eye drops that are very effective in controlling the eye's drainage.

Eye Drops Are Essential for Glaucoma. If eye drops are prescribed, plenty of people eventually get lazy about applying them. The result can be painless damage to the eye and impaired vision within not weeks, but days.

Don't become lax, if it is your responsibility to apply the drops, or remind others to do so. Eye drops have to be put in every day, and without fail!

Beyond making certain that eye drops are given according to the doctor's directions, other information about the medication is required.

• Medication can sting and irritate the eye when first dropped in. The older person should talk to the doctor to see if this reaction is normal. Discomfort should not become a consideration for skipping applications.

• Occasionally eye drops can cause side effects. Watch for dry mouth, dizziness, and the form of incontinence called urinary retention. Report such side effects to that the doctor can make changes in the drug treatment.

• Many doctors encourage patients not to wear tight elastic clothing, such as girdles and support hose. Hard to believe, but such clothing does affect the body's fluid system, including the intraocular pressure.

• Anything that can raise intraocular pressure should be avoided. The list of cautions includes lifting heavy objects, overexertion, and straining while constipated. Call the eye doctor for advice if your relative is ill and risks coughing, sneezing, or vomiting.

• Many over-the-counter drugs can make glaucoma worse, including antihistamines, appetite suppressants, and antidiarrhea medications. Don't let the older person take any medication whatsoever without the doctor's approval. Make sure your parent wears a bracelet to warn a hospital team in an emergency that glaucoma is an issue.

Macular Degeneration

Although macular degeneration is the leading cause of permanent impairment of reading and fine, close-up vision for people over sixty-five, it has been little publicized in the press and on television. The disorder was not understood until recently, because people rarely lived long enough for it to develop fully. Blonde, pale-eyed Caucasians seem most affected, and it is especially prevalent in the over-eighty-five age group.

Senile macular degeneration is just what the name describes, an age-related breakdown in the macula, a very small area in the center of the retina at the back of the eye. This small area is responsible for our straight-ahead sight, which is gradually lost as the disease progresses. A severely affected person sees only a blurry, dark ball at the center of the field of vision — a blind spot.

You can imagine how macular degeneration is perceived by the individual experiencing it by thinking of a dark splotch smack in the middle of a photograph. Because side vision is unaffected, walking around is not a problem. Driving and reading fine print certainly are problems.

Unfortunately, no treatment is available for most forms of the disease, so that sufferers simply have to learn to adjust as the disease progresses, using adaptive measures and low-vision aids such as magnifying and telescopic glasses.

It is extremely important that all older people become aware of the disease so that they can watch out for it. When a diagnosis is made sooner — rather than later — loss of vision is only partial, making it much easier to learn new coping strategies and how to use visual aids comfortably and efficiently.

Many doctors give their older patients grid-test stickers (Amsler tests) to take home and put on the bathroom mirror. The patient is asked to glance every day at the test, which is simply a grid with a dot in the middle. Macular degeneration is apparent when the line at the middle of the grid looks distorted. Generally people with macular degeneration see any straight line, near or far, as wavy.

Laser Treatment. Occasionally, in about 4 percent of cases, macular degeneration in the elderly is caused by a breakdown in the tiny blood vessels of the macula. For no well-understood reason new blood vessels grow beneath the macula and leak fluid that can irreparably damage it within a few weeks or a month.

If this form of degeneration is detected early, laser treatment performed by an eye surgeon can seal off the blood vessels so that they don't leak and cause further damage. The laser used emits heat that essentially welds fragile tissue.

Do Consult a Low-Vision Specialist. Make sure an older person you know who develops macular degeneration gets the benefit of consultation with a low-vision specialist. "Low vision" is a relatively new and little-known specialty in eye care; sometimes medical doctors (who often pick up eye problems in their older patients) are not up on it.

The low-vision specialist is an optometrist or an ophthalmologist who has taken special training in prescribing assistive devices for those who are severely impaired visually. They like to think of themselves as the specialists people should see when other doctors have told them, "There's nothing we can do for you" to treat an eye problem. Many of them like to say, "We don't think of what we can't do for a visually impaired person, but what we can do for problems that no longer respond to conventional glasses and medical or surgical treatment."

Contact the Lighthouse National Center for Vision and Aging for names of low-vision specialists across the country and for information about low-vision aids. (See the Appendix for this organization's address.)

HEARING LOSS

A Common Difficulty

Hearing is our most finely tuned sense, but it is also our most fragile. As the extremely delicate organs of the ear age and hearing is affected, communication channels are lost. The latest research shows that aging itself is the main risk factor contributing to hearing loss in people who are not exposed to extreme noise levels.

Many older people have mild to moderate hearing loss, and all the "very old" have some difficulty with hearing. It is said that about 10 million older Americans have age-related hearing impairment, their difficulty ranging from understanding words to hearing specific sounds to total deafness. Usually, hearing loss comes on gradually. For this reason, many people who don't go for hearing tests don't know they can't hear well.

Look for Clues

Besides encouraging your spouse, parent, or friend to have hearing tests, you need to be on the lookout for clues to hearing loss in their behavior. Even a slight loss can be terribly upsetting. You don't want the older person withdrawing from group gatherings and staying home for fear of embarrassing encounters with anyone who tries to start a conversation. And they will suffer by missing television dialogue, telephone talk, musical entertainment, and talk with family and friends. Furthermore, you don't want a hearing impairment to complicate the older person's ability to cope with difficult and stressful events, such as the death or moving away of friends. Finally, you don't want others to interpret superficial "dullness" and apparent lack of willingness to participate in social activities as signs of mental deterioration, if the reason is impaired senses.

You need to know that people with hearing loss may:

- Speak with inappropriate loudness or softness; the voice may sound monotonous or may have an unusual, "weird" quality.
- Accuse others of mumbling and not speaking clearly. "What?" or "What did you say?" are often responses to conversation.
- Cup hands to ears.
- Turn the head toward those speaking to them.
- Ask speakers to repeat words just said.
- Talk over others who have begun speaking.
- Have trouble following a conversation when two or more people are speaking together.
- Fail to respond to directions or remember directions.
- Fail to hear sudden sounds.

- Become easily distracted. The attention span often shortens, and as listeners they can seem uninterested in a conversation.
- Display paranoid behavior and suspicion when others are talking.
- Turn the television set or radio volume much too high.
- Not hear the doorbell or telephone.
- Find it easier to understand deep-voiced men than shrill-voiced women and children.

Types of Hearing Loss

Many of us assume that people with hearing loss experience the world as quieter, as we do when radio volume is turned down. Hearing loss doesn't always mean lowered volume; it can involve altered sounds or absence of specific sounds. Next, we examine the two general categories of hearing loss either alone or in combination, which commonly affect older people.

Presbycusis

The condition called presbycusis is always associated with aging, for it is universal among the "very old." This is a progressive hearing loss, caused by decline and death of the nerve and sensory cells of the inner ear that process and relay auditory signals to the brain.

The older person who has presbycusis generally hears low-pitched vowel tones loudly and clearly, but high-pitched consonants are distorted or unheard. The vowels, "a" "e" "i" "o" and "u" are heard, but consonants such as "th" "s" "sh" "f" and "p", being high-pitched, are difficult to hear.

Discriminating between words that sound almost the same can be especially difficult. The person with presbycusis may hear "fifty" and "fifteen" as the same word, or "choose" instead of "juice," or "fill" for "pill." High-pitched voices are also more difficult to understand.

Often we raise our voice when talking to an older person with presbycusis, but the increased volume only aggravates the confusion, because loud sounds can be painful and very irritating. Most of us also raise the pitch of our voice when speaking louder. You must have heard an older person say, "Don't shout, I'm not deaf!"

Talking more slowly, in a low voice, rather than louder, is usually a better way to communicate. Messages travel through the aging ear at a slower rate, and so the older person will appreciate slow, deliberate speech, but certainly not talking at a fast clip. If the older person needs time to process information, short sentences with pauses between them are better than long ones that are difficult to follow.

Conductive Loss

The type of hearing loss called conductive loss occurs when sound waves are blocked by obstructions in the middle ear. Too much wax can be the cause, as can scarring or infection in and around the eardrum. Sometimes aging changes can add insult to the injury of an already damaged and scarred eardrum, so that sound does not flow smoothly to the inner ear.

All sounds seem muffled if conductive loss has occurred, even though ability to distinguish and understand sounds is not impaired. The person with conductive loss will want you to talk louder. On the other end of the conversation, you too may want him or her to talk louder. Those who have conductive hearing loss often speak softly because their own voice is enhanced by the blockage in the ear.

Because older people have thicker and drier earwax, they often have hearing loss simply because the wax has become impacted in front of the eardrum. Men are especially prone to this problem because the ear hairs become thicker and more profuse.

Very often, all an older person needs to bring hearing back to normal is a good old-fashioned ear cleaning. Older people need to remove earwax regularly by instilling drops of over-the-counter earwax dissolvers, as directed by their doctor. Cleaning the ear with a cotton swab is not recommended, because the swab can further impact the wax, causing damage. If wax is impacted, an ear doctor should do the job of removing it.

Hearing Aids

Unfortunately, medical science has not found a way to cure most hearing problems, other than those caused by a removable obstruction or an infection. Nevertheless, incurable hearing problems can be helped. In some conditions, especially presbycusis, hearing aids can enhance hearing, but for others a rehabilitation program can make a big difference to the hearing-impaired person's quality of life.

The person suffering hearing loss must consult an audiologist after a medical diagnosis has determined the cause. Most ear doctors work in partnership with an audiologist, who is trained to precisely determine the level and kind of hearing loss; a program of rehabilitation can then be planned. The audiologist will run an audiogram, among other tests. Ask for a copy of the audiogram's paper printout. The record can be used to get a second opinion from another audiologist or doctor, if the need for one arises.

Beware the Quick Sell

Do not buy a hearing aid unless it has been prescribed by your ear doctor or an audiologist. Frequently, people go straight to a hearing-aid dispensary or shop without a prescription, buying a hearing aid that ends up in a drawer because it is useless or badly fitted to the ear, or because the person who sold the hearing aid gave inadequate instruction on how to use the device. Some audiologists work in places where hearing aids are sold, or themselves sell hearing aids to their patients.

Hearing aids can make big profits for those who sell them. For this reason plenty of hucksters sell hearing aids to people who don't necessarily need them, or who may be mentally confused and incapable of learning how to use them. Anyone can sell hearing aids, which are very expensive — the average price is around $600, and some cost as much as $2,000. In most states older people have to pay all costs for hearing aids out of pocket. Advocates for the elderly are attempting to get the industry regulated so that aids will be paid for by state and federal insurance programs.

A reputable hearing-aid supplier will sell the devices with a thirty-day, money-back return policy. If you are helping a family member buy a hearing aid, insist on such an arrangement. It will mean the supplier will have a financial incentive to carefully teach the older person how to use the device, or to try different ones. Again, ask the audiologist for a copy of the audiogram so that you can get a second opinion on whether or not a hearing aid will help the older person.

The Training Period

Bear in mind that hearing aids are indeed aids — they do not restore hearing to normal as glasses can with vision. Because the hearing aid amplifies all sounds, including background noise, the person wearing one will not hear normal sounds clearly. A hearing aid can be effective in correcting some kinds of hearing loss if the wearer is given careful instruction to persevere in getting used to it.

A period of adjustment to the hearing aid — as long as six weeks — is usually needed. Besides learning to listen through a hearing aid, those who first wear one have to get used to the feeling of the device in the ear, to turning it on and off as appropriate, to storing it properly, and to changing batteries frequently. Older people who have difficulties with vision and trouble with manual dexterity because of arthritis may become frustrated in a hurry unless they fully understand the complexities involved.

Wearing a hearing aid for only a short time (15 to 60 minutes) during a quiet time of day and gradually increasing the time over a month to 10 to 12 hours a day makes the adjustment easier. In the beginning the aid should not be worn at gatherings, or at noisy times such as a meal with pots and silverware clanging, because the older person will become exhausted and frustrated by hearing too many sounds amplified at once.

A hearing aid can become a tool in restoring communication for your family member, if you can work together during the adjustment period. The older person will need your encouragement, and if need be you should learn how to place the appliance in the ear, manage the controls, and maintain it.

Types of Hearing Aids

In-the-Ear Hearing Aid. The smallest, least-visible, and therefore most cosmetically appealing hearing aid is custom made to fit directly in the shell of the ear. Only people who are mildly impaired can wear one, however, because the size limits the amplification. This kind of aid is not a good idea for the older person who has arthritis or problems with vision, because the controls are tiny and the aid itself can easily be lost if dropped or set down.

Behind-the-Ear Hearing Aid. The behind-the-ear appliance consists of a small earpiece connected by plastic tubing to a battery holder and control box. The box hooks behind the ear with the tubing. These aids are recommended for people with moderate to severe hearing loss, and for those who would have difficulty fiddling with the smaller controls of the in-the-ear hearing aid.

Body Hearing Aid. The body hearing aid looks like a small radio with a long wire attached to an earphone. The radio part is worn around the body on a belt. This type is recommended for the severely impaired because the sound amplification is excellent, and also for those who need large, easy-to-use controls.

Hearing-Aid Maintenance
Like any other mechanical device, a hearing aid needs proper care. If you are responsible for the job, here's how to handle it:

- Before inserting the device, make sure it is working. Check any cording for kinks, twists, or breaks. Close the battery case and turn the volume to high — you should hear a feedback sound. If you hear no sound, change the batteries for new ones. If the problem is not with the batteries, the device is broken — you need to contact the hearing-aid dispenser.
- Turn off the batteries when the aid is not in use.
- Make sure the appliance is removed before going to bed, bathing, or showering.
- Clean the earmold daily with a damp cloth and once a week with mildly soapy water. If any part becomes clogged, clean it with a pipe cleaner. Never use alcohol for cleaning — it can dry and crack the mold.
- When the hearing aid is in use, keep it dry. A drop of water can muffle sound.
- Avoid exposing the device to extremes of temperature. Never dry hair with a hair drier while the hearing aid is in position.
- Keep all pump sprays and aerosol sprays away from the device.
- Store the aid in a clean, dry place; keep it in the bedroom, not the bathroom.

How You Can Help

You can do plenty more to enhance different listening situations besides setting the older person up with a hearing aid. You can investigate the many devices on the market for the hearing impaired and learn techniques for talking to someone who is hearing impaired.

Seek Special Products
Many low-cost, high-technology products have recently been introduced in electronics specialty shops and department stores. You will find amplifiers for the telephone ringer and the caller's voice, for the

doorbell, and for radio and television sound. Even alarm clocks with flashing lights and loud buzzers are on the market. In some states, telephone adapters are available without charge, once the telephone-company client provides medical verification of a disability.

A sound amplifier with earphones can be an enormous help in hearing for someone who is hard of hearing but unable to wear a hearing aid because of a confusion disorder or difficulty with manual dexterity. The amplifier is also good to use when someone is taking a break from a hearing aid. You can buy the device and earphones at most electronics stores, and a perfectly good one can cost around $25. The headphones are attached to the small radio-sized amplifier box, which can be placed near someone who is talking, or a television set or radio. Two-way conversation can be carried out if the hearing-impaired person listens through the earphones to someone speaking into a microphone in or attached to the sound-amplifier box.

Be Sympathetic
Many older people become alienated and demoralized by hearing loss, beyond being embarrassed by it as a sign of aging, because few people in their circle of family and friends know how to interact with the hard of hearing. Hearing loss is usually much more difficult to deal with for the affected person and more troubling emotionally than loss of vision, and yet it doesn't engender as much sympathetic understanding.

Although few older people become completely deaf, as Helen Keller was, we include this quotation from her works because it describes the consequence of hearing loss: "The problems of deafness are deeper and more complex, if not more important than those of blindness. Deafness is a much worse misfortune. For it means the loss of the most vital stimulus — the sound of the voice that brings language, sets thoughts astir, and keeps us in the intellectual company of man."

Learn How to Communicate
Here are some communication tips that apply to a listener with or without a hearing aid. Be sure to share them with everyone in the family, and with all friends who visit.

- Get the attention of the older person before speaking.
- Face him or her directly at eye level; position yourself 3 to 6 feet away. You do not need to talk directly into the ear.

- Position yourself so that light shines from above or toward you, rather than from behind you, into the older person's eyes.
- Speak clearly and just a little more slowly than usual, in a moderate, low voice.
- Do not shout. Shouting creates a booming effect and makes your voice difficult to hear. Shouting accentuates only the vowel sounds and obscures consonants.
- Use facial expressions, gestures, and objects to illustrate the verbal message.
- Do not exaggerate the movements of your lips. Overarticulation will distort your mouth and interfere with lip reading.
- Never talk with chewing gum, food, or a cigarette in your mouth.
- Decrease background noise. Turn off the radio and television set and close the windows if street noise is distracting.
- Allow longer intervals between sentences. It often takes an older, hearing-impaired person longer to absorb and understand a message.
- If the older person has a greater loss in one ear than in the other, direct your conversation toward the "good" ear.
- If he or she can't understand you, try other words by rephrasing your statement.
- Use short sentences.
- When giving important instructions, write them down as well as presenting them orally.

3

Recognizing and Dealing
with Memory Loss and
Diseases of the Nervous System

MORE DRAMATICALLY than any other part of the anatomy, the brain and nervous system change with age. Billions of nerve cells die out between adolescence and old age and the brain becomes smaller, lighter, and more water-filled than it was in youth. Some brain and nervous-system areas lose as many as half their original nerve cells by age ninety or so.

Amazingly, despite physiological evidence indicating otherwise, healthy older people are able to keep sharp minds and functioning bodies. These losses and aging changes in the nervous system do not mean that the system inevitably fails.

Healthy older people can remain intellectually acute, but some subtle inefficiencies affect the working of the brain and nervous system. They may find it harder to recall facts and figures quickly, and their body movements may respond less quickly. They may also sleep less, because the region of the brain that controls stages of sleep loses effectiveness. Then too, many older people have trouble adapting to especially hot or cold conditions, and to stress from overexertion, because the nervous system is no longer in optimal form.

It used to be widely thought that people became "senile" when they got old, but today we know that dementia is a disease, not a normal part of aging. Studies show very clearly that mental capacity can remain intact throughout life: of the 29 million Americans over age sixty-five, only about 15 percent have Alzheimer's and other irreversible dementing illnesses. As people age past eighty, however, a larger percentage contract these diseases of brain function.

In this chapter we discuss the normal kinds of changes older people experience with thinking and the overall behavior of the nervous system. We hope the information we provide will enable you to help your parent, spouse, or older friend understand how to manage these changes without becoming unduly alarmed by them.

You can do much to help an older person adapt to noticeable changes if you understand which problems are normal and how to handle them as they occur. Forgetfulness and slowness, changed sleep patterns, and heightened sensitivity to hot and cold are difficulties that can be tackled quite easily with self-help measures.

We discuss too the serious diseases of the brain and nervous system — Alzheimer's and other dementing illnesses — and how to go about getting them properly diagnosed and treated. An accurate diagnosis is essential to avert the tragedy of allowing a reversible condition to deteriorate, when it could be treated or cured. Geriatricians say that in about 25 percent of cases, confused mental behavior in an older person is not caused by a permanent dementing illness.

Normal Mental Changes in Old Age

"I keep forgetting what I went out to buy at the store."

Let's begin with the normal changes in an older person's thinking processes. Changes in thinking ability happen to everyone in old age, no matter how intelligent or capable. These changes are more bothersome than burdensome, especially if the older person expects them and learns how to compensate. Normal changes involve intellectual glitches — forgetfulness and slowness — but these in no way mean that the person's overall intelligence has faltered.

Forgetfulness
The big problem for many older people — causing consternation and embarrassment — is simple forgetfulness. The nagging details of daily living can become trouble, such as remembering to turn off the stove after cooking, where you parked the car, where you last put down the car keys, whether or not the bills were paid last week, and what needs to be bought at the supermarket. Recalling names of people recently introduced can also become more formidable, even to the consummate hostess.

People of all ages lapse into forgetfulness and difficulty in remembering new information, some people more than others. But with aging even people considered highly capable and organized notice increased forgetfulness.

If your parent or an elderly friend starts to have "memory" lapses, don't become unduly worried. Every little change in the older person's behavior is *not* the beginning of the end. Fear and worry about forgetfulness and absentmindedness can only intensify the condition.

Older people who are forgetful have *not* lost their memory, and we must distinguish clearly between forgetfulness and the much more severe memory loss. Someone older worried about forgetfulness should ask, "How did I know I forgot?" The answer, "Because I remembered later," should most often be reassuring. In a dementing illness memories cannot be recalled because they have been erased from the mind. Losing the car keys all the time is forgetfulness; not knowing that they are lost or why you need them is memory loss. Forgetfulness also involves remembering an occasion but not all the details. Not remembering everyone you met at a wedding is forgetfulness; not remembering that the wedding took place is memory loss.

Forgetfulness is best explained by looking at how information in the brain moves from short-term memory to long-term memory. Short-term memory is material that you "have in mind" for a few seconds before it dissolves. You can put a new telephone number into short-term memory before dialing and then lose it as soon as you say "hello." But if you concentrate on something that is in short-term memory, such as a phone number, the information can be transferred into long-term memory, where it is filed away. Long-term memory is lasting and permanently imprinted in the brain.

Many older people have noticeable difficulty, in varying degrees, with processing or memorizing information from short-term to long-term memory, unless they make a concerted effort to commit what they have in mind to the brain's storage. And, unlike younger people, older people are less likely to commit to memory information they did not consciously intend to retain. A person with excellent short-term memory can quickly walk through a room and two hours later describe all kinds of trivial details about the room. Details which seem important to someone, or which have highly charged emotional content, seem easier to remember, but day-to-day details are often easily forgotten and get us labeled absent-minded.

Problems with Hearing and Vision Compound Forgetfulness. "I for-got where I put my glasses and can't see to find them."

An older person who is burdened with physical problems and sensory losses, especially the double loss of hearing and vision, has a much harder time coping with memory problems. Such people have problem-filled lives and are especially prone to depression. Unless the older person lives under the wing of an alert, caring person — who is willing to organize helping strategies — life can be full of aggravating and disconcerting incidents.

Consider Joe Allen, a very old man who has difficulty with his vision. He has to rely on feeling for his glasses when they are misplaced or lost, and when they can't be found he stumbles to a chair and waits in a blurry haze for hours, straining to hear a neighbor he can summon from the open window.

Or consider Susan Shapiro, a woman who has great difficulty in moving around and preparing meals because of crippling arthritis and loss of vision. While climbing the stairs to her front door, exhausted by her shopping outing, she remembers that the bag with the dinner ingredients got left behind in the taxi. Defeated and upset, she gives up on eating that evening and spends the time hungry and despondent in front of the television set. When her neighbor calls to chat, Susan is short-tempered and rude with her friend, then bursts into tears and says, "Everything has become too much."

No wonder so many old people are cruelly labeled "senile," "helpless," "dotty," and "unreliable," when the run of their daily lives can be often full of calamities.

Slower Timing
"Don't worry. I'll get it done slowly, but surely."

When psychologists talk about "slowness" being a difficulty for older people, they mean older people's timing as they pull information out of long-term memory. The information is there, tucked away in the mind, but older people take longer to retrieve it for use in all situations, including mastery of new tasks.

Research on older people's thinking ability shows that slowness does not change general overall intelligence; on a self-paced test, older people can do just as well as younger people of comparable intelligence and aptitude. On some kinds of tests of accumulated knowledge, such as manipulating vocabulary and ability to put something in writing, people actually perform better as they get older.

The person who is a whiz at some subject — say history — is not going to forget it or how it can be used in a political argument. Slowness is a subtle change and usually not noticeable unless the older person is rushed, distracted, or generally under pressure while performing tasks, learning to do something new, or making conversation.

Older people just need enough time to concentrate on what they are doing, and the old saying, "you can't teach an old dog new tricks" is simply not true; it just takes longer.

How Memory Can Be Jogged

Older people can become quite resourceful in finding ways around lapses in memory by routinely putting things in the same place, writing notes as reminders, and trying memory-training tricks. With a little courtesy and extra time, forgotten names and items can be ignored for a while; they may surface a few minutes, or even hours, later. Encourage the older person struggling with forgetfulness to use any technique that works for each problem and to experiment with different approaches.

Be very careful to keep any praise and discussion about coping methods and tricks from turning toward teasing and mockery, or worry about memory becoming worse. Older people are easily embarrassed about forgetting, and embarrassment itself becomes a discomforting stress, inhibiting and interfering with clear thinking and the inclination to explore options.

Studies show that most people at any age respond to and remember pictorial directions better than written ones. If you find that your parent or any other older person still has trouble remembering what to do despite written reminders, then turn to picture labels and directions. Buy sticky-backed pads of paper and place written and pictured directions and reminders around the house — on the refrigerator, bathroom mirror, telephone, and other strategic spots.

Helpful Hints for Remembering Better

Use the following chart to help a forgetful older person simplify household routines and daily tasks and generally cope safely with living alone.

Problem: Loses keys, eyeglasses, dentures, and other common necessities.

Solution: Choose a permanent place in which to keep important objects. Make it clear that no one is to deviate from returning objects to their designated spots. Prominently place a hook or magnetic board near the front door for car and house keys. If keys still become misplaced, ask the older person to wear keys on a neck chain, or purchase an electronic key-ring device that whistles at the sound of a clap (ask at any hardware store). A spare pair of eyeglasses should be kept in a bedside or other table drawer. The older person can wear glasses on a string during the day. Keep dentures in a bright-colored container next to the bedside or in the bathroom. If the budget allows, keep spares of these in a designated spot.

Problem: Forgets to eat.

Solution: Phone at mealtimes and remind the person about prepared food you have left in the refrigerator or freezer. Written or pictured instructions about what to eat each day can be left on the refrigerator.

Problem: Forgets some household tasks, including stocking the kitchen.

Solution: Keep a calendar with a schedule of household tasks. Remind your mother or father to do these tasks every day. Keep a pad just for grocery lists in the kitchen. Put written reminders of daily tasks on the bathroom mirror or the refrigerator.

Problem: Overlooks and disregards bills.

Solution: Set up a file box or a drawer just for bills. Encourage the older person to pay bills only while feeling rested and to write all checks down in the check register. A special checkbook (most banks offer them) with built-in carbons will guarantee that all checks written are recorded. If bill paying becomes a problem, do it yourself or assign the job to a volunteer or paid helper.

Problem: Misplaces or does not record reimbursement for Medicare and other medical payments.

Solution: Keep a notebook that can be filled out by the doctor's secretary at every visit, including columns for these: (1) date and kind of medical service received (doctor visit, test, x-ray, procedure); (2) name of the doctor who ordered the service; (3) location of the service, amount of payment, including the check number and date of payment; (4) whether medical forms are completed (check yes if completed); (5) date and amount of reimbursement received.

Reimbursement for medical bills is a complicated business. If necessary, do it yourself or assign the job to a volunteer or a paid helper.

Problem: Forgets to turn off the stove after cooking, burns pots, and leaves food in the oven too long.

Solution: Ask your parent to always set a simple egg timer while food is cooking, or to wear a timer on a chain so that it can be worn away from the kitchen. If the older person forgets to use the timer, work out a system so that you or someone else will telephone at the time food needs to be put in and taken out of the oven. Provide a whistling tea kettle. Install a smoke alarm outside the kitchen. A microwave oven can make cooking considerably easier and safer.

Problem: Forgets appointments, birthdays, anniversaries, and the day of the week.

Solution: Put a large clock in every room and a calendar or appointment book next to the telephone. The older person can maintain awareness of each day by crossing off days on the calendar. Looking at a daily newspaper and television news programs will also help the older person know what day it is. Once a week, go over important appointments and dates and make a duplicate appointment book for yourself so that you can remind the older person of appointments and special occasions.

Changed Sleep Patterns

"I wake up several times a night and can't seem to go back to sleep like I used to."

Older people often complain that they can't get a good night's sleep. The problem is especially real for those who expect to fall asleep as easily and as deeply as they did when younger. On the average, the elderly need more time to get to sleep, experience less sleep in the deeper, most restorative stages, and have more frequent interruptions in their sleep. Altered sleep patterns can be explained by an estimated 20 to 30 percent of cells lost in the part of the brain responsible for sleep — the locus ceruleus.

Sleep is divided into four stages, the last being the rapid-eye-movement (R.E.M.) dream stage when the eyes flicker and the brain becomes perfused with an increased blood supply and a blissfully restorative flow of brain chemicals. Most older people experience less of this stage-four REM sleep and, by age sixty, some people lack it altogether.

Most older people sleep more lightly and know that they do so because they can easily be jarred awake in the night by noise or physical discomfort, to say nothing of having to get up one or more times a night to go to the bathroom. Once awake it can be frustratingly difficult for them to get back to sleep, and many people say they toss and turn in the middle of the night, or the early morning, when the world seems lonely and quiet.

Older people vary in their ability to adapt to changed sleep patterns. Most seem able to gain adequate rest from light sleeping as long as they do not fret over the expectation that it should be otherwise. Nevertheless, plenty of older people do become extremely frustrated that they can't sleep a full night through, and they worry that failing to get as much sleep as they think sufficient might contribute to poor health.

For a start, it may help the older person who is upset by sleep changes to know that sleep researchers have good evidence that older people generally need less deep sleep than younger people.

The older person may have to give in and accept lower standards about how long to sleep. Rather than tossing and turning and trying to go back to sleep in the middle of the night, or the wee hours of the morning, one can think of time in bed as time to pull out a favorite book or magazine, or listen to favorite music or books on tape. The best way for older people to know whether their sleep is adequate is to judge how they feel in the morning.

Medications Can Cause Insomnia. Many of the drugs commonly taken by the elderly can contribute to sleep disturbances. Any older person having sleep difficulties must ask the doctor to determine if any medications are to blame. Medications causing loss of sleep should be changed for others that don't shorten it, or must be dropped from the drug program if they are not absolutely necessary. Blood-pressure medications, diuretics, antidepressants, and even sleeping pills can cause undesirable side effects, including confusion, agitation, jitteriness, and drowsiness. Drugs that cause daytime drowsiness can make the older person nod off during the day and rob the body of its need for sleep at night.

Sleeping pills are not the answer. Used routinely for more than a few days, they can actually interfere with sleep as the body becomes

Ways to Promote a Good Night's Sleep

If your parent complains of not being able to sleep at night, make every effort to ensure a comfortable and pleasant bedtime so that the maximum gain can be had from the sleep that does occur. Here are ways in which an older person can get a comfortable night's sleep:

• Keep to a consistent sleep schedule, with the same bedtime at night and naptime during the day.

• Keep daytime napping to a maximum of two hours. If a nap is needed, schedule it after lunch, remaining dressed and on top of the bedcovers or on a couch.

• At bedtime keep the bedroom quiet and pleasant. Make sure the temperature is comfortable and keep the room in order. For consistency, keep familiar things where they belong, such as the same lighting, pillow, and bedcovers.

• Keep active during the day, both physically and mentally. If possible, fit active exercise into the day, but avoid such strenuous activity before bedtime.

• Be sure to eat dinner long before bedtime. The digestive process can hinder sleep. On the other hand, hunger can keep someone awake, and so a light snack, such as cheese or warm milk and crackers, is a good idea, especially because the tryptophan in milk products has a mild sedative effect.

• Avoid coffee, tea, and other caffeine-containing drinks and chocolate eight hours before bed.

• Drink liquor at least five hours before bedtime, and in moderation, if at all. Alcohol will cause drowsiness for about two hours after a drink, but it can interfere with sleep and provoke early wakefulness.

• Stop drinking fluids four hours before bedtime, if bladder fullness causes awakening and frequent trips to the bathroom.

• Form an association between bed and sleep. Turn in at bedtime and use a chair or another room for evening amusements, such as television, conversation, reading.

• Use sleeping medication for three days at most and only in a special circumstance, such as a time of extreme stress when sleep is difficult to achieve.

• Do keep in touch with the doctor if sleep difficulty persists. It is a good idea to keep a record of sleep patterns and share it with the doctor. Also keep and share a record of medications taken, and recognize that medications can cause havoc with normal sleep patterns.

used to them and alters their effects. Also, many sleeping pills eventually lose their potency, meaning that to remain effective the dose has to be increased. Sleeping pills also can make us sluggish and lethargic and prone to accidents and falls.

Heat, Cold, and Being Old

Older people, particularly those who are very old, who have heart or circulatory system disease, or who are on powerful medications, are very susceptible to extremes of hot and cold. The brain's thermostat starts to lose sensitivity in many older people and body temperatures can easily fluctuate to dangerously low or high levels on either side of the normal. The older person is frequently unable to feel that the body is extremely chilled or overheated.

Both accidental hypothermia, which is a drop in internal body temperature, and hyperthermia, also called heat stroke, which is an elevation of body temperature during hot weather, are extremely dangerous medical emergencies. As we often see in news reports, every year thousands of frail or infirm older people die during cold and hot spells because they are unaware of the threat of hyperthermia or hypothermia or do not take it seriously enough to take sensible precautions.

Heat Exhaustion Can Lead to Heat Stroke
An overheated young person can easily tolerate hot weather because heat transfers out of the body's inner core to the skin, which is cooled by evaporating sweat. But elderly people retain heat not only because sweating is often absent, but also because the circulatory system is unable to make the necessary adjustments to dissipate heat.

Older people who enjoy being active should be careful during hot weather and avoid being outside doing gardening or any other outside jobs. On hot and humid summer days, hospital emergency-room staffs almost routinely expect to receive patients who have stubbornly insisted on mowing the lawn or taking a long walk outdoors.

Even a sedentary older person can have difficulty tolerating the heat on a very hot day. An older person just sitting in a chair with too many clothes left on from the cool morning can become overheated and ill in an inside temperature approaching 80 degrees. They don't feel the heat enough to complain about it, though younger family members may be cooling off on the porch with cold drinks and light clothing.

Only when heat exhaustion starts to take its toll will the older person complain of headache, nausea, and weakness. The skin is ashen pale and perhaps slightly moist. If heat exhaustion does occur, slowly cool off the older person with a sponge bath of tepid, *not* cold, water and have him or her lie down in a cool room, offering plenty of cool fluids. Take the temperature, and if it is above the normal 98.6 degrees, call the doctor.

Heat stroke occurs when the older person goes into circulatory shock and unconsciousness because the body temperature rises higher than 105 degrees. Immediately call for an ambulance if you find an older person obviously hot to the touch, unable to speak and near unconsciousness, or actually unconscious. You must absolutely *not* try to quickly cool the individual down with cold compresses or a cold bath, nor should the victim be put in front of a fan or air conditioner. Of course take the older person from direct sunlight or an overheated room to a cooler one before the ambulance arrives; otherwise, leave the job of treatment to medical professionals, who know how to cool down a heat-stroke victim with the aim of preventing a fatal heart attack.

Hypothermia

The scenario of hypothermia that comes to mind for most people is of an old person freezing to death huddled against the cold in blankets, while winter rages outside. Although many older people do suffer hypothermia in badly heated living quarters during the winter, the condition can occur at any time of year, in any chilly atmosphere, at 65 degrees or less.

Those who have defective temperature regulation can lapse into hypothermia while sitting in front of an air conditioner, a fan, or in a drafty corner of a room. Extreme cold is not the only cause of hypothermia, then; older people can become hypothermic in temperatures that active younger people would find tolerable, if not comfortable. Quite a few people go along day after day, suffering the effects of mild hypothermia without recognizing that they feel the cold.

Symptoms of low-grade hypothermia include lethargy, vague-

ness and slow thinking, and pallor. The lethargy is the most dangerous symptom, for the older person will want to lie down frequently,
lowering the body temperature even further.

Low-grade hypothermia can be diagnosed by taking the older
person's temperature and feeling to see if the skin is indeed cold,
even on the abdomen. If the temperature is hovering just below 98.6
degrees, and the older person is obviously conscious and alert, then
call the doctor for medical advice. First, make the person comfortable in a warm room with a couple of blankets snugly wrapped around
the body, then offer a warm drink.

Hypothermia is always a medical emergency if body temperature drops below 95 degrees. As with heat stroke, an ambulance has
to be called so that the body can be brought back to normal temperature range under strict medical supervision. Although it will be
tempting to warm the person with direct heat from an electric blanket turned up high, a hot bath, or sitting in front of the fire, no direct
heat must be applied. Localized heat will cause a rapid increase in
flow of blood to that area and deplete the vital organs (heart, lungs,
brain, and so on).

Ways of Preventing Accidental Hypothermia

• Become aware of the symptoms of mild to severe hypothermia.

• If the older person you are caring for finds it necessary to save
on fuel costs, contact government-funded programs designed to help
low-income elderly people pay energy bills or to get emergency repairs of heating units.

• Keep indoor temperatures always above 65 degrees F (18 degrees C).

• Make sure adequate clothing is worn indoors and outside. For
inside wear, two or three layers of light, warm clothing are better
than one or more layers of thick, warm clothing worn close to the
body. Hats and gloves must be worn outside in weather below 60
degrees.

• Encourage the older person to be as active as possible, because
exercise keeps body temperature up.

• Make sure the older person is eating correctly; the body needs
calories to produce heat.

• Hypothermia can more easily start during sleep and repose.

Provide warm pajamas, adequate blankets, and, if the older person is especially prone to hypothermia, a hat to wear in bed.

• If you can't do it yourself, ask friends and neighbors to look in once or twice a day, particularly during a cold spell.

• Ask the doctor whether medications the older person is taking might affect control of body temperature.

Memory Loss and Confusion Disorders

Memory loss is a very different problem from the simple forgetfulness that we described earlier. When long-term memory goes because of disease that impairs brain function, an older person will start to show telling signs of dementia, or the condition doctors commonly speak of as confusion.

If the disease causing confusion progresses, drastic personality changes become evident, as well as complete inability to perform even the simplest tasks. Eventually the demented person may need to be spoon fed like a child and kept out of harm's way.

Probably no other disease involves families as much as dementing illness. The family becomes just as much a victim of the disease, for the caregiving is a relentless and extremely difficult twenty-four-hour job.

How Do You Know Memory Loss Is More Than Normal Forgetfulness?

At first, unless a sudden onset of memory loss occurs, which is a medical emergency, the memory losses of dementia are barely distinguishable from the forgetfulness and absentmindedness that everyone experiences.

How do you tell, then, if someone's memory lapses indicate a real problem that merits consultation with a doctor? These questions should help you assess whether or not you need to go to the doctor for an evaluation:

1. Does the older person forget well-known information?
2. Does the older person repeatedly totally lose recall of recent events, such as your visit the day before, or the food just served at lunch?
3. Are there signs of difficulty in doing tasks that have always

been done well, such as reading a book, knitting a sweater, or balancing the checkbook?

4. Has forgetfulness begun to cause significant troubles with safety, such as driving on the wrong side of the road, or leaving the cooking gas on repeatedly?

Acute Confusion Can Be Treated

Jane Simpson left her husband, James, at home in Oregon, while she helped take care of a newborn grandchild in California. One day when she called James he sounded far from normal. He couldn't remember why his wife had gone away, and when Jane asked if he felt ill, he giggled and hung up the phone. Naturally being extremely worried, Jane called the family's doctor.

James was hospitalized. After extensive tests Jane was told he had a thyroid condition that had come on without the characteristic protruding eyes and hyperactivity seen in younger people. Within several days of drug treatment, James started to feel and act like his usual self.

Acute confusion in an older person usually means that something is drastically wrong with the body. Because older people are often so frail physically, with few physical reserves to fall back on, a number of conditions and illnesses can easily throw the body off so that the brain and nervous system are tipped out of balance.

Often the only way you can tell that an older person is suffering a physical crisis is that his or her behavior changes over a week, day, or even an hour. If symptoms come on suddenly, it is more likely that they are caused by a reversible disease.

For you and those who know the older person well, understanding that something is wrong should be obvious. If you call your mother one day and she sounds odd, perhaps even does not know who you are, then you are up against a medical emergency.

Any change in an older person's behavior indicates trouble. If he or she suddenly starts to appear disheveled and sloppy, this too may be a sign of mental confusion and an underlying health problem. The acutely confused person will typically appear disoriented about time and place, mistaking one person for another, and common objects for others. Restlessness, unusual aggressiveness, or a dazed expression may be noticed.

A number of conditions can cause temporary confusion in the elderly — temporary if they are swiftly diagnosed and treated. In the hands of an expert doctor who fully understands the complex differences between older and younger patients, a condition can be reversed and the older person can be back to normal within days or weeks.

The commonest causes of temporary confusion, not specifically disease-related, are drug toxicity, a blow to the head in a fall, or a bump into a door or a wall.

The brain has no storage reservoir for oxygen, which is essential to healthy brain function, and so any number of conditions that impede normal and efficient oxygen transport are likely to cause confusion, such as heart failure, a small stroke, malnutrition and anemia, any kind of infection, dehydration, and many other conditions. The body's endocrine glands — the thyroid, pancreas, adrenals, pituitary, and ovaries and testes — are responsible for keeping the body in homeostasis or composure. These can easily go awry as hormone levels wax and wane in the aging body.

If you find yourself taking care of someone who is acutely and temporarily confused, you need to know how to help this person manage behaviors that are self-destructive, potentially embarrassing, or harmful to others. It can take weeks after a cause for confusion has been pinpointed for the brain to calm down and fully accept treatment, or withdrawal of a drug. The chart "Ways of Managing Confusion Behaviors" at the end of this chapter describes behaviors that can occur and how you can manage them.

You Must Find a Doctor Who Fully Understands Confusion
Doctors often say that nothing is as confusing as confusion in the elderly. When sitting in front of a seemingly demented older person in the office, the doctor is faced with the taxing task of pinning down a cause. More than a hundred reversible and treatable conditions, some of them acute and some of them not, can mimic any of the symptoms of the serious dementing illnesses such as Alzheimer's, and these must be ruled out before a diagnosis of permanent dementia is possible.

A scrupulous diagnosis is essential; a mistaken one and too quick a verdict of permanent dementia is not just a mistake but extremely dangerous. The underlying cause of confused behavior can turn a reversible condition into a permanent disability, or worse, a slide into a life-threatening illness.

You Need to Take Charge. If you do need to take your relative to a doctor for an evaluation of confusion, make sure the doctor is willing and able to devote the time you should expect for an accurate diagnosis, and, particularly important, time alone with you and other family members. More than in any other condition, other than looking out for the best interests of someone who is unconscious, you need to be an advocate. It is up to you to present the case and make sure that everything possible is done to get to the bottom of the condition. The doctor will want to find out from you how your family member behaves normally, when behavior became obviously "off" the normal, and what behavior is prevalent now.

Your confused relative will not be able to present an accurate history. Typically, even a mildly impaired person cannot do so because pride gets in the way, along with the confusion. Confused older people often know they are confused, and they will go to great lengths to disguise their disorientation and memory loss. Often charm and humor are used as coverups. The older woman who can't remember her age will say to the doctor who asks her age, "What's a young person like you doing asking me a question like that?" Or the man who can't recall how he got to the doctor's office will respond to the question, "Do you know where you are?" with the coy answer, "Here with you, of course."

Getting to an Accurate Diagnosis. Your usual doctor may be able to do the evaluation or send you to a specialist who can. If you do not feel confident about finding a good doctor in this way, contact the Alzheimer Disease and Related Disorders Association (see Appendix). They are an effective national group and can supply you with names of doctors near you, as well as information about dementia and caregiving.

Not all doctors are able to take the time to thoroughly look at a demented patient, especially those with crowded practices, and some may not be skilled enough to do the specialized job. Also, it is a deplorable fact of life that you can come up against a doctor, or more than one, who is unsympathetic and lacks interest because of personal anxieties, even abhorrence, about dementia. Someone with these limitations may quickly label the person "senile" and deny them an extensive examination to seek the cause of the dementia.

Here's what an evaluation should tell you and the doctor — do not settle for anything less:

- the exact character of the underlying illness
- the extent of the disease
- whether or not the illness can be treated and reversed
- whether or not other health problems, including vision and hearing disabilities might be making the confusion worse
- whether or not extraordinary stresses, such as grief and isolation, could have contributed to severe depression
- what the long-term picture looks like so that you can start arranging plans and assistance for the future

To make a diagnosis the doctor should start with the complete history that involves you, or another family member. Right away, the history may reveal that the confused behavior comes from a drug-induced brain dysfunction that may have taken months to form; drugs very often cause mental changes and confusion in the elderly. The history could also reveal that depression is causing profound behavioral changes. A depressive illness can totally change one's personality, contributing to lack of attention to personal hygiene, insomnia, and a pervasive feeling of being no good. Depressed people often forget what happens to them from one day to the next.

Even the basic early steps in the examination may bring up abnormalities that could be causing the confusion. An abnormal pulse and blood-pressure reading could indicate that the brain is getting too little oxygen because of a blood-pressure disorder, or a urine test could show a urinary-tract infection.

A complete battery of tests should be conducted and a process of elimination started before a diagnosis of a permanently dementing illness is put in the record. In the final analysis a computerized axial tomography (CAT) scan test or a magnetic resonance imaging (MRI) test may be warranted. These tests are costly if insurance coverage is not available, but worth the expense. An efficient doctor will want to run more tests on the patient even after a suspected cause of dementia has been pinned down, to be sure that other causes are not present to add insult to injury.

The Two Commonest Incurable Dementing Illnesses

Late-life dementia is the name for a number of diseases that cause tissue damage to the brain and permanent, progressive confusion, or dementia, in a person over sixty-five. Most people who become demented with an incurable condition have either Alzheimer's — now as well known as the common cold — which accounts for an estimated 60 percent of cases, or multi-infarct dementia, a blood-vessel disorder responsible for about 20 percent of cases. About 15 percent of demented older people have both Alzheimer's and multi-infarct dementia. Approximately 5 percent of the cases are traced to a few very rare diseases.

Any late-life dementia presents a tragedy, a hell on earth, for its victims and their families, because with it personality gradually disintegrates, often in an otherwise healthy body. The breaking down of personality, not being a psychological disorder, has nothing to do with a person's previous personality, intelligence, or education.

Alzheimer's Disease

The media attention to Alzheimer's disease in recent years has been so widespread that everyone has become aware of and dreads it. Although the disease afflicts around 4 million unfortunate people, and is the fourth leading cause of death among the elderly, it is not as prevalent as many people think, especially among the young old. About 10 percent of those over sixty-five suffer from the condition, and the likelihood of developing the disease increases with age. In the over-eighty-five population, about 47 percent suffer from Alzheimer's and it is the commonest reason for someone to be admitted to a nursing home. The disease does not discriminate between races, but it does seem to affect more women than men, for the uncomplicated reason that women are likely to live longer.

Although the cause of Alzheimer's disease is still a medical mystery, much is known about how the disease damages the brain. In the early stages, strings of the brain's nerve cells start to clump and tangle together and abnormal waxy formations — amyloid plaques — form around nerve cells. A brain chemical — acetylcholine — responsible for transmitting information between cells also decreases in concentration. These damaging developments first occur in the parts of the brain that control performance, memory, mood, and sleep; the signs of the disease usually involve gradual changes in these functions.

Alzheimer's is commonly divided into three stages. Symptoms often become so extremely difficult to deal with toward the end of the second stage that families place their relatives in a skilled nursing home despite any financial hardships.

The earliest stage may last from two to four years. Subtle changes occur, such as lack of "spark" in a person with a previously sharp sense of humor; lack of energy and enthusiasm for life; or decreased interest in family, friends, and favorite pastimes. The victim's personality change may come out in behavior that is a caricature of the previous personality; an extrovert may become a bombastic show-off, and an introvert may become extremely shy and afraid of new people and situations. This first stage includes progressive loss of short-term memory, though events of the distant past may remain relatively clear and understood. Toward the second stage the victim will not be able to hold a job, carry out most daily tasks, or organize time and dates.

The middle stage may last several years, and is characterized by extreme confusion and difficulty in coping with new situations, as long-term memory fails and is gradually erased from the mind. Driving must of course be given up because Alzheimer's sufferers at this stage become unable to sort out signals and cues, such as sounds, lights, and signposts, and they can easily become lost, even in familiar places close to home. The individual may babble in conversation and not remember from one sentence to the next. Immigrants who have spoken a second language for decades may revert to their native tongue. Wandering, especially at night, can occur, as well as agitated repetitive behavior. "Sundowning," a phenomenon associated with extreme restlessness, agitation, and wandering, may become a daily occurrence at about four o'clock in the afternoon.

During the middle stage, victims will still recognize familiar people. Trying to find security in their Alice-in-Wonderland tangled world, they will latch on to one or more favorite people, so that sharing the task of caregiving among a family and friends can become complicated.

The final stage of the disease usually is fairly short, one to two years at most, although it can be longer. The suffering patient will become emaciated and thin, and reach a virtual vegetative state. Memory traces are so thoroughly erased that the victim recognizes no one, not even his or her own face in the mirror. And the overall nervous system controlling body functions starts to show it is damaged by incontinence, difficulty in coordinating body movements, and sometimes seizures.

The facts about Alzheimer's disease are hard and most cruel, and no one can provide total care to an Alzheimer's victim in the middle to final stages of the disease without help. Those who try usually become physically exhausted and emotionally drained. If you do find yourself caring for a relative who has been diagnosed as having Alzheimer's disease, do start early to ask for help and understand where you can get it. In Chapter 15 you will find a thorough look at the various services available to caregivers.

If you are caring for someone who has Alzheimer's disease you need to recognize and learn how to handle the specific problems of the disease. Contact the Alzheimer's Disease and Related Disorders Association in your state or community. They will offer you information about the disease and support you in finding out about nearby programs for Alzheimer's disease. The disease has become so well known in recent years that well-funded programs have cropped up in all large and medium-sized cities across the country, and in many small towns as well.

Multi-infarct Dementia

In this disease, sufferers gradually lose their long-term memory traces — in effect, their mind — just as someone does with Alzheimer's. But here the brain becomes damaged by frequent ministrokes, often so small and painless that they do not show up in the sophisticated tests usually applied in diagnosing strokes.

These ministrokes occur because blood vessels supplying the brain are fragile and diseased, and they often rupture, causing tiny amounts of blood to leak into brain tissue, or they block up with accumulated atherosclerotic material — fatty plaques — so that oxygen-rich blood cannot perfuse the brain. Brain tissue may be destroyed in just one area at first, but as more strokes occur many small scattered areas of the brain are affected.

The disease is three times commoner in men than in women because men are more prone to diseases of the vascular tree and heart. Risk factors include atherosclerosis, previous strokes, heart attacks, angina, high blood pressure, and diabetes.

The disease is preventable to the extent that everyone can ward off heart disease, strokes, and diabetes by not smoking and by drinking alcohol in moderation, exercising regularly, and eating a low-cholesterol, sensible diet. Those who get early and proper treatment for high blood pressure can also bring their blood pressure into normal range and ward off ministroke destruction.

As ministrokes occur over and over, the sufferer may start to show the same general intellectual deterioration and episodes of confused behavior that are characteristic of Alzheimer's disease; however, insight and personality remain intact longer with this disease. For this reason the sufferer may easily become despairing and severely depressed about the gradual loss of reasoning and inability to keep a grip on the "self."

Ministrokes are not always recognizable when they happen. The older person may appear clouded and disoriented and complain of dizziness, but not always. All such symptoms must of course be reported to the doctor.

The mental deterioration that gradually occurs cannot be placed into definable stages, as it more typically can with Alzheimer's. As strokes occur, mental functioning deteriorates in a more erratic and more steplike way. Sometimes mental state improves within a few weeks of a stroke, but always some disability is left. Although not much can be done to repair a disease-ravaged network of blood vessels, treatment is generally aimed at keeping blood pressure down.

Ways of Managing Severe Confusion Behaviors

If the cause of confused, generally odd, and even "wacky" behavior is temporary, the brain can sometimes take several weeks to settle down to its normal functioning after corrective medical treatment. If the cause is a permanent illness the confusion will gradually get worse.

While taking care of a confused person, be as understanding as you can of the cause behind any behavior and use patience and repetition in your communication. Memory-impaired confused people need more time to comprehend what others are saying. They respond better to positive statements: it is easier for them to understand what you "want" them to do than what you don't want them to do.

This list will help you manage several behavioral patterns often exhibited by older people who are confused and disoriented by drug side effects, or a temporary or permanent dementing illness. The behaviors are examples of disturbed brain function and therefore are much more pronounced and severe than the so-called normal problems we address in the list of helpful hints beginning on page 34.

Confused behavior: Agitated, purposeless, hurried conduct.
How you can manage it:

- Try to determine why the confused person is agitated. Is he or she too cold, too hot, hungry, frightened, in pain?
- Establish eye contact and approach the confused person slowly from the front.
- Maintain an atmosphere of calm, and keep the household orderly.
- Play soothing music.
- Try to direct the person to a purposeful activity or chore, such as watering plants, putting photos in an album, or helping prepare meals.

Confused behavior: Overreacting and aggressive, hostile behavior "over nothing at all."
How you can manage it:

- Simplify tasks and requests.
- Keep noise and activity in the household low.
- Understand that an emotional outburst can be triggered by the confused person's being frightened because he or she does not know what is going on at the time.
- Fear of something whether real or imagined and illusory, can cause overreaction. Is something frightening the confused person, on television, outdoors, a stranger, an animal?
- Make the person as physically comfortable as possible. Is there pain or constipation?
- Avoid scolding and arguing.
- Calmly remove the confused person from any stressful situation, and divert him or her to another activity or a "treat." Soft music, holding hands, and even gentle rocking or going for a walk may help calm the person. (Most confused people can easily be diverted.)
- If the confused person becomes dangerously violent, get several people, if possible, to stand around the person, but out of reach. He or she may calm down when his or her violent actions seem futile.
- Do not hesitate to leave and call for help, if your safety is in jeopardy. Usually, violent outbursts are temporary and quick. Call the police, however, if this is the only option. (But explain that illness is the cause of the violent behavior.)
- Avoid arguments and explanations about the overreactive behavior; it is generally beyond the confused person's control.

Confused behavior: Suspiciousness.
How you can manage it:

- Whenever possible, keep to a predictable daily routine and explain deviations from the normal.
- When appropriate, always explain what you are doing and give simple, accurate information.
- Never whisper in front of the confused person, or talk about the person while you are in the same room.

Confused behavior: Hoarding objects.
How you can manage it:

- Find out where objects are being hoarded (may be in several special spots). Look in dresser drawers, boxes, coat pockets, shoes, and wastebaskets.
- Accept the behavior if it is safe and not too inconvenient.
- Keep important and valued items locked up.
- Limit hiding places by locking cupboards and rooms that the confused person does not use.
- If the person shows attachment to and holds on to a dangerous object, replace it with something harmless.

Confused behavior: Rummaging for "lost" items.
How you can manage it:

- Help the older person "find" whatever is being sought, and then try to redirect him or her to a constructive activity.

Confused behavior: Sees illusions — distortions of things that are there.
How you can manage it:

- Respond calmly to whatever the confused person is "feeling" (remember that the person's beliefs are based on his or her reality).
- Touch the person gently and offer reassurance that you will see that things are all right.
- Remove disturbing objects from the room, if possible.

- Make sure distorting losses of vision are corrected with appropriate glasses and proper treatments.
- Provide adequate lighting that eliminates shadows and dark areas in the room.
- Keep furnishings simple.

Confused behavior: Wandering out of the house.
How you can manage it:

- Look for possible reasons for wandering behavior and determine if you can offer solutions to the problem.
- Try to reduce wandering by taking the confused person on frequent walks, or by providing other exercise, such as raking leaves or sweeping the house or the driveway.
- Install a high fence with locked gates so that the confused person can freely wander outdoors.
- Alert neighbors to the problem so that they can call you if they see the confused person beyond safe boundaries.
- Never leave the memory-impaired person alone in a parked car.
- Provide a Medi-Alert identification bracelet with name, address, and telephone number.
- Attach a bell to exit doors, or a photoelectric device that rings when the confused person goes outside.
- Lock doors with deadbolts placed at the top of the door.
- Keep a recent photograph of the older person readily available so that it can be used if a police search is needed.

Confused behavior: Disorientation at mealtimes.
How you can manage it:

- Keep mealtimes and meal routines consistent, and menus familiar.
- Do not use patterned tablecloths or dishes.
- Provide one utensil at a time.
- Cut food into bite-size pieces.
- Serve soup and stew in a handled mug or bowl.
- Use bendable straws for drinks.
- Leave condiments off the table.

Confused behavior: Choking while eating.
How you can manage it:

- Confused person must eat in an upright sitting position.
- Serve moist foods: applesauce, puréed vegetables, scrambled eggs, cottage cheese.
- Serve thick liquid drinks (clear liquids are easy to choke on) — milkshakes, or fruit or vegetable purées.
- Offer clear liquid only through a bendable straw.
- Check if dentures are properly fitted.
- Learn the Heimlich lifesaving maneuver for choking.

Confused behavior: Fear of splashing and spraying water and bathtime procedures.
How you can manage it:

- Fill the bathtub with three to four inches of water before the confused person enters the bathroom.
- Don't drain the bath while the confused person is in the tub (commonly creates anxiety).
- Initiate bathtime slowly and methodically while the household is calm and the bathroom warm and uncluttered.
- Keep to a routine bathtime, consistent with the person's lifelong routine.
- Never force bathing. If you meet resistance, wait until a suitable time. You may have to lower your expectations about how many times the confused person should have a bath.
- Have towel, soap, cloths together at the start and show each, so that the confused person can use them in sequence.
- Showers usually are more disturbing than baths. If neither works, try seating the confused person in a plastic bath chair placed in the tub. Next, give a slow, gentle sponge bath while explaining each step.
- Install grab bars, a nonslip mat, and a shower head on a flexible hose.
- Keep bathing as private as possible. Allow the confused person to do as much as possible. But most important, never leave the person unattended in the bathtub or shower.

Confused behavior: Wears inappropriate clothing.
How you can manage it:

- Remove off-season clothes from closets and drawers, and edit the wardrobe to the appropriate basics.
- Put suitable clothes out every morning and for bedtime.
- Use clothes, such as sweat pants and tops, that can be put on and taken off easily and that help the confused person dress independently.

Confused behavior: Difficulty in finding the bathroom.
How you can manage it:

- Put bright, glow-in-the-dark colored tape on the floor leading to the bathroom.
- Place a sign or a picture on the bathroom door.

Confused behavior: "Sundowning" or increased confusion in the late afternoon and evening, as confused person becomes unable to cope with any more stimulation and with the surroundings.
How you can manage it:

- Evaluate the person's day and determine if it is too tiring and stimulating.
- It may help to alternate activity (including dressing, meals, and so on) with quiet periods, and generally to gear down daily activity.
- Encourage a scheduled one-hour nap after lunch, and reduce all noise and distractions during this time (music may be the exception).

Confused behavior: Problems with the sleep-wake cycle. Inability to settle down for sleep, disorientation at night.
How you can manage it:

- Have a consistent wakeup time, no matter when the confused person goes to sleep.
- Make sure the person dresses soon after awakening.
- If possible, use the bedroom for sleeping only.
- Keep the house brightly lit both day and evening.
- Establish a bedtime ritual: place nightclothes on the bed before changing into them, toileting, washing, offer a soothing backrub.

- Don't offer liquids in the three hours before bedtime and do make certain the confused person has urinated before bed.
- Discuss medications with the doctor. It may be helpful to discontinue inappropriate medications, or change to alternative medications.
- Offer a stuffed animal for comfort (many confused people will accept one).
- Avoid caffeine, excess sugar, and alcohol in the diet. Be sure the diet is sensible.
- Offer any prescribed pain medications half an hour before bedtime.

4

Beating Out Depression

DEPRESSION IS THE MOST common mental-health problem for older people, but it's often overlooked.

Few people realize that depression should be looked at with the same concern as stroke, cancer, or heart disease. We worry about getting proper medical treatment for these problems, but don't think of depression as the serious disorder that it is. Too often when an older person goes to the doctor, his or her emotional state gets short shrift compared to all the things that can go wrong with the body's nuts-and-bolts physical functions.

All of us feel down sometimes in reaction to major disappointments and losses, and we all go through the terrible pain and sorrow that mourning the death of someone we love brings. But depression as an illness is something different.

Depression is a mood disorder that can range from prolonged feelings of sadness to the pain and despair of a severe depression, where every experience is felt as mental pain. In more severe forms depression can be life-threatening.

Severely depressed people can feel so much suffering that suicidal thoughts enter their minds as the best way out from a world they see as a deepening sinkhole of despair. Suicide is disturbingly common among the severely depressed elderly; in fact, elderly white men have the *highest* rate of suicide — three to four times that of the general population.

Depressed people can also experience worsening in any of their previous health problems. For older people, poor appetite, lost sleep, constant fatigue, and constipation, among other physical signs of depression, can bring on illnesses or tip any others they may have over the edge. Muddled thinking, negativism, and inertia can make it difficult for the older person to remember, or see the point in taking, helpful medications on time — if at all — or to carry out any other health-promoting measures that are part of a treatment plan.

Old Age Does Not Necessarily Mean Despair

One great misconception about aging is that to be old is depressing. This myth walls off older people from proper treatment for depressions that they are unable to pull out of on their own. Plenty of older people don't get depressed as a matter of course, despite the frequent blows they usually get hit with at their stage of life.

Many older people do indeed become depressed as hardships stack on top of each other. Losses can occur in rapid succession, without adequate recovery time before the next loss hits. An older person can watch several friends — those who are left — die within a year or two of a beloved spouse's death. Wearing and disabling illnesses can also occur along with diminished senses.

But despite the extraordinary hardships, many people in their eighties and nineties are able to ride through the despairing and sad times and find the wherewithal to cope. Plenty of older people do remain quite happy in their final years, and they somehow achieve a sense of wholeness and integrity.

Eric Erikson, the well-known psychologist, put together a theory (while in his mid-eighties) explaining why some older people are able to overcome despair. With this theory he expanded his model of the life cycle as a series of developmental stages each of which we must successfully master to go on to the next one. He does believe we can successfully reach and go through old age, if we achieve "ego integrity" — realize who we are and who we have been — versus "despair" at being old. To find integrity an older person must grapple with the positive and negative experiences of a lifetime so that this lifetime has meaning. The older person must use the past to bring meaning to the present.

A lifetime of loving relationships and a sense of effectiveness make coming to terms with integrity easier. Also important is that the older person believe he or she has a place among the generations, with the idea that his or her life will have a positive bearing on future generations, not just within the immediate family and circle of relationships, but in the world at large.

As family or as a friend, you can help the older person experience this idea of generations. Do all you can to help make the person feel important, not just now, but in the lifetime context. Encourage your mother or father to reminisce about the past with storytelling and photographs. If possible, help your parent arrange visits to old friends and places that continue to hold special meaning.

Reasons for Depression

Although depression is by no means a normal part of growing old, many, many older people do suffer depression. The elderly of all types and temperaments are at high risk. Several factors predispose older people of any personality type to depressive illness.

For a start, extensive evidence now shows that aging changes in the nervous system — altered quantities of chemicals secreted by the brain — have some influence. Although these changes by themselves probably don't cause depression, they probably can do so when combined with factors such as falling ill, or distress from an upsetting circumstance, be it the death of a friend or the diagnosis of a dreaded disease.

Plenty of illnesses — to which the elderly are prone — create depression as part of their disease process by altering the brain's balance of chemicals that control mood. Stroke, Parkinson's disease, rheumatoid arthritis, and brain tumor are prime examples. Many hormonal disorders can cause depression, and almost everyone who develops hypothyroid disease feels depressed and irritable. Anemia also causes alterations in mood. Some types of cancer can bring on depression. Beyond specific diseases better known as causes of depression, any disease that upsets the body's metabolism can set it off. Fluid imbalances, lack of oxygen, or depletion of body salts such as sodium and potassium, are all culprits.

Any disease that produces fear, chronic pain, disability, and dependence — let alone social isolation — can cause someone to react to these stresses with depression. A slowly developing disease may bring out an evolving depression, and one with sudden onset can bring on a more dramatic psychological response. The person with a serious cancer condition, a disabling heart attack, or a stroke is at especially high risk of becoming severely depressed.

Another major and often-overlooked cause of depression is medication. Hundreds of drugs that are given to treat disorders other than those of the brain enter it anyhow and tamper with its func-

Medications That May Cause Depression

Tranquilizers or sleeping pills

Dalmane	Librium	Valium
Halcion	Restoril	Xanax

Heart and blood-pressure medications

Aldomet	Lopressor	Norpace
Catapres	Minipress	Procan SR
Corgard	Moduretic	Tenoretic
Inderal		Tenormin

Ulcer medications

Tagamet	Zantac

Antiparkinsonian drugs

Dopar	Parlodel	Sinemet

Steroid medications

Aristocort	Decadron

Antiseizure medications

Dilantin	Luminal	Zarontin
	Mysolin	

Arthritis medications

Advil, Motrin, Nuprin	Feldene	Nalfon
	Indocin	Naprosyn
	Clinoril	

tioning. Drugs known to cause depression — sometimes — include blood-pressure medications, some antibiotics, many heart drugs, diabetes control pills, and steroids. Even drugs given to help people with psychiatric disorders or physical disorders of the brain are also known to flip in their intended effects and cause depression.

Alcohol can also strongly contribute to depression in people of any age, but especially the elderly. Most elderly people can't hold their drinks as well as they could when younger, because they become more sensitive to alcohol's effects. Alcohol and depression actually combine in a vicious-circle relationship. The depressed person can turn to drinking and then feel more depressed, which in turn can lead to more drinks and eventually alcohol abuse with its three-ring circus of problems.

Symptoms Are Not Always Easy to Identify

It is often quite tricky to tell if an older person is indeed depressed. The label "masked" depression — which could also be called "missed" depression — means a depression that is not manifested in the usual way with outward expressions of sadness and dejection.

Depressed people at any age often feel ashamed of being depressed and try hard as they can to cover up their pain, for fear that owning up to it will be interpreted by others as weakness of character. Often people hang in there, believing and hoping that their anguish will go away by itself. And even when it doesn't, they suffer in silence rather than seek help from a psychiatrist — a specialist for "crazies" or self-indulgent neurotics, they may well think.

But aside from covering up and not admitting to suffering, elderly people sometimes don't even know that what they are feeling is depression. Many grew up in a family atmosphere and at a time when it was *not* socially acceptable to outwardly and frankly express emotions such as sadness, guilt, and anger. In such people, emotions are replaced by physical complaints because they can't express disturbances in their mood.

Such manifestations of depression are often reported to the doctor as vague complaints about aches and pains. "It's not my headaches that are bothering me this time, doctor, but the pains in my side" or "My neck's stiff all the time." Other symptoms can include constipation, sudden shortness of breath with no apparent cause, or chest pains. Weight loss is another common symptom.

Often older people who are depressed give the initial appearance of being mentally confused. Consider Joan Harman, an eighty-two-year-old who was brought to a geriatric psychiatry clinic at the local medical center by her daughter, who was worried her mother had Alzheimer's disease. While her mother sat in the waiting room, the daughter told the psychiatrist how her mother had recently stopped taking care of herself and going out of the house. Mrs. Harman, who had always gone to the beauty parlor and loved to dress up, hadn't washed her hair in weeks, hardly even took a bath, and paid no attention to her wardrobe. She had also become very forgetful about where things were in the house and how to do simple everyday tasks. One day, the daughter reported, Mrs. Harman overflowed the bathtub water, and when a visitor heard the water dripping down the stairs from the floor above, Mrs. Harman didn't seem to care.

In the psychiatrist's office, Mrs. Harman fidgeted and looked down at her feet and answered every question with a slow "I dunno." Hearing this response over and over made him think his patient was more likely to be depressed than suffering a dementing illness. He knew that people who are suffering from such an illness usually go to great lengths to keep from admitting they don't know the answers to questions.

If your parent is not obviously letting anyone know he or she is severely down, you may have to pick up hints that something is wrong. You know your mother's usual way of doing things and her usual temperament and how she usually takes care of herself. When she visits the doctor, he may miss her depression and instead look only at the physical symptoms she complains about.

Obvious signs of depression are easy to spot. Your parent may come out and say he or she is depressed, with expressions such as "I'm old and tired and what's the point of going on?" or "everyone is waiting for me to die, so why should I keep going to the doctor?" Your parent may also become sad-looking and teary over every little irritation, even about events that happened years ago, perhaps in childhood. Anxiety, irritation, worry, and grouchiness all the time can also be signs of depression. The person in a deep depression may not even want to talk about it, but may show marked depression with a dejected expression and a slow, sorry, stooped way of walking.

Psychiatrists these days generally agree that depression has become a mood disorder if someone feels low, empty, and down in the dumps *for more than two weeks* with four or more of these classic symptoms:

- lack of appetite and significant loss of weight (in younger people, weight gain can also be a problem)
- sleep disturbances, including insomnia, early-morning awakening, or oversleeping

- hyperactivity or a slowdown in activity
- loss of interest in everyday activities that formerly were enjoyed
- tiredness and lack of energy
- expressions of pessimism, feelings of worthlessness, guilt
- indecisiveness, muddled thoughts, and inability to concentrate
- frequent talk and thoughts of death and references to suicide, or even a suicide attempt

Treatment

Treatment starts when the older person sees a doctor who understands depression in older people: how to look for it, how to rule it in or out, and how to treat it — if it is indeed present. The primary doctor is the best person for your parent to see first because he or she can start examining your parent to find out if any new illnesses are causing the depression, or, for that matter, any illnesses already there. This doctor, as commander-in-chief of your parent's medications, will also be the best person to have a good look at all the medications your parent is on, to see if any of these are the crux of the depression, or a contributing cause. The doctor will probably want to run a full battery of basic tests, as well as specific tests to help determine the cause of any physical symptoms your parent may be complaining about.

Evaluation of the depression is best left up to a psychiatrist interested in working with older people.

Your primary physician should be able to diagnose that a depression is there; but the psychiatrist will know best how to do a thorough workup of the depression, as a psychological illness, and from there prescribe treatment that can be continued either with the psychiatrist, or with the primary doctor. Any good primary physician will know names of psychiatrists who treat problems peculiar to the elderly. If, for any reason, you need to find a psychiatrist on your own, try a local medical center to see if it has a geriatric psychiatry clinic, or staff specialists in geriatric psychiatry.

Depression is not just one illness, it is a broad name for a number of depressive illnesses that affect the normal chemistry of the brain. Treatment depends on the psychiatrist's determining the kind of depression the older person has, as well as its severity.

Older patients who have mild depression are not routinely put on a course of daily antidepressant medications, for these usually have side effects that can impair daily functioning worse than the disorder does. Antidepressants may also not work for some of the more moderate forms of depression.

Mildly depressed older people more frequently are helped by talk therapy to expose self-defeating behavior and problems that can be resolved. Many psychiatrists refer mildly depressed older people to group-therapy sessions led by psychologists and psychiatric social workers. Often these groups are put together to help people who have similar problems, be it adjustment to widowhood, incapacitation of a spouse, or a specific disease.

Support from family and friends is also indispensable for the mildly depressed person. As a family you need to help your parent try to get out of the trap of depression in any way possible. First, you need to solve any immediate problems — let's say getting your parent a hearing aid or proper eyeglasses — and then take steps to ward off imminent problems within your control.

More severe forms of depression are usually treated with anti-depressant medications — not tranquilizers — and talk therapy combined, either one on one with a psychiatrist or in group therapy. The severely depressed person is suffering a drop in any number of brain chemicals responsible for his or her depressed mood. Most antidepressant medications jump-start the manufacture of such chemicals in the depressed person's brain so that they start building up to normal levels. When a patient is severely depressed and unwilling or unable to communicate, talk therapy is held off. When the medications have started to work, the patient is usually much better able to benefit by talking about the illness and what may have brought it on.

Today, psychiatrists agree that talk will not help the depressed person as quickly and effectively as medications do. In fact, medications are thought to be life-savers, because they can spare the severely depressed person months of suffering so intense that it can throw them over the brink into dangerously poor health or even suicide.

Medications are a terrific help after they have started to take hold. But because they usually take from two to six weeks to start lightening the depression, they are not always the best choice for someone who is terribly depressed. Such a person is capable only of moving from the bed to a chair all day — if that — and is in such bad shape that he or she may not be able to withstand many more days in this state, not eating, sleeping, or washing. Take this person right to the closest hospital that has a psychiatric department, preferably one that has a geriatric psychiatric staff. Once there, the depressed person needs thorough examination for medical causes of the depression, such as thyroid disease, severe anemia, medication side effects, or a brain tumor or other brain damage.

If the state that looks like severe depression is indeed that, the psychiatrist may decide electroshock therapy (ECT) is the best choice. This treatment shows results almost immediately, certainly within a few days to a week. This statement may surprise you if you saw the movie or read the novel *One Flew over the Cuckoo's Nest,* which portrayed ECT as frightening, if not gruesome; it often was that bad until recently. Today the procedure has been drastically refined, and it is now a gentle procedure with few risks. It is considered so safe that even older patients who have medical conditions that contraindicate antidepressants are given ECT.

The person receiving ECT is given anesthesia and muscle relaxants and a brief electric current from a machine. The current causes a controlled seizure in the brain, while the rest of the body remains relaxed, although the muscles of the hands and feet do usually twitch a bit. After ECT the patient is confused and may not know where he or she is, but after a few hours this disorientation goes away. The therapy works only when treatments are given several times a week. The number of treatments is determined by the patient's response.

Numerous antidepressants on the market work very well to help elderly people recover from clinical depression. These medications are the reason for today's high cure rate for depressive illness (80 to 90 percent). Even though it has been proved over and over that these drugs do help people, plenty of patients and their families and even their primary doctors are skeptical that they really do work. Even patients who are in terrible despair are known to balk at taking medication.

You can be a big help to your parent, if a carefully chosen psychiatrist decides that medication is the best treatment. Be supportive of the decision and learn all you can about what drug therapy involves. Here are some basic questions to ask the psychiatrist before drug therapy begins:

1. What kind of depression does my parent have? What do you think caused it?

2. What drug is my parent being given? What classification of drug is it: tricyclic antidepressant, lithium, minor tranquilizer, major tranquilizer, monoamine oxidase inhibitor, or stimulant?
3. How does this drug treat depression?
4. How long does the drug take to work? (Many antidepressants take as long as six weeks, although some positive effects may show up within two weeks.)
5. What are the side effects of the medication? Common ones are dizziness, constipation, drowsiness, urinary retention and incontinence, dry mouth, Parkinson's-like symptoms, rapid heartbeat, and difficulties with memory.
6. Does my parent need to avoid other medications?
7. Should my parent avoid any foods?
8. How will you follow up in prescribing medication? How many visits to you are needed? Do you recommend psychotherapy or counseling?
9. How long do you think my parent will need to remain on this drug?

The psychiatrist will prescribe the drug with an eye to minimizing side effects. Older depressed patients are usually given one-third the normal adult dose, and as days go by sometimes the dose is upped gradually, while side effects are carefully observed. To help make the medication therapy run smoothly at home, here's what you should know:

- The medication must be taken every day on a schedule (most antidepressants are taken as one pill a day).
- Encourage your parent to ask the physician what time of day to take the medication. Some drugs need to be taken at bedtime because their hypnotic effects may cause daytime drowsiness.
- If dizziness occurs, report it to the psychiatrist. While dizziness continues, encourage your parent to get up from a chair and to change positions slowly.
- Encourage your parent to drink fluids and to eat a nonconstipating diet.
- Watch for expected side effects and learn how to manage them.

- Call the psychiatrist when side effects, including peculiar or unusual behavior, occur.

Grief Is Not a Disease

Anne Edwards's husband of fifty-nine years died suddenly of a heart attack on a Thursday afternoon. Mrs. Edwards went home from the hospital with her daughter in profound shock. Once home she went to bed and wept inconsolably through the night. Throughout the next day she would talk to no one and was so tearful, weak, and distressed that she could hardly move around the house. Her daughter, despairing at her mother's pain, decided to call a doctor for some Valium pills for her mother to take, just for a few days, so that she could calm down enough to attend the funeral service on Sunday and "pull herself together."

At the funeral, Mrs. Edwards didn't cry; in fact, she showed little emotion. To her children's relief, she sweetly greeted the numerous relatives and guests who were there, though she appeared dazed and shaky.

In the weeks after the funeral, Mrs. Edwards slowly tried to enjoy life. She was getting better all the time, but slowly. It was extremely difficult for her to do much of anything. One evening while they were talking about the funeral, Mrs. Edwards tearfully admitted that she had no memory of it. This lapse, she said, was a source of deep regret, especially because she would have liked memories of the eulogies special friends and relatives had given.

Grieving for the death of a spouse or a dear friend involves despair. The person suffering profound grief experiences many of the feelings and symptoms that characterize a depression. The grieving person will feel sadness, tearfulness, a sense of unreality, and possibly distance from other people, as well as lack of strength, exhaustion, poor appetite, and digestive symptoms. The grieving person will also have an intense preoccupation with the person who has died.

We include Mrs. Edwards's story as an example of how difficult it is for the family of an older person to watch and bear the suffering that a grieving relative feels. Too often, well-meaning family members take steps to hurry parents out of grief, either by encouraging them to take medication, or by too early trying to take steps to cheer them up. The suffering of bereavement is necessary. Those who investigate the subject of grief and work with the elderly will tell you that the elderly — like people of any age — should be allowed to cry and feel their suffering after the death of someone much loved or needed. For someone to move on, they must feel the pain and sadness of acute grief.

The period of profound grief can go on for weeks, according to how dependent the person grieving was on the deceased person and the quality of the relationship that they shared. The grief can be a function of missing the dead person, or it can have to do with unresolved and ambivalent feelings about the marriage or friendship that was.

How long someone should suffer the despairing stage of grief is a difficult question. Some people never get over their grief and remain morbidly preoccupied with the person who died for the rest of their lives. People who never resolve their grief and who are unable to move on to enjoy friendships and other pleasures are said to be clearly abnormal in their reaction.

What then is normal grief? How do you as a concerned child of your parents, or a friend to someone suffering grief, determine when you should encourage this person to seek help from mental-health professionals? We have no quick answer; grief is a complicated emotional state to qualify. But we can say that mental-health professionals usually judge someone's mourning by its length. The acute stage of despair and preoccupation with the deceased is said to be normal if it lasts four to six weeks, although if the relationship lasted most of one's life, this despair can carry on even longer and be accepted as understandable. Six months of relentless grief seems to be the limit that most mental-health experts allow before they call the grief abnormal and pathological.

The most important role for you to take as a child of a grieving parent, during the acute stage, is to be there as much as possible to help with daily tasks and to love and to listen as best you can.

5

*Common Skin Problems
and How to Cope with Them*

SKIN IS THE BODY'S largest organ, and yet it gets poor press outside of fluffy advertising and beauty magazines.

All of us care about cosmetics because, naturally, we want to look attractive. But thorough information on skin care in the older person is critical. People don't really expect to get skin problems as they age, and so they do little to prevent them.

When skin problems do occur in the older person, however, family and friends are often less than sufficiently sympathetic. Few people think of the skin as a place where serious disorders originate. And yet, problems such as dry, itchy skin, infections, cancer, and shingles are common among elderly people. These are some of the chief complaints taking elderly people to their doctor's office. In fact, 40 percent of people sixty-five and older suffer from skin disorders that are severe enough to merit referral from their usual doctor to a dermatologist.

Any disorders of the skin can be terribly irritating, painful, and unpleasant, affecting the older person's ability to sleep, to walk out into the sunlight, or even to be comfortable sitting still and talking to a friend. If the problem persists, it can be depressing and can deeply affect the older person's self-esteem and sense of well-being. Shingles, which commonly flares up on the older person's torso or face, is in a category of its own, for it can be excruciatingly painful and can become a critical, sometimes life-threatening illness if the pain is so devastating and lasting that it leaves the person malnourished and depleted.

An older person's skin is extremely sensitive to outside forces —

even to bacteria that normally sit on the skin without causing problems. For years, doctors and nurses have seen that an older person's skin is usually quick to bruise, abrade, and form rashes, and that it's slow to heal and susceptible to skin cancers. They have seen that aged skin usually becomes wrinkled and marked by dark spots of pigmentation; it gets thinner and looser, and looks less firm than younger skin.

But only in the past few years have researchers analyzed the intricacies of aging skin and discovered *why* it's so different from younger skin. The reason, they've found, is that aged skin has lost large numbers of cells in specialized categories. The loss in thickness — the quality that makes a very old person's skin appear paper-thin and almost translucent — happens because from 20 to 50 percent of the skin's original cell content may be gone. These cells may be in the epidermis or dermis, the skin's outer layers: the collagen, a gluey substance that gives skin its elasticity, consists of the immune cells or the melanin cells, which are produced in response to the sun's burning rays.

Even the tiny blood vessels that transport nourishment to the cells and carry wastes away from them start to atrophy as we get older and thus trigger a vicious cycle, diminishing other structures such as hair follicles and sweat and oil glands. As less oil is produced, the skin becomes drier, and sweat glands respond less actively to stimuli, from either an overheated body or an emotional affront. The skin also becomes less protective because fat drops away from the bony prominences of the body, such as the elbows, knuckles, hips, knees, and even hands. The body then has less padding between skin and bone.

Many things can be done to protect an older person's vulnerable and sensitive skin, and if problems arise, to address and correct them. You as the child or friend of an older person must be aware of and alert to how serious and bothersome some of these problems can really be.

Itching

Itching is not generally thought of as a scourge of old age; it is, after all, a rather plebeian-sounding complaint. And yet, pruritus — or "feeling itchy" — is the most frequent skin problem among the elderly. A great annoyance to many, it disturbs sleep and enjoyment of just about everything, except that which relieves the itch. If the older person you are caring for tells you itching is troublesome, take the complaint seriously, and see if you can find the cause and what can be done about it. Even an easygoing person can become irritable and weary under the torment of pervasive, prickly itching. It can occur with or without a rash, and may be caused by the aging skin's reacting to its own loss of cells and oils, or to degeneration of nerve endings in the skin. Other causes may be: irritation by chemicals in soaps and other household products, internal problems related to a number of diseases to which the elderly are prone, a drug reaction, or emotional stress.

Dry-Skin Itching

People over seventy inevitably have drier skin, and, as we have said, thinner, more-sensitive skin. Those who have not wised up to measures for preventing dry skin start to have itching problems. Once skin is dry, few can resist scratching, and the itch, scratch, cracked-skin cycle starts.

The cornerstone of dry-skin prevention is moisturizing with emollients. Although younger people can usually rely on the skin's natural oils to lock in moisture so that the skin remains soft, supple, and comfortable, older people have to rely on artificial replacements. Most women are used to applying body lotion, and so, for them, dry-skin care is routine. But men usually need to be told to apply moisturizer by their doctors or nurses, as a matter of medical prescription.

The best time to coat the skin with moisturizer is after a bath, while the skin is still slightly damp, to trap the underlying moisture. Too much bathing is actually bad for the skin, especially in very hot water, for the heat is drying and water draws moisture away from the skin's deeper layers. When dryness is a severe problem, long soaks in the tub or long showers need to be curtailed, and bathing should be done only three times a week. A good way to hydrate the skin on the days when baths or showers are not taken is by gently rubbing it with a moist cloth, followed immediately by an application of moisturizer.

Soap should be chosen carefully. The thinner, drier skin of the elderly is a less effective barrier to irritating chemicals, which can actually enter the skin and irritate it easily. The older person should use superfatted or glycerin soaps — with no strong perfume or al-

cohol added. We recommend Dove, Tone, Basis, Evcerin, and Neu-
trogena dry-skin soap, which is glycerin-based. Also, clothes and bed
linens need to be carefully rinsed; residue can be very irritating.

In winter, when the weather outside is cold and dry and the indoors heated, insult is added to the injury of dry skin. Nurses talk
about their patients having "winter itch" or "winter skin." Beyond
paying extra attention to moisturizing the skin, humidifying the air
may help. If you buy a humidifier for the bedroom and other rooms
of the house, remind yourself every day to change the water and clean
out the machine. Mold spores and other germs can quickly build up
in an untended machine, and float around the room to cause pneumonia, a disease to which the elderly are most susceptible.

When Itching Skin Merits a Call to the Doctor
If you can determine the cause among yourselves, and get rid of this
cause, you can save yourself a trip to the doctor. When itching seems
to come from dry skin or "winter skin," proper moisturizing and
limits on soaks in the tub will usually take care of the trouble. Otherwise, do some quick detective work to find anything that has been
newly introduced to the household or the older person's drug regimen. Consider possibilities such as having switched to a new deter-
gent, a dye in an unwashed new garment or blanket, or an over-the-
counter medication never taken before. While an itching problem is
subsiding, over-the-counter preparations with hydrocortisone should
provide the necessary relief.

If itching is extremely intense, or accompanied by a rash that
keeps flaring for more than a day, get medical attention. The doctor
will want to run tests if the cause is not obvious, and if necessary
prescribe antihistamines and steroid medications for relief of itching
discomfort. Always call the doctor, too, if a new prescription drug
brings on a skin reaction.

Swollen Extremities and Stasis Dermatitis

Many older people have swollen legs because of circulatory problems caused by a weak heart, varicose veins, or diabetes. The swelling comes from pooling of fluids that are not easily draining out of
the body's soft tissues into the circulatory system.

The heavy, turgid feeling of swelling itself is a discomfort, but
not nearly as disturbing as stasis dermatitis, an unpleasant skin dis-

order that occurs because swelling blocks the exchange of nutrients and wastes in the skin. People who have stasis dermatitis have dry, itchy, cracked-looking legs mottled with bluish red discoloration beneath the skin surface. When the problem becomes severe, blood vessels of the skin and legs can easily develop cellulitis, an all-over painful and dangerous infection. Or nasty-looking, painful ulcers, which are difficult to treat and very slow to heal.

Preventing stasis dermatitis requires the double-pronged approach of good nutrition and local treatments that cause fluid to move through the legs. A diet high in protein and tissue-sustaining vitamins is recommended, because protein deficiency causes fluid to seep from the tissues into the circulation. Sadly, those who suffer stasis dermatitis most are chronically ill elderly people who live alone with no one to help prepare, or to bring in, nourishing meals.

Good venous return, which is the shifting of fluid out of the tissues into the blood stream, can be enhanced in a number of ways. As a matter of course, the person with circulatory problems must elevate the legs several times a day so that pooled fluids can flow backward with the force of gravity; and while sitting during the day, take the opportunity to prop the legs up on a stool or chair. Also, while sleeping, slightly elevate the legs on a pillow or two. Although older people must keep taking exercise, standing still for long periods needs to be avoided. Elastic support hose are effective at keeping swelling down and can be worn during the day and put on when the legs are at their least swollen while still elevated in bed. Elastic hose are usually not satisfactory unless made for the individual by a special fitter in a surgical supply store; this kind is expensive and rarely covered by insurance. If the cost of special hose will make a significant dent in the older person's budget, a good alternative is to use elastic (ace) bandages according to a doctor's instructions.

Fungal Infections: Prevent Them in the First Place

Elderly people are especially prone to fungal infections because their skin lacks its full force of immune cells, as well as good circulation. Also, older people, far more than younger people, overdress in a way that creates the hothouse environment fungi need for rapid growth. Various invading organisms can cause the athlete's-foot type of fungal infection, which, given the chance, grows on the feet, in the armpits, or in the groin, where moisture is trapped by shoes or clothing.

We all "catch" the fungus at one time or another, and it can live as a dormant infection in the nailbeds or some other cranny for years until conditions are just right for it to make itself a bother.

Steps should be taken to avoid the unpleasantness of a fungal infection, because getting rid of it, once it has set in, takes an all-out assault.

The first step is to create a hostile environment for fungal growth, by keeping the feet clean and dry and exposed to the air — if it is warm enough — for some hours during the day. Athletes, who keep their constantly sweating feet in closed shoes, avoid athlete's foot by changing their shoes often and letting their feet air out. Older people need to practice the same kind of routine prevention by changing their shoes once or twice a day, and in hot weather by wearing mesh, canvas, or open-toed shoes or sandals. Socks should also be changed once a day. Cotton or wool socks should be worn, not those made of nylon and other synthetics, which cause the feet to sweat. In hot weather, women should wear nylon hose with open-toed shoes, or even better, no hose at all. Although most older people sweat less than younger people, they still do sweat, especially around the feet.

A second step is to keep the feet clean, which means at best washing them every day with soap and water, and carefully drying the spaces between the toes before putting on shoes and socks. The older person who has difficulty bending over should use a hair drier, on a cool setting, to dry between the toes. A cool setting is important, because warm air from the drier would promote fungal growth. Preventing fungal infection anywhere else on the body requires good hygiene and loose clothing so that the skin can breathe.

An infection can assume one of three forms, all of which take weeks to cure, if not much longer. Fungi are so tenacious and resilient that sometimes it is impossible to get rid of a colony despite all-out antifungal tactics.

Fungal infections usually sprout between the toes, causing intense itching, scaling, and often cracking of the skin. In this form the infection can often be thwarted with the steps just mentioned and with over-the-counter antifungal preparations, which are just what a dermatologist would prescribe for someone seen in the office. If the cracks become infected with bacteria, a foul-odored "pasty foot" results, which is a sure sign that the problem should be looked at by a doctor so that an appropriate antibiotic cream can be prescribed.

A second form is often chronic and leaves the skin on the soles and sides of the feet itchy, thickened, and scaly. This type too is best treated by a physician, who may prescribe oral as well as topical antifungal agents.

The third and most tormenting type forms itchy, fluid-filled blisters on the heel and base of the foot. This type also should be cared for under a doctor's supervision so that appropriate medications can be prescribed. Usually the patient is told to soak the feet several times a day in warm water and otherwise to rest with the feet elevated.

Shingles Is Not Just a Skin Disease

Shingles deserves a more impressive name to express how grindingly painful it can be, especially for older people, whose experience with the disease is usually much more painful than that of younger people. Until recently, shingles was considered a pariah of a disease, not prevalent or even serious enough to merit dedicated research. But as the population ages, shingles is much better known and drug companies are aggressively competing to find an effective cure. It affects people primarily in the fifty- to seventy-year range, and we have a 50 percent chance of contracting it by age eighty-five. Fortunately, shingles usually strikes only once, although about 10 percent of shingles sufferers experience a second episode.

Shingles is caused by reactivated chickenpox virus (herpes zoster), which may lie dormant for decades along a nerve pathway, most commonly one that strings through the torso, but also through the arms, legs, and sometimes the neck and face. The virus can resurface and rapidly reproduce when the immune system is weakened during or after an illness, during a stressful event, or when the immune system weakens with age just enough that the virus can no longer be kept at bay.

When the disease is manifest, the proliferating virus travels up and down the affected nerve pathway, in a sense eating away at it to cause pain. Often the pain is so intense that someone will mistake it for a slipped disc, pulled muscle, appendicitis, or even a heart attack, depending on where it originates.

Usually shingles can't be diagnosed until the characteristic shingles rash appears around the area of skin where the infected nerve pathway ends. The rash looks just like chickenpox — fluid-filled pustules that itch for several days before drying and forming scabs. Typically, shingles is first characterized by a feeling of malaise; within two to four days the severe, deep pain takes over for up to four weeks. The telltale rash can erupt up to two weeks after the severe pain, but usually does so within three days.

Unfortunately, the disease does not always stop hurting after the acute phase of pain and the rash have subsided. At least half of shingles sufferers over age sixty experience a less intense but still devastating residual pain called postherpetic neuralgia, and this next phase of pain can last up to two months, sometimes even longer.

The person who gets shingles needs a lot of loving support during the phase of acute pain, and in the time it takes for the postherpetic neuralgia to resolve. Often the shingles sufferer is too exhausted and uncomfortable to prepare his or her own meals and carry out daily routines. Most people who go through the painful stages of shingles need help in taking care of themselves. Sufferers who are provided with nourishing meals, support, and sympathetic understanding generally heal faster. Those who become increasingly debilitated can contract a disseminated and life-threatening form of the disease that spreads to the internal organs, even into the eye if the affected nerve is on the face.

Any signs of a shingles outbreak on the face, particularly around the eyes or on the nose, signal an eye emergency that needs prompt treatment, with the aim of preventing permanent eye damage.

If someone you love suffers from shingles, you must make sure he or she is well taken care of during the painful, incapacitating period. We can't emphasize enough how wearing and painful shingles pain can be. We have seen patients describe it as "up there with childbirth, but without the breaks between pains," "like a terrible toothache," or "a gnawing, searing pain."

If aspirin or Tylenol (acetaminophen) do not help mask the pain, patients are sometimes given stronger pain medications, even narcotics. Some people are so incapacitated that they are hospitalized for pain management. During the acute phase, pain medications must not be delayed or withheld. But, as the pain subsides, every effort should be made to wean the shingles sufferer from medication stronger than aspirin, for all painkillers have side effects, especially constipation, mental disorientation, and dependence.

No one has a quick, knock-it-out cure for shingles, but clinical trials show that the drug acyclovir, approved by the FDA for herpes simplex (a distant cousin of shingles), shortens the disease and lessens the acute pain and postherpetic neuralgia. The drug works best if it is given as soon as the rash appears. At major medical centers across the country, large doses of the drug are being given to shingles patients in the initial phase of the disease and current research shows that the drug has no side effects. Until the FDA approves acyclovir specifically for shingles, some doctors are still prescribing the anti-inflammatory drug prednisone to help ease the inflammation along the affected nerve pathways. Some prescribe acyclovir and prednisone in combination. If your doctor seems less than sympathetic about the seriousness of shingles pain, and poorly informed about current drug therapy, we suggest you quickly shop around for a dermatologist working through a major medical center who has had experience in treating the disease. Waste no time; remember that treatment is most effective when started early.

How to Help Someone Through Shingles
Keep the person you are taking care of from becoming exhausted, weakened, even incapacitated by the pain. Here are some suggestions to help you in this job:

The Skin Rash

• The lesions can be easily irritated by clothing and by moisture trapped under clothing. Ask the person who has shingles to wear loose, comfortable clothing made from a soft fabric, preferably cotton.
• Avoid ointments and creams, which prevent the skin lesions from drying out and healing.
• Applications of calamine lotion, cornstarch, or baking soda hasten drying.
• Temporary application of ice packs or cool, clean compresses may help palliate the itching and pain.

The Deep Pain

• Provide pain medications on time, as prescribed by the doctor.
• Try to promote a good night's sleep. Give pain medication prior to bed, and see the section, "How to Promote a Good Night's Sleep," in Chapter 3.
• Keep the apartment or house calm and pleasant.
• Turn on soft music, if the person who has shingles enjoys soothing sound.
• Distracting pursuits can divert us from feeling pain. Try con-

versation, games, television, or visits by sympathetic friends. If the pain is not severe, arrange for simple outings, such as a drive (with you driving) or a trip to the movies.

• Provide constant reminders that the painful stage of the disease is self-limiting.

• Some herpes sufferers report that compressing the affected area seems to help ease the pain. Pressure from a pillow and even from tight clothing or pantyhose are worth trying, unless circulatory problems or some other condition prohibit such measures.

• Make sure nourishing meals are eaten on time every day. Good nutrition bolsters the immune system so that it can vanquish the active herpes zoster virus.

Skin Cancer

More frequent than any other kind of cancer, skin cancer strikes just about everyone over sixty-five who has spent time outdoors enjoying the sun. Sooner or later a skin cancer will need to be removed. Although most skin cancers form slowly, without spreading to other sites in the body, and can easily be removed in a doctor's office, some forms of skin cancer can be disfiguring, or even deadly, if not treated early.

Most skin cancers are basal-cell cancers affecting the outermost layer of the skin, the epidermis. This kind usually progresses slowly on sun-exposed parts of the body — head, neck, and hands — as a raised, red, quick-to-bleed, firm-looking area of skin with a flat, scaly center and a rolled-looking border. Although basal-cell cancer does not travel through the blood stream, it can extend beneath the skin to the bone, causing extensive destruction. Squamous-cell cancer, also prevalent, appears most commonly on the ears, face, and lips as red, scaly, platelike patches. This form of cancer can grow and spread throughout the body, though it rarely does so. Both squamous-cell and basal-cell cancers are curable in 95 percent of the cases, and are always curable if the cancer is treated early by a competent physician.

Malignant melanoma is a serious, life-threatening skin cancer that necessitates prompt surgical removal. Melanoma is a cancer of the melanin cells, which produce the skin's dark pigment. Most melanomas develop from moles; others arise elsewhere, spontaneously. A malignant mole looks changed in color, larger or thicker, and irregular in outline. It may also itch, hurt, erode, or bleed. People who have many moles dotted on their skin from birth are at especially high risk for melanoma. The disease used to be rare, but worldwide the incidence of melanoma doubles every decade, as more and more people tan in the sun.

Checking for cancer is slightly more complicated on the skin of an older person, because aged skin often is rife with dark pigmented areas, skin tags, and bumps of one kind or another, all brought on by aging and cumulative sun exposure. The skin should always be thoroughly checked by the doctor who does the annual physical, and the older person should of course look out for changes in moles, birthmarks, and any other kind of skin bump. Any skin growth that alters in size and appears pearly, translucent, tan, brown, black, or multicolored should be suspect, as well as sores that do not heal.

The "it is never too late" cliché holds true for preventing skin cancer. Older people should practice as much "sun sense" as younger people do to protect their skin from cancer and premature aging:

- Protective clothing should include long-sleeved shirts made of a closely woven cotton fabric.
- Wear a hat with a brim to deflect the sun from the ears and upper cheeks.
- Cover the ears with a hat, hair, or sunscreen.
- Use a sunscreen with the highest skin-protective factor on all exposed areas. Apply it at least half an hour before sun exposure.
- Try avoiding the sun between 10:00 A.M. and 3:00 P.M., when the sun is most intense.

6

Oh, My Aching Bones!

YOUNG OR OLD, we all have vague complaints about creaky joints or aches and pains in our muscles and bones, especially when we overdo some activities. But in later years such complaints can become much more frequent and pronounced as bone, muscle, and connective tissue begin to wear out after many decades of normal use.

No one in old age is exempt from some alterations in skeletal frame or muscles and connective tissue. Bones lose calcium and become brittle and more easily broken. Cartilage thins, especially on the joints that endure the weight of the body: the knees and the hips. With age, muscles lose some of their strength as well as mass, and body movement becomes slower and more sluggish. Smaller stature, stooped posture, and the inability to move rapidly are as characteristic of old age as graying hair and wrinkling skin.

Not that everyone becomes doddery and decrepit. Some older people remain spry in movement and able to carry on all normal activities — well into their nineties. Such people are blessed with especially good genes, as well as a disposition that spurs them on throughout life to be physically active. But most people, by the time they are eighty, are not so fortunate as to remain free of mobility problems. The aging body is especially prone to disorders that affect comfortable ease of movement, and quite a few people, even in their sixties, have difficulty carrying on the activities the rest of us take for granted.

We bring you now to the common disorders of the muscles and bones. Understand these and you will be able to make a real difference in the independence maintained by the older person you care about. You can help prevent this person from becoming unnecessarily racked and worn down with miserable aches and pains, as well as the fear of falling down and breaking bones. It helps to know the responses to these questions: What are the common disorders? Why do they occur in the aging body? Can they be prevented? Who provides treatment? What are treatment options? Where does self-help come in?

Yes, Basic Problems Have Typical Treatments

Most older people have a low expectation of help from the medical community when it comes to stiffness and pain with movement. Sad, for many new treatments are available for muscular skeletal problems, as well as self-help techniques, from properly selected doctors and health professionals.

Unfortunately, such labels as "rheumatism" and "arthritis," and even "old bones," are often applied indiscriminately to any kind of joint pain, stiffness, and limitation of movement. Older people who use these descriptions accept just about any ache or pain — unless it is excruciating — as normal functions of aging. Then too, doctors who are not educated in or sympathetic to the physical problems of the elderly can be downright flippant about their older patient's complaints of creaky joints, aches, and pains. "What do you expect, at your age!" is a retort too many doctors offer older patients.

The label for a disorder must be correct, and anyone suffering an ache or a pain that gets no better after six weeks of tincture of time should go to a doctor for a diagnosis. Of course, any older person debilitated by pain should be in touch with a doctor for medical advice as soon as possible. (See the next section in this chapter, "When to Call the Doctor.") So many categories of muscular skeletal problems affect the elderly that you should expect the doctor, after an examination, to tell you in which category your relative's problem fits. Here are the commonest categories that we discuss in this chapter. We have simplified a complex picture so that you can see clearly how each problem differs from the next.

A Quick Anatomy Lesson

Most mobility problems bothering the elderly have to do with joints. Before going any further, look at the following definitions describing the parts of a joint.

Category	What is it?	Places affected?	Sudden onset?	Morning stiffness?	Typical treatments
Osteoarthritis	Breakdown of joint cartilage, usually in one part of the body	End of finger, joints, knees, hips, neck, low back	No	No	Aspirin, *low* dose, Tylenol
Rheumatoid arthritis	Systemic disease causing inflamed membranes, usually of many joints (mostly women)	Fingers, wrists, knees	No	Definitely	Aspirin, *high* doses, sometimes gold, methotrexate
Gout	Chemical crystals in the joint fluid that cause excruciating pain	Great toe, knee, ankle	Yes	No	Colchicine, Allopurinol, adrenocorticotrophin (ACTH), steroids
Polymyalgia rheumatica	Painful muscle inflammation	Muscles, not joints; often the shoulders and neck, but elsewhere, too	No	Some	Prednisone
Osteoporosis	Bones lose calcium and become brittle, easily broken (mostly women)	All bones	No	No	Supplements of elemental calcium, along with proper diet. Accident prevention. (Estrogen replacements if started within ten years after menopause.) Etidronate, Calcitonin

Cartilage. A tough, resilient material, the cartilage protects and cushions the ends of bones. Also known as gristle, it is the rubbery stuff we do not like to eat in meat. You can feel some of your own at the tip of your nose and in your ear lobes.

Synovial membrane. This fluid-filled sac balloons around each joint. It protects the joint and contains the synovial fluid, a marvelous slippery solution that makes the joints into nearly frictionless surfaces.

Bursa. A much smaller sac that sits outside the synovial membrane. It secretes the slippery stuff that allows muscle to move across muscle and muscle to move across bone.

Muscles. You know them well. They move you around by picking up your bones, which they surround.

Tendons. Fibrous cords that attach muscles to bones. You can almost pluck them at the back of your knee.

Ligaments. Fibrous cords that attach bone to bone within the joints.

When Do You Need a Doctor?

Usually, Most Problems Respond to Tincture of Time

Young or old, we cannot go through a year without episodes that seem to be pulled muscles and stiff joints. Just consider the anatomy lesson above and it's obvious how many bits and pieces in any joint can go out of whack. All kinds of "-itises" or inflammations can occur, including bursitis, tendinitis, sinovitis, and inflamed tense muscles (fibrositis). Most of these episodes can be taken care of by home treatments, without a doctor's care (but do alert the physician about any worrying muscular skeletal problems). Warm baths, heating pads, rest, and moving the affected part more cautiously will usually help to resolve the maladjustment.

Also, massage can do wonders in relaxing tight muscles when tenderness is not present. Older people need to be touched, as we all do. Massage is a wonderful way to add touch — and sensuality — to the older person's routine. Often, soothing touch is left out of their lives, especially those who are widowed or who live alone.

Natural mending usually takes from two to six weeks. In the beginning, if pain is oppressive, aspirin or an aspirin substitute can be taken if the doctor approves. For this degree of trouble, though, generally drugs are not a good idea. They can't accelerate natural healing, and older people, already taking medications, certainly can do without adding to their usual regimen.

If a joint or muscle problem that is not terribly uncomfortable or which seems trivial does not get better after six weeks, it should be looked at by a physician who knows how to diagnose muscular skeletal disorders. The problem could well be a form of localized arthritis that simply does not go away, at least at present. The wait should not cause harm — in fact, the test of time is usually a necessary part of diagnosing disorders of joints and muscles. Do seek medical attention, however, if general achiness and inflammation of joints occurs in more than one part of the body. An all-body illness could then be setting in that might respond to medical treatment.

Emergencies Need Quick Medical Attention

Some conditions are true emergencies, for which medical help should be sought that very day, either by calling the doctor or by going to the office for an examination.

Relative emergencies are: (1) fractures, (2) nerve damage, (3) infection, (4) a joint that is frozen into rigidity, and (5) gout. The first four emergencies can result in serious if not permanent damage to the body if the problem is neglected, even for a few days. Gout is not considered dangerous as a disease, and an attack runs its course over a couple of weeks. And yet, the attack is so horribly painful that no one should have to wait for help any longer than it takes to see a doctor, who can start immediate treatment to stop the pain and resolve the disease.

Be aware of these emergency situations:

- Pain from a known injury or fall that might have caused a broken bone. Not all fractures look especially deformed.
- An obviously broken bone. You can see deformity and swelling and the affected person is unable to move the affected part below the break, and probably above it, too.
- A joint that will not move, or that can't be used because of pain. You do not want the joint to permanently stiffen.
- Possible nerve damage may be occurring if pain runs down the side of the leg to the foot, if numbness appears in the fingers, or if numbness is felt in the head when the neck is moved.
- Fever of more than 100 degrees and a joint that is warm to

the touch, stiff, and exquisitely painful may indicate a severe infection of a joint.

- A throbbing, excruciatingly painful, tender-to-the-touch big toe, knee, or ankle often signifies an attack of gout, unless a fall or injury to the painful part has just taken place. The same condition may mean a joint is severely infected.

Degenerative Joint Disease (Osteoarthritis)

Degenerative joint disease is, technically speaking, not arthritis, although it is often called osteoarthritis by doctors who are used to that name. Most forms of arthritis include inflammation, but osteoarthritis has very little, if any inflammation. In the word *arthritis*, the *arth* part means joint, and the *itis* means inflammation, a reaction of the body that causes swelling, redness, pain, and loss of motion in a joint.

Osteoarthritis involves the wearing down and disintegration of cartilage, the shock-absorbing, cushioning material that sits on the ends of the two bones making up a joint. The not yet well understood process that underlies this joint disease occurs in everyone, and in fact is found in all animals that have bony skeletons. In x-rays, joint degeneration is easily seen, as cartilage frayed, split, and much thinner than normal. In some cases, cartilage can be seen worn all the way down to the bone. Some people also form abnormal growths of bone, called bony spurs, on the bone directly underneath the places where cartilage is thinnest. Although osteoarthritis used to be thought of as primarily a wear-and-tear disease, it is now felt to have a more complicated explanation. Researchers are finding more and more information leading them to believe that osteoarthritis is also an active disease, wherein joint tissues are broken down by biochemical changes in their composition.

Disease is said to have set in at a joint only when one feels stiffness and pain as a result of the degenerated cartilage. Interestingly, research comparing x-rays with people's health complaints reveals that many people have severely degenerated joints without apparent discomfort. About 40 million people are said to have degenerative joint disease, and about 16 million of them need medical care. So far, researchers have come up with no easy answer as to why some people develop joint degeneration that they can feel, whereas others do not.

Few people are bothered by symptoms before middle age, unless they have injured or overused poorly fitting or damaged joints. Injuries at any age can cause poor alignment and wearing of joints, as can being overweight and diabetic. A few people are born with joints so far out of alignment that their cartilage quickly starts to rub abrasively against bone. Athletes, especially dancers, can wear down their joints, but only if they carry on repetitive, harsh activities most of every day.

Joint health depends on plenty of use and exercise. Besides keeping the cartilage of a joint supple and nutrified, exercise strengthens the muscles surrounding a joint so that muscles carry more of the stress load. Careful studies of athletes and others who put lots of stress on their joints have shown no correlation between sensible, intense activity and osteoarthritis.

Osteoarthritis is primarily a problem of older people. Typically, people start to complain of truly bothersome symptoms in their seventies. Discomfort is usually mild, and relatively few people have severe pain and stiffness. Degeneration of the cartilage in the hip and knee joint is generally the most troublesome.

Pain begins to creep into joints slowly and comes and goes. Often pain comes only with motion or overuse, or even with underuse, as during a bed-bound illness. An older person may find going up stairs slightly painful in the hip or knee joints, or picking up heavy bags a strain on the back, the elbows, or the fingers. Opening a jar may provoke discomfort in the fingers or wrist. Usually stiffness, creakiness, and pain go away if the joint is rested for a while, although a few people have constant, wearing pain, even at rest.

A Look at Five Usual Places for Osteoarthritis

Arthritis can occur in any joint, but it is rarely seen in the jaw, elbows, or shoulders unless at some time an injury damaged the joint structures. Osteoarthritis usually gives trouble at five places in the body: the hands, the spine, the hips, the knees, and the feet, and some people are affected in more than one place.

Hands Usually Look Worse Than They Feel. You have probably seen older women with knobby, bony bumps on the joints of their hands. These are called Heberden's nodes if they occur in the end joints of the fingers, and Bouchard's nodes in the middle joints. The bumps are in fact bony spurs, the abnormal bone growths we described earlier as a complication of osteoarthritis. Spur development is primarily a problem of older women, especially if their mothers also had the problem.

If your mother forms bony spurs, understand that they usually look far worse than they feel, at least for most women with this form of hand arthritis. Be sympathetic whether or not they have pain, for the bony spurs are a cosmetic nuisance for any woman who cares about her appearance.

Usually the bony enlargement occurs slowly over several years, and is seen but not felt. Some women, though, do indeed bear symptoms of swelling, tenderness, and aching, even numbness and tingling. Most women bothered by these symptoms still have good use of their hands and usually do not need to take painkillers.

Is Pain in the Back Really Arthritis? The spine changes dramatically throughout life. In fact, we are an inch or so shorter by our old age, because the spine compresses along the way. On x-rays of older people, the spongy disk material between the vertebrae almost always looks degenerated. Amazingly, however, most people do not feel these changes. If a doctor tells you that an older person's pain in the back is caused by arthritis, it may well be so. Nevertheless, make sure the doctor has done a thorough examination to rule out other causes.

Osteoarthritis can cause neck or back pain, but usually pain in the back is from an injury — a torn muscle or a sprain that needs time to heal, often at least six weeks. Injuries to the back are almost always incredibly painful, and so not even the most stoical individual waits to call the doctor. Take no chances with back pain, and always consult a doctor; nerve damage or a fracture may have occurred.

Some older people grow bony spurs on their neck vertebrae and those of the lower back. Again, these spurs may or may not become painful. If they do compress a nerve or irritate surrounding structures, pain can usually be relieved with painkillers, local heat with warm compresses or a heating pad, and lots of rest. Sometimes a neck brace or a corset worn around the lower back will support muscles and bone, relieving pain. Occasionally the problem is so disabling and unpleasant that surgery is considered.

All older people should practice measures to prevent back problems, and do all they can to keep the back comfortably straight, whether lying down, standing up, walking, or lifting.

Hips and Knees Take the Brunt of the Body's Weight. As we have said, the hip and knee joints seem to undergo the most serious degeneration. These joints take the full weight of the body and, in time, some do wear out. Surgery can be dramatically effective for people with severe osteoarthritis of the weight-bearing joints, especially hip joints. Surgery is an option to consider when one can't move around without great difficulty and pain, or if sleep is constantly inhibited.

Mild to severe osteoarthritis is managed with conservative measures. Devices such as canes, splints, walkers, or crutches can be used to take weight off affected joints and protect them from further damage. Pain-relieving drugs can be prescribed, including those with anti-inflammatory action.

Pain and stiffness generally wax and wane in these joints; they may remain constant and then go away completely. If pain seems to miraculously disappear, it is usually because of eburnation. Eburnation happens when two bones wearing against each other polish the surfaces so that the joint again moves smoothly and without pain. Even without complete eburnation, use can sometimes mold joints into a more functional state.

Feet: The Forgotten Stepchildren. Osteoarthritis can also show up in the feet, especially in the big toe and the other toes. The joint where the toe bones meet the next set of bones (the metatarsals) is the point of greatest stress when we walk. A little osteoarthritis can make walking difficult even with a cane or walker.

Often pain will subside if stress is taken off the painful part of the foot. A device called a metatarsal bar can be glued into shoes an inch behind the contact point where the sole of the foot puts most of its weight. Although doctors know when to recommend one, a cobbler should be able to do the job. Compare the area of greatest pain with the place of greatest wear in the shoe: this is the place to put the bar. Comfortable shoes with a wide toe box are critical for someone who has foot arthritis of any kind. Arthritis of the foot is showing up especially in older women who have spent most of their lives in shoes with pointed toes and high heels.

General Foot Problems

Anyone unable to take care of his or her own feet should go to monthly foot-maintenance sessions with a podiatrist. Some podiatry costs are paid by Medicare. Diabetics and people who have vascular disease in their legs should see a podiatrist as a matter of medical necessity (see Chapter 9 for diabetic foot care).

All kinds of problems can agonize the feet, from bunions to corns and calluses. In the table on page 90, you can see what an older person can do to prevent them and keep them from getting worse.

Helpful Ways to Manage Osteoarthritis

Even in the worst cases, osteoarthritis takes years to form. It is not a condition that creates excruciating pain, and if unpleasant aches and pains do come, usually plenty of time is available to try different treatments and medications for discomfort. When hip pain and difficulty with movement become apparent, the decision to have surgery can be made sensibly and carefully.

Joint Protection. We can protect our joints by carefully using them in ways that will not add stress and damage. Joints should be put through their full range of motion every day; protection doesn't imply immobility — quite the opposite. Joints need to be protected so that they can be used as comfortably as possible. Here are tips that anyone with arthritis should know about.

• Being overweight puts much strain on the joints; it's like carrying a heavy package at all times. Encourage the older person who is overweight to lose weight under the doctor's supervision.

• Use the strongest and largest joints for the specific task. If hands are arthritic, push with the hips or thighs and use both arms to move clothing from closets or take objects down from shelves.

• Use body leverage correctly. Objects feel much heavier held away from the body, and much lighter when held close. Grocery bags should be held against the chest, rather than in one arm to the side. A purse or shoulder bag is best carried with the strap across the body.

• Avoid keeping a joint in one position for a long time. Change will reduce stiffness and contractures (permanently stiff and deformed joints). Get up and stretch frequently from a sitting position. To prevent fatigue when sitting for a long time, frequently bend and point toes and change position of the legs.

• If writing with pen or pencil, with long-sustained grasp, be-

Help for Nagging Foot Problems

Problem	Cause	Treatment
Ingrown nails, which become painful as the sides of the nails press into sensitive toe tissue	Nails cut too short and curved at sides	Trim toenails straight across; do not round off corners.
Horny nails, so thick they are difficult to cut	Years of trauma from poorly fitted shoes	Wear properly fitted shoes. File with emery board several times a week.
Dry, cracked feet that are prone to infection	Fewer oil glands with aging	Apply cream to top and bottom of feet, not between toes. Rub pumice stone on dry, flaking skin. Check feet for cracks and signs of infection.
Corns and calluses	Too-tight shoes rubbing against skin and bone	Wear properly fitted shoes. Apply moleskin to protect area. Do not remove corns or calluses yourself.
Bunion, an unsightly and often painful deformity of the big toe occurring when bone at base of toe slants outward	Heredity. Prolonged wearing of tight, narrow shoes and high heels	Wear properly fitted shoes and stockings with plenty of room in the toe box. Minor surgery can be performed on advanced cases.
Hammertoe, a hooked or clawlike deformity of the toe joint, usually the second toe	Years of tight-fitting stockings and poorly fitted shoes contract the toe joint and cause it to bulge upward	Wear properly fitted shoes that are not too tight at the toe box. Soak feet if bunions become irritated and painful. Wear special orthotic device in the shoe. Minor surgery may be needed to realign the toe.
Painful arches	Inherited "flat feet," years of wearing shoes with inadequate arch support, for people who are susceptible to arch problems	Wear shoes with good arch support and a wide enough toe box. Custom-designed orthotic arch supports can be worn in shoes.

comes difficult, the person who has arthritis in the hands can use a typewriter or word processor.

• Use wheels around the house and for outings. Shopping carts are great for transporting things from room to room, tea tables for moving snacks and meals back and forth to the kitchen, and luggage carriers for traveling with suitcases and other heavy loads. Trash cans are now available with wheels.

• Use canes and walkers if prescribed by the doctor. Each needs to be specially fitted, to take weight off an arthritic joint, protecting it from damage. Bend the elbow and hold the cane at hip level, positioning the hand comfortably below the elbow, *not* above it.

• All kinds of assistive devices are available for arthritis, including eating utensils with large handles, special kitchen aids, adapted tools for home repairs and gardening, aids for unzipping and zipping clothing, hairbrushes and combs with long handles, and pronged object grabbers. Ask the doctor, nurse, or your local drugstore for names of catalogues offering devices. Or write to American Association of Retired People (AARP) for their catalogue.

Exercise. Arthritic joints need to be used. If they aren't they can become so stiff that movement may become more difficult and even more painful. Also, surrounding muscles will atrophy. If your spouse, parent, or an older friend becomes arthritic, he or she needs to start a sensible, regular exercise program. It will strengthen bones and ligaments around the affected joints, keep the joints flexible, and protect joints against further damaging stress. Another reason to exercise a joint, even if it is painful, is that continuous use may smooth it to a more comfortable shape (eburnation).

If the older person is fit and able, a regular program of walking, swimming, and bicycling is excellent. These activities are continuous, not jerky, and can be modified according to how the older person feels each day. These kinds of activities are often fun to do with other people as a social activity. Also good to consider is a walking or bicycling club, or a swimming program at a local pool.

Less-active, homebound elderly people need to follow a program of exercises that are limited in number, easy to remember, and simple to perform. Exercises for specific joints need to be recommended by the doctor, nurse, or physiotherapist according to the older person's ability and tolerance. Turning and raising motions are introduced to put a joint through its full range of motion, and isometric tightening motions are introduced to strengthen muscles.

Be sure prescribed exercises are done every day on a schedule. So that they won't be forgotten, sit down with your parent and work out easy-to-remember times for the exercises. Good times are after getting dressed in the morning, before breakfast, or after meals, during a favorite television show or radio program. If the older person is reluctant to start exercising, do the routine together, or find someone else in the family to join in, so that the experience can be companionable and fun. The payoff of exercises will be well worth the effort: your parent will have a sense of control over the arthritis and feel better physically as well as mentally.

Rheumatoid Arthritis

Rheumatoid arthritis (RA) is a whole-body disease, but osteoarthritis is a localized condition bothering one or only a few joints. In rheumatoid arthritis the immune system goes wrong. Its cells, which normally protect the body, turn against the joints, and also against other connective tissues in the tendons of the joints, the heart, the lungs, and the arteries.

The main problem with RA is inflammation of the synovial membranes in the joints. This normally thin membrane around each joint becomes unnaturally thicker, as millions of tiny inflammatory cells from the immune system invade it. The resulting inflammation causes the joints to feel boggy and warm to the touch, and often painful. If the disease carries on for many years, this inflammation can slowly digest the healthy parts of a joint and cripple it.

Although the disease varies tremendously from person to person, usually the onset is much more dramatic in older people, though for them the outlook fortunately is much better than for younger people. Rheumatoid arthritis can flare up and wane with dramatic ups and downs of pain and stiff joints in middle-aged people, before settling down. The older person with RA typically has the painful, most difficult cycle of the disease from six months to a year. Most often it strikes people between ages twenty and sixty, but is fairly common among the elderly. Older women are six times more susceptible to the disease than men of equivalent age.

Diagnosing Symptoms
Early in RA most people notice such flulike symptoms as fatigue and sore, stiff, and achy joints. Some people may also have a slight fever.

Joints of the hands and feet are especially stiff in the morning and after long periods of sitting or lying still. Often, the same joint on both sides of the body will become affected — both hands, both feet, or both shoulders.

A doctor will suspect RA if the symptoms above are present, especially those of pain and morning stiffness in joints for more than six weeks. Several blood tests can help confirm the diagnosis, although no one test can determine it. One test is for rheumatoid factor, an abnormal antibody found in the blood of about 80 percent of adults with RA. Another test, for red blood cell sedimentation rate, can measure extent of inflammation. Damage to the bones or cartilage can be partly determined by x-rays. It is unusual for changes to be seen on an x-ray in the first few months, and so many doctors wait to do an x-ray.

What triggers the disease is still a mystery. For years researchers have looked at possible causes, such as a viral, bacterial, or fungal infection, or a hereditary factor. The hereditary factor looks like the most promising explanation, because the disease does run in families.

Managing Rheumatoid Arthritis
Although the pain and difficulties of "mild" rheumatoid arthritis are usually treated in much the same way as we describe for osteoarthritis, we will not delve into the complexities of rheumatoid arthritis. It is a serious disease, usually dotted with flareups and remissions. Although a mild onset can be managed at home, often the patient will need to be hospitalized initially under supervision by a rheumatologist, who will know more than any other specialist how to treat various stages of the disease with medications and physiotherapy. If the person you are caring for got the disease in younger years, it will probably have been put under control, also with help from a rheumatologist.

If you have difficulty finding a rheumatologist, contact the nearest chapter of the Arthritis Foundation, which has chapters in all major cities, and in many smaller places as well. Chapter volunteers or personnel will be able to provide names of doctors as well as arthritis clinics. The organization has proven extremely helpful to rheumatoid arthritis sufferers and their families, by offering many informative written materials, help in finding home health care, classes on self-care, exercise classes, and clubs or support groups for people with the disease. If you can't easily locate a local chapter, call the national office information line at (800) 283–7800.

Medications

Two main forms of drug treatment are applied to osteoarthritis and "mild" phases of rheumatoid arthritis. They are aspirin, which has been around for centuries, and a new class of aspirin substitutes with the lengthy name nonsteroidal anti-inflammatory agents, or NSAIDS. (Acetaminophen [Tylenol], by the way, is referred to as an aspirin substitute. Understand, however, that it is only a pain reliever. Because acetaminophen has no anti-inflammatory properties, it is not recommended for someone who has an inflammatory form of arthritis.)

Aspirin

Because aspirin is used so commonly for everyday headaches, most people don't think it is distinguished enough to use for arthritis pain. Drug companies have been very successful in making people believe that far more expensive but similar brand-name drugs are better choices for arthritis. But in fact, plain, ordinary aspirin is the drug recommended by rheumatologists for osteoarthritis, "mild" rheumatoid arthritis, and the pain of temporary "-itises" such as bursitis, tendinitis, and "pulled" muscles.

Used properly, aspirin is one of the safest drugs around for arthritis, both for relieving pain and reducing inflammation. In rheumatoid arthritis, suppressing inflammation is a big factor, for the inflammation causes damage to joints. But in osteoarthritis, because inflammation is slight, aspirin is usually taken for its painkilling results, which can be achieved with much smaller dosages than those required for anti-inflammatory effects.

When it comes to effects, dosage does the work. Painkilling has a limit of two tablets (650 milligrams), which can be repeated after four hours. Taking more than two for pain is futile. In contrast, the anti-inflammatory action requires about three to four weeks to take effect, but only by ingesting a whopping dose of 12 to 24 tablets (325 grains each) a day. Of course, anyone taking this much aspirin most certainly needs to do so under careful supervision by a doctor.

If the older person has been told by the doctor to use aspirin to relieve arthritis pain, here's what each of you needs to know.

• You are perfectly safe in buying the cheapest USP standard brand in the drugstore, or from a discount mailing service. The abbreviation USP means United States Pharmacopoeia — the tested legal standard for drug strength and purity. A standard tablet is 5 grains or 325 milligrams.

• If the older person has stomach irritation — generally a rare problem at low doses — consider buying aspirin that is buffered or combined with an antacid (Bufferin, Ascriptin).

• Other ways of easing stomach irritation: take aspirin after meals, or with a glass of milk; try coated aspirin, which dissolves in the intestines (Ecotrin is best absorbed, Enseals is next best); drink eight ounces of water after each dose to dilute the aspirin in the stomach (this method is not suitable for coated aspirin).

• When aspirin smells like vinegar, or is broken, it has gone bad. Throw it out.

• Side effects are rare when aspirin is taken in doses for pain relief only. Common side effects at high doses include nausea, ringing in the ears, and decreased hearing — all usually reversible within a few hours if the dosage is decreased.

NSAIDS (Nonsteroidal Anti-inflammatory Agents)

This newer class of anti-inflammatory drugs includes Advil (ibuprofen), Butazolidin (phenylbutazone), Teandearil (oxyphenbutazone), Clinoril (sulindac), Dolobid (diflunisal), Feldene (piroxicam), Indocin (indomethacin), Meclomen (Meclofenamate), Motrin (ibuprofen), Nalfon (fenoprofen), Naprosyn (naproxen), Nuprin (ibuprofen), Rufen (ibuprofen).

Most of these drugs are available only with a doctor's prescription. Pills with 200 mg of ibuprofen are now available over the counter, however, with the brand names Advil and Nuprin, and are sold generically as ibuprofen.

Over-the-counter ibuprofen is now widely used because it has been promoted heavily as gentler on the stomach than aspirin. It is a good drug for those who cannot tolerate aspirin; however, studies are showing that it too can disturb the stomach if used for more than occasional relief. Those who have continuous episodes of arthritis pain should take the drug only under careful supervision by a doctor. Over-the-counter versions of the drug are not suitable for most people who have painful arthritis, because they may need at least 2,400 milligrams of ibuprofen daily. No one should use the availability of ibuprofen as an excuse to stay away from the doctor and continuously self-medicate for arthritis pain.

The older person who uses daily doses of an NSAIDS must be careful to take it only according to the doctor's prescription. Too much of the drug will greatly increase potential side effects, which include lightheadedness, dizziness, drowsiness, skin rash, itching, swollen face and extremities, and stomach discomfort. Because the medicine can upset the stomach, it may need to be taken with food, milk, and other liquids. The doctor should be consulted about how to take the drug without causing stomach irritation, for individual brands of NSAIDS have different patterns of absorption in the stomach. Aspirin or acetaminophen should not be taken at the same time.

RED ALERT: Aspirin, NSAIDS, and Ulcers

People who take aspirin or NSAIDS regularly risk developing stomach ulcers. According to the Federal Drug Administration, two to four in every 100 people taking these drugs form ulcerations in the stomach. Such ulcers from aspirin and NSAIDS usually are painless, because the drug masks pain signals.

An effective stomach-protecting drug, Cytotec (misoprostol), was approved in January 1989 by the Federal Drug Administration (FDA) for preventing stomach damage such as that caused by aspirin and nonsteroidal anti-inflammatory drugs (NSAIDS). Widely used in Europe, Cytotec is beginning to be prescribed by doctors in the United States. The drug is considered useful for those who have a history of ulcers caused by NSAIDS or to prevent such ulcers. Because it can cause diarrhea and stomach discomfort in the first few weeks of use, a low dosage is prescribed; it is usually taken four times a day, and the dosage is raised gradually for those who tolerate the drug.

An over-the-counter antacid that contains magnesium (Maalox or Mylanta) should *not* be taken with Cytotec, for the combination can cause diarrhea or make it worse. If stomach discomfort is intolerable, the person taking Cytotec should ask the doctor if it is a good idea to use occasional doses of an aluminum-containing antacid (Gelusil, Alternagel, or Amphogel). It is best, however, to avoid antacid use and to take the drug with a meal or a snack. Two doses should not be combined if one is missed.

Ulcer complications can be very serious. See the section on ulcers in Chapter 7, "Helping Digestive Disorders."

Total Hip Replacement

Encourage anyone who suffers relentless pain from a bad hip to talk to the doctor about surgery for hip replacement. An arthritic hip can become so annoyingly painful and problematic that the affected individual has difficulty sleeping and performing basic tasks. Many older people put surgery off, fearful of it and the ordeal of recovery, only to say after recovery, "I wish I had gone in for the operation sooner."

A major 1982 conference on the subject at the National Institutes of Health (NIH) concluded that hip replacement, "when done for incapacitating pain and dysfunction . . . gives a predictably excellent result in the vast majority of patients." The risk of death from the operation is less than 1 percent, as is the risk of infection. Clearly, risks are drastically diminished if you have hip replacement done by an orthopaedic surgeon who has extensive experience with the operation. Hip replacements are done 60 percent of the time for osteoarthritis, 7 percent for rheumatoid arthritis, 11 percent for hip fractures, and the rest for other disorders.

The big issue for hip replacement, beyond whether the patient can withstand the surgery, is that replacement parts do not usually last longer than ten to fifteen years, and then loosen. An older person who expects a long life, say beyond ten to fifteen years, should be aware that another surgery may well be in the future. This prospect may be a reason to delay surgery until pain and difficulties become truly intolerable. A great deal of promising research is under way to make devices last longer in the body; conceivably, longer-lasting prosthetic devices will be available before long.

The older person thinking about having surgery should know that the operation is successfully performed on healthy individuals of all ages. People of advanced age who are not considered at high risk for complications usually do well after surgery, although they generally recover and get back to normal activities less easily and quickly than those much younger. Many orthopaedic surgeons recommend that their older patients have spinal anesthesia, because recovery is usually pleasanter and safer than with general anesthesia.

Hip replacement became available in the United States in 1968, ten years after first used in England, where it was pioneered. The operation sounds rather like a carpentry project. The surgeon replaces the hip socket with a specially designed cup. Then a stainless-steel ball and connecting stem are fitted into the cup. The ball and cup form the new hip joint and the stem is inserted into the top marrow cavity (inner core) of the thigh bone. The stem end is fixed there with the help of bone cement, or bone is allowed to grow into the metal of the stem.

The recovery takes time, resolve, and hard work under guidance by a physiotherapy team, first at the hospital and later at home. The usual hospital stay is about two weeks, although patients are usually out of bed and in a chair one or two days after the operation. About the fourth postoperative day, patients are taught to start walking again with an assistive device. For about two months the patient needs help with meals, bathing, dressing, and getting to the toilet, and a great deal of kindness to support the will to do prescribed exercises. Movement is subject to very definite do's and don'ts. As a caregiver, get a list of these from the doctor for the older person to follow, as well as for everyone helping with the convalescence.

The hospital's social-work department can help you arrange for a short stay in a rehabilitation facility, if no one in the family can provide the necessary "hands-on" support. Medicare or Medicaid will pay for a limited stay for convalescence, as well as some hours of in-home physiotherapy and assistance by home health aides.

Polymyalgia Rheumatica

Poly What?
You are not alone if you haven't heard of polymyalgia rheumatica (PMR): quite a few physicians are little aware of it. The recently recognized rheumatic disease affects only older people. A geriatrician will certainly know about it, as well as any rheumatologist.

You should know something about this disease, which is often misdiagnosed as early rheumatoid arthritis. A sad mistake for the misdiagnosed person, who may receive inappropriate treatment for an easily treated disease that is somewhat unusual, but by no means rare. Doctors should definitely rule it out before confirming a diagnosis of rheumatoid arthritis.

What Is PMR?
No one really knows why, but PMR can strike older people, at an average age of seventy, as an inflammatory disease of the tiny blood vessels weaving through muscles. Although technically a cardiovascular disease, it comes within the rheumatologist's domain because

those affected complain of painful muscle aches and stiffness of muscles and joints.

The illness starts with viral-like symptoms, consisting of fever and sometimes extreme weight loss. Afterward, pain begins in the neck muscles and spreads to the muscles of the shoulder and down to the pelvic area. Pain can be on one side of the body, or both. Often sufferers feel terribly stiff in the morning, and painful areas also feel tender to the touch.

Some people experience inflammation of the large blood vessels of their temple (called PMR arteritis). Their temples will hurt to the touch and chewing may bring on pain. Rarely, the artery to the eye is affected, and then blindness can occur. This is the severest complication of the disease.

Without treatment the disease goes away by itself in two to three years. Proper treatment should be sought; the disease is very wearing and unpleasant for any older person, especially someone coping with other disabilities.

Treatment

The brightest fact about PMR is that it can be controlled promptly, within forty-eight hours. The response to treatment is so dramatic that hale and hearty older people may call their doctors within three days of treatment to gleefully say they are doing active yard work, or back on the golf course.

The treatment consists of appropriate low doses of prednisone, an anti-inflammatory corticosteroidal drug. A trial run of the drug for two days is now established as a diagnostic test for the disease. The drug is soon tapered to low levels and given usually for eighteen months or longer. The drug does not cure the disease, although certainly it does block symptoms from expression.

Prednisone in small doses does cause some side effects, loss of calcium being the one most relevant to the elderly. Many doctors prescribe calcium and vitamin D supplements, and recommend lots of walking to prevent osteoporosis.

Gout

It Is Called Crystal Arthritis

A gout attack brings on very sudden, very painful inflammation to a joint — so painful that even the touch of a sheet will send waves of pain through the foot, or any limb that is struck. Most attacks occur

---

Foods to Be Avoided in Gout

This list comes from the Arthritis Foundation. These foods contain a high purine concentration — about 150 to 1,000 milligrams per 100 grams.

Liver	Mussels	Wine	Heart
Brains	Kidney	Herring	Beer
Sardines	Broths	Gravies	Sweetbreads
	Anchovies	Fish roe	

---

in the big toe, the ankle, or the knee. Gout is arthritis in the strictest sense of the word. Fortunately, gout is now one of the most successfully managed forms of arthritis; only in classic novels do old men live in dread of yet another crippling attack.

An attack hits when uric acid crystals (called tophi), formed from an abundance of uric acid in the body, build up in a joint to irritate and jab the joint's lining (the synovial membrane). An inborn error in uric acid metabolism seems the cause in those who get the disease, mostly men. Uric acid is a waste product of substances called purines, which are found in some foods (see box).

Left untreated, an attack will ease off in two or three days to gradually fade out over a two-week period. Treatment reduces the chance of other attacks, although it cannot be guaranteed to prevent them. In severe cases attacks can come on six times a year.

Can Attacks Be Prevented?

Not everyone who has high levels of uric acid has gout. Although a simple blood test can check for high levels, geriatricians do not generally believe it makes sense for someone to bear the cost of medications to lower uric acid unless an attack has occurred.

About half of those who have attacks are over sixty-five. Gout attacks can start at any age, although people who get them will have had elevated levels of uric acid in their blood for a number of years, perhaps twenty or more.

Beyond medications, susceptible individuals have ways of warding off an attack, possibly preventing one altogether. Keeping a reasonable weight by proper diet and exercise helps, along with avoiding alcohol. The diet should exclude, not include, high-purine foods such as organ meats (although these days few people eat liver, brain, pancreas, and heart) and the other foods on our list. Drinking at least eight glasses of water a day is also helpful to flush built-up uric acid from the body, and especially from the kidneys, where crystals can form, along with kidney stones related to the disease. Occasionally the first sign that someone has high uric acid levels may be kidney stones.

More older people than ever may be contracting gout as a complication of drugs they are taking. You know the story by now: typically these days, as people get older they use more drugs. Some drugs can elevate uric acid levels, especially water pills or diuretics (particularly the commonly taken thiazide diuretics, such as Divril or Esidrix). The prospect of gout is another reason to help older people manage their illnesses with as few drugs as possible.

Treatment
An acute attack is usually treated with colchicine, which can enable someone who is writhing in pain to be up and free of it within a few hours. A time-honored drug, colchicine is derived from the autumn crocus or meadow saffron, used since the sixth century to treat gout. But it can be toxic, and as little as 7 milligrams of the stuff may be fatal. Your father and you as observer must be alert for signs of toxicity. Look for diarrhea, nausea and vomiting, and stomach cramps, and if they occur stop use of the drug and call the doctor immediately. Other drugs such as nonsteroidal anti-inflammatory drugs (NSAIDS), phenylbutazone, and steroids are a frequent choice for people who cannot tolerate colchicine.

After an attack has abated, further drug therapy may be a good idea for those who have especially high levels of uric acid in the blood stream and many crystal tophi. Lower, maintenance doses of colchicine can be given to those who can tolerate the drug. Probenecid and allopurinol are also used to treat acute attacks.

Many doctors recommend self-medication treatment for those likely to suffer future gout attacks. For instance, a painful attack can come on just an hour or so after the person has gone to bed for the night. Just knowing that colchicine is at the bedside can be a tremendous psychological relief to those who suffer repeat attacks (in severe cases they can occur up to six times a year).

The drug has to be taken at the very first sign of trouble; colchicine works best when given early. Do talk to your father and the doctor about this self-medication option. It can save a lot of aggravation, to say the least. Obviously, self-medication should not be handled alone by an older person who is confused in any way. Remember, colchicine can be fatal if taken in higher than prescribed doses. Caregivers for the confused elderly need to safeguard the patient, and learn from the doctor how to give it in an acute attack. Colchicine should be taken with meals to prevent stomach irritation.

Osteoporosis

Osteoporosis, or bone thinning, is one of those miserable conditions that used to be considered an inevitable consequence of aging. It is mainly a women's problem, correctly associated with broken hips, fractured wrists, and "dowager's hump" or "widow's hump." Now bone researchers tell us the condition is most often preventable and partly treatable, especially if preventive strategies are started well before middle age. These measures include paying attention every day to a calcium rich diet and plenty of exercise, among other changes in life-style, including making sure one's physician keeps checking on risk factors for the disease and whether these indicate that testing for it should be done.

The trouble is that women who are older today missed out on this new thinking. Most of them never gave a thought to osteoporosis or its prevention in their younger years. As a result, osteoporosis is very common and it is devastating and a major health problem. It is well known among doctors that at least one in four women over sixty-five have the disorder so badly that they will inevitably suffer a broken bone, or other osteoporosis-related breakdown of the skeleton, by the time they reach eighty. Indeed, studies in recent years show that a third of women who reach age ninety will have hip fractures related to osteoporosis.

You certainly need to know how to help keep your mother from developing osteoporosis, or making it any worse than it is if she already has it. You also need to be sure that the general practitioner and gynecologist she goes to is interested in preventing and treating osteoporosis. As we have said, prevention during younger years is the most effective approach to the problem, but much evidence suggests that it is never too late to start.

What Is Osteoporosis?

Osteoporosis is a disorder leading to brittle, porous bones, which break all too easily. In the Latin roots of the word, *osteo* means bone and *porosis* means porous. As we age, the bones normally lose minerals, especially calcium, and new bone is not formed as effectively. Those who have osteoporosis have lost so much mineral that their bones are extremely thin and a slight fall, or sometimes even normal walking, can leave them with fractures.

Bones are constantly changing structures, adding and subtracting calcium and other bone-building minerals under the influence of hormones, the quantity of calcium in the diet, our physical activity, and stresses to the body, including illnesses and some drugs taken to treat them. Once significant bone loss has occurred, bones cannot build themselves up to normal density and strength. Some new bone can be made, but very little. We must therefore prevent minerals from seeping out of bone in the first place.

Osteoporosis Is Not Easy to Diagnose

No one can feel gradual bone thinning, which is insidious and silent. Those who have osteoporosis usually find that they have it only after they have easily broken a bone, or when their spinal vertebrae collapse upon each other after sudden bending, lifting, or a fall.

When the back collapses, a "wedge" fracture is said to have occurred and the sufferer will feel sharp pain in and around the back. Sometimes the back vertebrae can fall into each other less precipitately, causing aching and tenderness while the spine shortens. But pain is not always felt as the vertebrae gradually collapse; some women just become stooped in posture and slightly shorter with no pain at all. The older person who feels prolonged discomfort around the spine or rib cage should be tested for osteoporosis.

No simple tests will diagnose the disease before a bone breaks. Blood tests for calcium can be normal. And x-rays can reveal the disease, but only after 30 to 50 percent of the woman's bone density has withered away.

Among the methods for detecting osteoporosis, dual photon absorptiometry is accurate and the most widely used. Unfortunately, nearly everyone who has the test does so only after they have broken a bone and the doctor treating it suspects it may have been severely weakened by osteoporosis. Because the cost of absorptiometry ($200 to $300) is not covered as a diagnostic screening test, doctors and patients usually rely on looking at a woman's health history and her profile of risk factors for bone loss before ordering the test. The woman who is postmenopausal and seems a likely candidate for osteoporosis fractures is then persistently encouraged to practice lifestyle measures that will keep her bones as strong as possible.

The older person at risk for osteoporosis, and worried that she may have it, can benefit enormously from having the test. Its evidence will clear up any doubts and provide a basis for future prevention, and if necessary for treatment. The out-of-pocket expense may be well worth it.

Why Is Osteoporosis an Older Woman's Problem?

Nature is not on women's side, when it comes to keeping strong bones throughout life. Women are far more likely than men to have more and more fragile bones, by a ratio of 6 to 1. Most women start out with bones much thinner than those of men, who can lose a lot more calcium and other minerals before their bones become fragile. Men usually have a larger skeletal frame, so bone loss is not as critical. Some men do suffer osteoporosis, but far fewer than women. Although men who are alcoholics or who need to take medication that causes bone loss are exceptions, generally men get osteoporosis at much more advanced ages than women.

It's certainly most unfair, but *all women* after menopause lose bone mass more rapidly than men of comparable age, especially in the first ten years after menopause, the time of greatest loss. Men do not have the sudden decline in sex hormones that women do. After menopause, women may begin to lose bone at a rate of 1 to 3 percent a year until death as the hormones that promote bone density wane. The white woman who lives to age eighty may lose from 30 to 60 percent of her bone mass. Generally, black women start with stronger bones and are less prone to bone loss as they age.

Estrogen — the hormone that declines most — can be given as replacement therapy to prevent bone loss in women who are experiencing menopause. To work effectively, though, the drug replacement has to be started in the years immediately after symptoms begin. Ten years after the onset of menopause is generally considered too late for estrogen replacement, which therefore is not usually a choice for most older women who have osteoporosis.

Then there's childbearing and breastfeeding. Although high estrogen levels during pregnancy may be a protection against bone loss, both biological events can raid a mother's calcium stores, unless she has taken in enough extra calcium to make up for the baby's needs beyond her own. Many women in their seventies and eighties today were indeed urged to drink more milk during childbearing years, if they had good midwifery or obstetrical care. But not all of them followed this advice, nor were they offered the megacalcium pills their contemporaries take today, as insurance against calcium depletion.

Who Is at Greatest Risk?

A number of factors increase a woman's chances of developing fragile bones. If your mother has even one of these risk factors in her history she needs to start immediately strategies for preventing osteoporosis.

Chronically low calcium intake. The National Institutes of Health and the National Osteoporosis Foundation recommend that a woman take in 1,000 milligrams of calcium a day before menopause in order to set down dense bones. After menopause she needs 1,500 mg of calcium. Most women do not come close to consistently taking in the amounts they need each day. You can get 1,500 mg of calcium in about one and a half quarts of milk, or in other dairy-food equivalents. How many women do you know who drink even one glass of milk every day?

Being Caucasian. In general, the fairer the complexion the greater the risk of getting osteoporosis; white women get it much more often than black women.

Being thin and petite. The condition is rarely seen in women with a large body frame, for they have more bone to begin with.

A family history. Because osteoporosis does seem to have a hereditary connection, go over family photos to discover if anyone in earlier generations was pictured with curved back and rounded shoulders. Also, ask family members to find if aunts or grandparents have the disorder.

Early menopause. A strong predictor, especially if menopause is sudden, early, and a result of gynecological surgery, is a drop in a woman's estrogen levels. Estrogen-replacement pills can prevent much bone loss, but the current medical consensus is that treatment must be started within ten years of menopause, and the earlier the better.

Sedentary life-style. People long bedridden or sedentary actually lose calcium from their bones.

Smoking. Cigarette smoking is now known to increase chances of losing bone mass and breaking bones. A higher proportion of women cigarette smokers have osteoporosis than those who do not.

Excessive drinking. Alcoholics undergo bone thinning, and more than two drinks a day may up someone's risk for osteoporosis. As we have said, the few men who have osteoporosis are predominantly alcoholics.

Prednisone. The anti-inflammatory steroidal drug prednisone is known to cause bone thinning. It should be prescribed only when absolutely essential.

Three Strategies for Osteoporosis Prevention in Later Life

For women who are well past the menopause, and not on a lifetime program of estrogen replacement, bones are very difficult to actually thicken up again once significant amounts of calcium have been lost. But bone thinning can be slowed down, and in some cases halted, by late-life prevention strategies, and, in selected cases, by carefully administering one of the drug-therapy regimens developed in recent years.

Research on drugs for treatment and prevention of osteoporosis looks promising, as research advances and drug companies work hard to come up with a safe drug to strengthen weakened bones.

If your mother or father is at high risk for osteoporosis, or is definitely known to have the disease as shown in absorptiometry testing, or a CAT scan, then you need to encourage her or him to talk to a doctor about drug therapy. Preliminary studies show promising results in some cases. If your parent's usual doctor is not well informed about osteoporosis drug therapy, consider making an appointment at an osteoporosis clinic. More and more hospitals and most major medical centers have such clinics. And increasingly, doctors are specializing in the disease. For information about where to go for osteoporosis diagnosis and treatment, write to or telephone the National Osteoporosis Foundation, which is listed in the Appendix.

Calcitonin, a hormone that occurs naturally in the body, has been shown to slow bone breakdown in those who have excessive bone loss. It is also being used to prevent bone loss in high-risk women who cannot take estrogen. At present, the only form of the hormone approved by the Food and Drug Administration is salmon calcitonin. Patients are taught to inject the drug themselves three times a week, or have caregivers do the job.

One new drug therapy has proved successful in replacing lost calcium in some women who undergo the therapy during the immediate postmenopausal years. The drug etidronate is taken for fourteen days, followed by calcium for seventy-six days, either in the diet or as a supplement. The drug continues in use, although long-term use still needs to be evaluated. Your mother may want to talk to her doctor about the therapy, because a few very preliminary studies show it is promising for restoring bone mass in older women. It is presumed too that the etidronate-calcium regimen will benefit men.

Beyond medications, we list here what an older person can do to promote healthy bones.

ONE: Eat Calcium-Rich Foods. This is very important. All older people should try to get 1,500 milligrams of calcium from the many good food sources available. That quantity is a lot more than most people are used to taking daily. But the job should not be too difficult once they have learned which foods are high in calcium.

The easiest way to get calcium is in nonfat dairy products, and especially milk. Older people generally need some nudging toward milk — they may think of it as an unpalatable children's drink. And yet skim milk is light, low in calories, and dense in nutrients, and it can be drunk as a thirst quencher or an accompaniment to meals. A cup of skim milk contains approximately 300 mg of calcium, and so making a habit of drinking three glasses a day takes care of most of the daily requirement. Yogurt, hard cheeses, and cottage cheese are also excellent sources of calcium. Lactase-treated milk and cheeses are available for people who are lactose intolerant — unable to digest milk products.

Five cups of milk, three to four cups of yoghurt, and seven ounces of hard cheese provide the recommended 1,500-milligrams daily of calcium.

Another excellent source of calcium is nonfat powdered milk, the kind sold in boxes on supermarket shelves. The stuff is as nutritious a source of calcium as fresh milk, and a convenience for older people who have to do their own shopping. Every teaspoon gives 33 milligrams of calcium. A standard-size box will last a long time, for just a few tablespoons mixed with water will make up a quart of milk. Powdered milk doesn't discernibly change the taste of food, and it can be sprinkled into just about any recipe — soups, stews, baked goods, and desserts.

Calcium and Caloric Content of Some Common Dairy Foods

	Calcium (milli-grams)	Calo-ries
Milk and Milk Beverages		
Milk, whole (3.3%), 1 cup	291	150
Milk, low-fat (2%), 1 cup	297	120
Milk, low-fat (1%), 1 cup	300	100
Milk, skim, 1 cup	302	85
Buttermilk, 1 cup	285	100
Chocolate milk, low-fat (1%), 1 cup	287	160
Cheeses		
American pasteurized process, 1 oz	174	105
Cheddar, 1 oz	204	115
Cottage, large-curd, creamed (4%), 1 cup	135	235
Cottage, low-fat (2%), 1 cup	155	205
Monterey Jack, 1 oz	212	106
Mozzarella, part skim, low moisture, 1 oz	207	80
Swiss, 1 oz	272	105
Yogurt		
Plain, low-fat, 8-oz container	415	145
Plain, nonfat, 8-oz container	452	125
Fruit, low-fat, 8-oz container	345	230
Coffee or vanilla, low-fat, 8-oz container	389	194
Desserts		
Ice milk, vanilla, hardened (about 4% fat), 1 cup	176	185
Ice milk, vanilla, soft-serve (about 3% fat), 1 cup	274	225
Ice cream, vanilla, hardened (about 11% fat), 1 cup	176	270
Sherbet (about 2% fat), 1 cup	103	270
Some Other Good Sources of Calcium		
Almonds, whole, 1 oz	75	165
Broccoli, frozen, chopped, cooked, ½ cup	47	25
Collard greens, frozen, chopped, cooked, ½ cup	179	30
Kale, frozen, chopped, cooked, ½ cup	90	20
Salmon, pink, canned, with liquid and bones, 3 oz	167	120
Sardines, canned in oil, with bones, 3 oz	371	175
Snap beans, frozen, cut, cooked, ½ cup	31	18

SOURCE: National Dairy Board, 1989.

TWO: Take Supplements. Food is the best source of calcium. For someone who is not getting enough from food, however, supplements are an acceptable way to ensure that enough is being taken in. No woman should rely on supplements alone as a source of calcium, because food sources are more easily absorbed in the digestive system. Anyone with a history of kidney stones should take calcium supplements only under a doctor's supervision, because they can cause stones in susceptible people.

Calcium carbonate pills are one of the best types to buy because they contain the highest percentage of elemental calcium. Although calcium citrate has less elemental calcium, it is a good choice for those who get gas and constipation from calcium carbonate.

When reading labels, look for the words "elemental calcium"; the older woman needs 1,500 milligrams of elemental calcium, not 1,500 mg of whatever is in the pill. A 750-mg tablet of calcium carbonate, for example, will provide only 300 mg of elemental calcium, 40 percent of the mg dosage. Ask your pharmacist which brand will give you the most elemental calcium for the lowest cost, and also ask how many supplements to take daily to accompany food sources of calcium.

It makes sense to spread out calcium supplements during the day. The body will excrete any excess from a large dose taken all at once. To help absorption of calcium, calcium carbonate is best downed in a sip of orange juice, calcium citrate with water on an empty stomach.

THREE: Practice Daily Weight-bearing Exercise. Weight-bearing exercise combined with attention to calcium in the diet is the most promising nonpharmaceutical way to retard bone loss. The purpose is to get the muscles to exert themselves against gravity and to put stress on the long bones. Swimming, although a top aerobic activity and excellent for putting joints through their range of motion, is not considered a preventive exercise for osteoporosis because it does not stress the long bones. And yoga is not a weight-bearing form of exercise, but rather one to develop coordination and toning of muscles.

Walking is the best form of weight-bearing exercise for older people. At least an hour of brisk walking four times a week makes for good, safe prevention of osteoporosis. If your mother has been sedentary, she can begin walking slowly for short periods every day and eventually build herself up to walking briskly for an hour. Walk with her yourself, or encourage a grandchild or other member of the family to do so, if she has difficulty mustering the impetus to start a walking program. Make walking for exercise fun and enjoyable. More rigorous choices, but only for those who can physically handle them, are tennis, aerobic dancing, ballroom dancing, cross-country skiing, and treadmill walking.

Most communities have walking clubs for older people. They organize group walks in school gyms and on outdoor athletic tracks, and for the hot weather in air-conditioned malls.

If anyone in the family becomes bedridden or able to move about only at low speed, be sure he or she still gets some exercise. Two weeks in bed can cause bone loss equal to that of a year's normal aging. Do ask your doctor, or your local association of visiting nurses, to provide a program of weight-bearing exercises to be done in bed, in a chair, or in a standing position. Also, refer to Chapter 14, "Caring for the Convalescent at Home."

Falls

Falls Are a Very Serious Matter

Because of bone thinning, a fall for an older person can be disastrous. Children and young adults can fall down and not harm themselves, give or take a few bruises, but for elderly people falls carry a heavy penalty to themselves and to society. Each year 200,000 Americans over age sixty-five fracture their hips in falls, and 20,000 to 30,000 die of complications, especially pneumonia, related to bed rest and immobility during recuperation. For hip fractures alone the cost of direct care is $7 billion a year. Other bones too break easily in falls: the wrists, the legs, and the spine.

Broken bones can be life-threatening, and can also dampen an older person's ability to live independently, as well as the sense of vitality and will to go on living. The elderly who experience a broken bone can easily become frightened to move and sedentary for fear of another damaging fall. A sign of their timidity is resistance to the arduous work of physiotherapy and the effort it takes to recuperate completely. It is said that 50 percent of women who experience a broken hip do not recover their full independence after surgery. Studies show that often about a third of the elderly who break bones enter nursing homes and remain there permanently.

Why Do Older People Fall?

The kinds of health problems the elderly commonly experience tell us why they are prone to dangerous falls. Consider the visually impaired person who has a stiff knee because of osteoarthritis and a tendency toward forgetfulness. Unless her staircase is well lighted day and night, she is almost certain to overstep a stair edge while descending. She is also likely to trip over loose cords, bumps, or ridges in carpet or flooring.

Not being able to see well probably puts one at greatest risk of falling. But just about all impairments associated with aging increase the risk. Diseases that affect gait and ease of movement, such as Parkinson's and painful arthritis, and cardiovascular problems that cause dizzy spells and fainting, all contribute to the possibility of falls. Likewise, medications impose a high risk of falling, especially antianxiety drugs, antidepressants, and other sedatives. Also likely to fall are those who are so weak from sitting around that they feel unsteady as they get up from a chair or bed.

Finally, some older people experience a change in their righting reflex — the capacity to restore balance after a minor stumble. A young person may stumble momentarily after missing a step or tripping on a carpet, but the body rights itself. In an older person, the righting reflex can be slowed and muscular agility lessened, so that any imbalance can quickly spiral into a disabling fall.

You Must Safeguard Surroundings

Safety in preventing falls is a top priority. As a family, *you must safeguard surroundings*. If you haven't already done so, do the work now! If no one in the family can handle the necessary handiwork, hire a carpenter. If cost is an issue, contact the local Area Agency on Aging to find out if volunteer-based or low-cost programs to safeguard disabled and older people's homes are available in the community.

Most falls occur because of hazardous conditions in the home. The three commonest places are stairs, bathrooms, and kitchens. Inadequate lighting in stairways, lack of strong handrails, and rickety steps are hazardous. In the kitchen, slippery waxed floors, water, grease spots, and dropped food can cause a slip, a slide, and a nasty fall. In the bathroom, wet floors, slippery, soapy tubs, and lack of convenient grip rails are all well-known setups for older people's falls.

Here are some specific tips for safeguarding.

• Make certain lighting is adequate on stairs, in every room, and outdoors. Follow all our "Adaptive Help and Safety Tips for Failing Vision" in Chapter 2.

• Be sure handrails are on both sides of stairways. They should be round, positioned about 30 inches above the stairs, and set far enough from the wall to be grasped firmly.

• Examine all rugs and step runners for loose threads and torn areas that could cause a trip or a stumble.

• Consider low-pile, monotone wall-to-wall carpeting for maximum safety. Or fasten rugs securely at the edges with thick, durable tape. Remove all unnecessary scatter rugs.

• Remove or flatten door sills to prevent stumbling.

• Remove low-lying pieces of furniture, footstools, stepstools, and magazine racks from all rooms. Check whether coffee tables are a safety hazard. Also, put radios, stereo equipment, and other appliances on high shelves.

• Keep rooms tidy; clutter is likely to topple off surfaces and get under foot.

• Tack all appliance cords to the walls and out of walking areas.

• Encourage the older person to use chairs that are easy to get out of. Chairs equipped with armrests, about seven inches above the seat, increase leverage. The seat height is appropriate when the user can sit with feet planted firmly on the floor and knees flexed 90 degrees. Avoid seating the older person in a chair that has a crossbar spanning the legs in front, for it will hinder the older person from sliding the legs under the seat for leverage.

• If the older person can't safely get in and out of standard chairs, purchase an electric-powered pneumatic spring chair at a surgical supply store. It will go up and down and gently forward, allowing the user to stand without effort. Medicaid may reimburse the cost in your state.

• Mount horizontal handrails around the bathtub, and if showers are preferred, install vertical rails along the walls of the shower stall.

• Place a wall-mounted liquid-soap dispenser on the bathtub or shower wall. The older person might slip on a bar of soap or have to retrieve it in the shower.

• Put a nonslip mat in the bathtub.

• Mount handrails on the wall next to the toilet. One should run parallel to the floor at a height of 33 inches.

• If getting on and off the toilet presents difficulties, buy a raised toilet seat with armrests. One type looks like an armchair and can be bought at any surgical supply store or large drugstore.

• Stick nonslip strips on the floor in front of the toilet.

• To prevent slipping, consider covering the bathroom floor with wall-to-wall carpeting designed for bathrooms and kitchens.

• Consider installing wall-to-wall kitchen carpeting, or low-luster cushioned linoleum to soften falls. Otherwise, clean the kitchen floor with waxless cleaner.

• Place shelves and other storage areas within easy arm's reach.

• Provide safe kitchen seating at work areas to prevent fatigue.

Beyond Safeguarding, What Can You Do?

Seek Help Early for Problems. At least half the falls that harm the elderly are traceable to medical conditions. Therefore a vital measure for preventing falls is to make sure that the older people you love get proper treatment for medical problems. Encourage them to go for medical checkups and to follow the treatments prescribed by general practitioners or specialists, including eye specialists.

Notify the doctor if you notice that an older person you are with is not moving around normally, and of course if you spot mental changes and obvious symptoms of illness. Look out for signs of dizziness, faintness, tottering, and unsteadiness while walking, getting up from a chair, or bending over. Also, observe if the person is walking steadily with feet firmly planted on the ground. Many aged women have a narrow gait that can make them tottery and quick to stumble. Aged men with no gait-affecting disorder may have a much broader gait that keeps them stabler.

Besides treating any problem medically, or changing medications that may be contributing to a problem, your doctor may decide that a cane or a walker will help the older person move around more safely. Sensible shoes, or even specially prescribed shoes, may also be recommended. The doctor may decide to refer you to a neurologist who works at counseling and rehabilitating people with balance and gait difficulties, or to a geriatric rehabilitation center, with staff trained to teach people how to move about safely. Such centers are usually found at major medical centers and community hospitals.

Encourage Use of Canes or Walkers. Many older people resist using canes and walkers out of sheer embarrassment, unless of course they can't get around without them. If the doctor has recommended an assistive device, encourage its use, but negotiate sensitively. Somehow work out a happy way for your parent to use the devices the doctor has recommended; they will be bone savers.

Unfortunately, many people buy canes and walkers on their own without proper instruction, or hurried practitioners give them assistive devices without proper preparation. There is no such thing as a standard cane or walker; each needs to be measured to an individual's size, posture, and ability to grip. A properly selected and fitted device can make a huge difference in its user's ability to move safely and comfortably.

Many falls happen on the way to the bathroom, especially if one has the common problem of having to "go" suddenly. Be sure light switches are within easy reach of the bed, and keep a cane next to it.

At all times, keep a cane handy. Also, tune your sensors to the older person's need for assistance. Sometimes a helping hand or supportive arm is appreciated as a gesture of attention and love, as well as a substitute for an assistive device.

The Broken-Hip Emergency

Hip fractures are the commonest fractures in the elderly, especially among women who have osteoporosis. Here's what to expect in the event your mother or father breaks a hip. Anyone who breaks a hip cannot get up, and so one who lives alone and is prone to falling should wear an emergency response system button (see Chapter 15, "Help and Where to Find It").

You can easily recognize that someone has broken a hip bone. First, no one breaks a hip without obvious pain and total inability to stand up. Second, a look at the sufferer's affected leg will show that it has rotated to the side. Toes tell all: they will not point to the ceiling as they normally do.

You should *not move* the individual before the ambulance has arrived. Before calling the ambulance, of course, be reassuring and say that medical help is coming. Also, cover the individual with a blanket, unless it is a very hot day, and place a thin pillow under the head.

The Surgery. Emergency-room personnel are used to having people come in with broken hips. After x-rays have been taken, the patient is wheeled to an operating room for surgical repair.

Most hip fractures can be put together with a "pinning" procedure. The broken bone is bound together with pins so that the patient can be out of bed much sooner than if the bone were simply set and enclosed in a cast. Pinning is usually done if the injury is a trochanteric fracture, which is a break below the part of the upper leg bone (femur) that is called the neck of the femur. This neck juts away from the upper leg bone into the hip socket.

In large hospitals and major medical centers, orthopaedic surgeons usually are on call to operate on broken-hip patients, but in smaller community hospitals general surgeons may do the job. Hip pinning is a tried-and-true operation with a low rate of complications; it has been in use for around thirty years. Advanced age generally does not preclude surgery; it is performed routinely on patients in their eighties and even nineties.

Many surgeons will perform the procedure with the patient under spinal anesthesia, a good option for elderly people who may not so easily withstand the effects of general anesthesia. Do ask about the pros and cons of this option for your parent.

Pinning may not be adequate if the break occurs in the neck of the femur. Instead, the femur neck may need to be removed; an artificial replacement is then attached. The procedure is a hemi-hip replacement, which is similar to total hip replacement for people who have painful arthritis of the hip, as described earlier in this chapter.

The hospital stay is about the same for both pinning and hemi-hip replacement, around ten to fourteen days. Recuperation time is about the same, too. In the best circumstances the bone usually takes about two to six months to heal enough that a walker or cane is not necessary. Physiotherapy, started in the hospital, needs to be continued throughout the recovery period. Successful rehabilitation depends on the patient's general health and ability to understand and cooperate in all the hard work that has to be done. Consistent support from family and friends certainly can positively influence the older person's determination to start walking again. Medicare or Medicaid will pay for a physiotherapist's home visits, although the number of visits varies from state to state.

If you are unable to take care of your parent or friend at home during the recovery period, consider finding a place in a good nursing home set up to rehabilitate those who have had hip surgery, just for the convalescence. The hospital social worker will help you decide if this is the best choice, and which home to select.

7

Helping Digestive Problems

ALTHOUGH PLENTY of age-related changes have been identified at various places along the digestive tract, they seem to exert relatively little adverse effect on the overall processing and absorption of food. It does indeed take longer for a meal to be digested and pass through an older person's intestines; some digestive juices are less well produced, and the muscle tone of the gut does slacken. Marked changes are not usual and normal, however, for someone who is healthy and eating a sensible diet. The entire system remains able to meet most reasonable demands.

Proper diet, adequate exercise every day, sensible bathroom habits, and careful drug taking make a huge difference in the health and functioning of the digestive system. Many problems that arise result from a breakdown in such measures. Fortunately, most problems can be quickly taken care of with common-sense changes in diet and self-help remedies. Going off a medication or changing to another can also bring about an immediate change. Often, medications cause a dry mouth, stomach upsets, diarrhea, and constipation.

The digestive system, though, is by no means invincible. Diseases and problems in this body system are widespread among older people. We all know someone over sixty-five who has complained at some time or other about heartburn, constipation, diverticular disease, or ulcers. Ulcers are a big worry, especially for those who take arthritis medications or preparations that are injurious to the stomach.

Everyone needs to be alert for the signs of cancer in various organs so that quick and effective treatment can be provided whenever necessary. With every decade, cancers of the digestive tract are more likely to start. Any changes in swallowing, digestion, or elimination that vary from the pattern that is established as normal for the individual must be brought to medical attention, even if such changes are subtle.

Digestive-tract disorders can be thorny to diagnose, because often the symptoms are similar. This parallelism seems to be the rule rather than the exception, whether disorders are just annoying or serious. Unusual symptoms must be reported to a doctor if they carry on for more than a few days. Don't let your relative or friend self-diagnose symptoms as trivial; they may not be. Only a doctor can determine their origin and the appropriate action.

Your job is to recognize both warnings and frank expressions of problems so that you can encourage the older person you are caring for to seek medical advice. In this chapter you confront common problems and disorders and see how they can be treated, either medically or by self-help relief methods in which you can be involved in administering at home.

Dry Mouth

Many old people suffer the extremely disturbing annoyance of a dry mouth. A slowing of the saliva-producing glands used to be considered a normal consequence of aging, but recent studies on healthy people in their eighties and nineties show that their saliva production does *not* eventually run dry.

The problem is common and caused by a number of illnesses, or of medications, especially those designed to benefit circulatory-system disorders, diabetes, allergies, and anxiety. Do inform the doctor if your parent or older friend is suffering a dry mouth, and discuss whether or not drugs that may be causing it can be stopped and other drugs or treatments substituted.

An untreated dry mouth is much more than an annoyance, it is a debilitating preoccupation. If you have ever experienced a dry mouth from stage fright before making a speech, you can remember how uncomfortably dry your mouth became and how difficult it was to speak in a normal voice. Older people who endure a dry mouth have to do so around the clock. Besides altered speech, they have a hard time eating, swallowing, and tasting food. The mouth also becomes vulnerable to inflammation and sores and dental disease, such as cavities and sore gums.

A number of treatments are possible. The aim is to stimulate any saliva left within the salivary glands and to moisten and clean out the dry mouth. Drinking at least eight glasses of fluid each day is helpful (unless fluids must be limited for a medical reason) and moist foods should be served at mealtimes along with water, juice, or milk. Citrus drinks such as orange juice and lemonade will temporarily stimulate saliva, and they seem to be a favored mouth-refreshing drink for those with the problem. Rinsing the mouth out frequently with salt and water or a glycerine-based mouthwash will also help.

A number of artificial-saliva products — including 10 percent glycerine in distilled water — can be bought over the counter in drugstores. These squeeze-bottle preparations are very effective in lubricating and protecting the mouth.

RED ALERT: What to Do When a Pill Gets Stuck in the Throat

Anyone looking after an older person with a dry mouth should be alert to the potential danger of having a pill become stuck in the throat. A lodged pill can painfully irritate the esophagus and even ulcerate it.

If a pill does get stuck, ask the older person to sit upright and relax; next, reassure him or her that you will stay there until the pill has passed down to the stomach. Offer a few sips of a carbonated drink, which may disintegrate the pill. Try using water if no carbonated drink is in the house. If the older person can still feel that the pill is stuck after fifteen minutes, call the doctor for advice or calmly go to an emergency room after half an hour. Usually, relaxation and carbonated water will do the trick.

Swallowing Difficulties

Research shows that subtle changes occur in the muscular aspects of swallowing and movement of food down the esophagus of older people, particularly those in the very-old age group. Because of such normal changes in the mouth, throat, and upper digestive tract, it may be necessary for an older person to chew and swallow more slowly so that food goes down comfortably without causing sputtering, coughing, or belching.

Marked changes in swallowing and discomfort in the esophagus are not at all normal and need to be examined by a doctor. Numerous illnesses, including Alzheimer's disease, Parkinson's, stroke, depression, and dental disorders can contribute to such problems, as can cancer. The cause of swallowing difficulties and any uneasy feelings in the esophagus must be determined so that the problem can be treated medically, and the person can have proper professional advice on how to manage eating.

An uncontrolled swallowing problem can easily tip an older person over the edge into malnutrition and spiraling physical deterioration. It can also put them in danger of choking on food and liquids, or inhaling these into the lungs to cause irritation and subsequent pneumonia. In fact, doctors routinely check for difficulty in swallowing if someone has repeated bouts with pneumonia.

In looking for a cause, the doctor will do a physical examination and if necessary run a barium-swallow x-ray series or look down the throat with an endoscope. Often the x-ray series is done first, for it can record on moving film how the muscles of the throat and esophagus look and move. To enhance the image the patient usually swallows a marshmallow or piece of bread that has been dipped in radioactive liquid barium, or is given barium liquid to drink. If obvious changes are not apparent on film, the doctor may then decide to do an endoscopic examination to check for cancer.

Swallowing problems can sometimes be treated simply by modifying the way in which food is prepared and eaten, or with medications or surgery.

Don't allow your spouse, mother, father, or friend to dismiss as trivial or normal any changes in their usual way of swallowing. Seek medical attention if you notice them coughing while eating, drooling, belching, or having difficulty eating some textures of foods and drinking liquids. Another sign of a swallowing disorder is a change in voice quality. A "frog in the throat" could mean that solid foods and liquids are pooling above the vocal cords. Pain and discomfort and the feeling of food stuck in the throat are other clear signs of trouble.

A disorder in the esophagus may show up as soreness down through the middle of the chest and the sensation of food being lodged. An esophageal problem can also cause small amounts of food to spit up into the mouth.

Once you have a medical diagnosis of a swallowing difficulty and treatment — if necessary — is begun, do make sure the person you are caring for, as well as you as caregiver, are getting practical advice on how to work around the problem during and after meals at home. Occupational therapists usually are the professionals doctors call in to work with patients who have swallowing difficulties, although sometimes speech therapists or specialized nurses do the job. Such professionals can tailor a program to an individual's problem and offer suggestions for compensatory eating techniques, as well as how to prepare food so that it is manageable and palatable.

Tips for Safe Eating
These tips apply to the person who is having swallowing difficulties.

- It's best to eat sitting upright in a chair.
- The person eating in bed (if necessary) needs to be propped up on pillows to a sitting position, or as close to that as possible.
- After eating it's a good idea to stay sitting up for at least 20 minutes. Gravity helps the cough reflex.
- Allow coughing — do not suppress the cough reflex.
- Keep conversation to a minimum between bites. If necessary, keep the mealtime atmosphere quiet all during the meal.
- While swallowing, keep the chin down to a natural level — don't throw the head back.
- Keep food bites small, about a teaspoonful.
- If necessary, serve ground meat and soft foods, such as mashed potatoes or squashes with gravy, yoghurt, applesauce, and pasta with nourishing sauces. Try flavorful vegetable and fruit purées.
- Keep food attractive and tasty. Flavorful food stimulates swallowing and is easier to swallow.
- Alternate sips of liquids and solids if liquids are tolerated.
- Water may be particularly difficult. Seltzer and carbonated drinks *may* be better tolerated.
- Liquids are often the most difficult to swallow; talk to a professional about adding thickeners to clear liquids so that they will go down the throat more easily. One good product is Thick-It, which can be ordered as a free sample, or in bulk, from Bruce Medical Supply: (800) 225–8446.
- Drinking from a flexible straw may make swallowing liquids easier.

Lactose Intolerance

Although older people never outgrow their need for milk, many out-grow their stomach for it.

Lactose intolerance or inability to digest milk products is a common condition that affects approximately 75 percent of the world's people by the time they have reached old age. Those who have lactose intolerance have a deficiency in the stomach enzyme lactase, which digests lactose, a complex sugar component of milk. People of northern European stock appear to have the best tolerance for milk at all ages, although many are exceptions. But the majority of people eventually have the problem, if they are from one of these populations among others: American Indians, Asians, blacks, Mediterraneans, eastern European Jews, central Europeans, and South Americans.

The deficiency takes years to form, but once it starts to be felt the affected person will experience indigestion, including gas, a "rumbling tummy," cramps, and maybe even diarrhea. The turmoil comes from gas- and acid-producing intestinal bacteria, as they feed on undigested lactose, which is normally broken up in the stomach by the now-deficient enzyme. Intolerance to milk and milk products can vary in degree.

Some people have indigestion only when they overdo it with milk, ice cream, or cheese; others are intolerant only of milk, but not cheeses and ice cream, which contain less lactose. Then too, a few have trouble when they unknowingly eat food prepared with just a trace of milk solids. Hundreds of medications use lactose in their formulation as a carrier for drugs. Temporary milk intolerance can follow a stomach flu, or occur if one is on antibiotics or an anti-inflammatory drug for arthritis.

Lactaid, an artificial lactase enzyme, allows those who can't tolerate milk to keep it in their diet. A wonderful invention is Lactaid, because milk is such an efficient way to gain calcium in the diet, along with other essential nutrients.

Lactaid-treated milk can be purchased in most supermarkets, or you can make your own by buying Lactaid drops at a drugstore and following the directions on the bottle. Usually four drops are added to a quart of milk and 70 percent of the lactose sugars are digested in twenty-four hours. The enzyme works in low-fat or whole milk, cream, and half and half. Most milk intolerant people can eat yoghurt without indigestion. For people who can't digest cheese, Lactaid-treated cheese is available in most supermarkets.

Constipation

Laxatives Are Not the Answer

Those tiresome advertisements for laxatives, shown every day on television, are designed to make people believe that constipation is as natural a part of aging as gray hair. Attractive older actors, glowing with good health, are often shown riding bicycles and playing golf while telling audiences that happiness comes with "regularity" and having a bowel movement every day, brought on of course by taking the laxative they are touting. Such advertisements are a sham, ridiculed by those who know about constipation.

Although older people are five times as likely to report trouble with constipation, healthy older people who eat a sensible diet, and especially those who exercise, should not have that problem. Constipation is a frequently overemphasized ailment associated with the elderly; perhaps because the myths in laxative advertising have succeeded in convincing so many of them that their digestive systems become sluggish and that to be healthy they must have a daily bowel movement.

Constipation is indeed a symptom of trouble in the bowels, and it occurs when one goes several days without having a bowel movement, which is then very hard and a strain to pass. Older people who suffer from it do so not because their digestive processes have slowed, but because they are ill, not eating correctly, sedentary, on bed rest, or on constipating medications.

Even those who do have constipation because of an illness and medications can usually prevent further episodes without resorting to laxatives. A laxative is not a cure for the underlying causes of constipation. Use one only after trying other methods of relief, and when you are uncomfortably constipated.

Laxatives are self-perpetuating if used habitually: they are one of the common causes of constipation because the bowel eventually relies on the laxative to "empty" itself, and before too long the bowel loses the ability to function. On the other hand, some people respond to laxative misuse with diarrhea, not constipation.

Plenty of other problems come with habitual use of laxatives, depending on the kind. Mineral-oil types coat the intestines and block

Medications That Cause Constipation

The medications listed here are frequently part of an older person's schedule. If the person you're caring for is taking any of these, he or she risks constipation.

The older person should ask the doctor if any medications can be eliminated. If none can be, then the doctor needs to recommend self-help measures to prevent constipation.

These medications are constipating:

Antacids containing aluminum or calcium — Amphojel, Gaviscon, Maalox, Mylanta, Tums

Antihistamines — Actifed, Benadryl, Contac, Dimetapp, Seldane, or any over-the-counter medicines containing diphenhydramine hydrochloride or promethazine hydrochloride

Antidepressants — Elavil, Norpramin, Pamelor, Sinequan, Tofranil

Antipsychotic drugs — Haldol, Mellaril, Prolixin, Stelazine, Thorazine, Triavil

Beta blockers, blood-pressure drugs — Corgard, Inderal, Lopressor, Tinoretic

Calcium channel blockers, heart and blood-pressure drugs — Colan, Isoptin

Eye medication — Mydriacyl

Gastrointestinal anticholinergics, irritable bowel — Donnatal, Librax, Pro-Banthine

Iron supplements

Narcotics — Dilaudid, Codeine, Percodan

absorption of vitamins A, D, E and K, and may also interact with other drugs we are taking. Magnesium-based products, such as milk of magnesia, may eventually push the food through the digestive tract so fast that nutrients are not completely absorbed, and they should *not* be used by those who have kidney disease. And habitual use of enemas leads to loss of normal bowel function. Many laxatives also contain sodium phosphate and so should not be taken by anyone who is on a low-sodium diet for such conditions as congestive heart failure or kidney disease.

Many doctors prescribe laxatives for their elderly patients because so many older people assume they need them and would rather take a quick dose of medicine than alter their diet. Besides, it is easier for a busy doctor to write a prescription than take the time to encourage and help the older person make adjustments in diet and lifestyle.

If you discover that an older person you are helping is taking daily doses of over-the-counter laxatives because of constipation, the laxatives themselves may well be causing the constipation. Encourage the older person to taper off the preparations gradually, while improving eating and exercise habits.

Safe Prevention

Bouts with true constipation make a person feel bloated and uncomfortable. But, besides temporary discomfort, constipation causes structural changes in the intestinal tract. Eventually, hemorrhoids become a companion disorder. Worse, constant straining and pressure against the bowel can weaken it and lead to outpouchings (diverticuli). When these tiny ballooned areas of the bowel become dangerously infected, one is said to be having an attack of diverticulitis.

Everyone needs to prevent constipation and tackle it wisely when it occurs. Poor diet, including too little water, is the main factor to consider if it occurs. We need one to two quarts of liquid every day for efficient digestion, although those who have circulatory and kidney problems may have to modify this recommendation. Then too, everyone — young and old — is better off eating a high-fiber, low-fat, low-sugar diet. Studies show over and over that high-fiber diets (fiber is the indigestible part of fruits and vegetables) result in larger stools, more frequent bowel movements, and therefore no constipation.

Many older people, especially those who live alone, choose soft, processed foods for convenience; these also contain little, if any, fiber. Quite a few older people become intimidated by fresh fruits and vegetables, believing they are difficult to digest. Loss of teeth and badly fitted dentures will also cause an older person to turn to these kinds of food choices. The average diet is also overloaded with animal fats (meats, dairy products, and eggs) and refined sugars (rich desserts and sweets). Anyone who wants comfortable, healthy digestion has to modify this kind of diet.

Ways of Avoiding Constipation
Each of us can find plenty of natural ways of avoiding constipation without resorting to medication. Diet is especially high on the list, as are good bathroom habits and staying active throughout the day.

The Diet Factor. Most experts agree that adults ought to aim for 25 to 35 grams of fiber daily, taking in about 15 grams per 1,000 calories of food.

• Ask your parent, spouse, or friend to keep a diary of everything eaten over a three-day period. Compare the foods in the diary to the list of high-fiber foods on page 126.

• Start including fiber slowly, if it does need to be added to the diet. Gas and a feeling of bloatedness may occur if you rush the adjustment.

• Notice that bran cereals have the highest fiber content, and poultry, meats, eggs, and dairy products have none. Fruits and vegetables vary tremendously in their fiber.

• Plain bran, often called miller's bran, can be bought in most supermarkets and health-food stores. As a supplement to other sources, an ounce a day is an excellent source of fiber. (Remember, however, that bran is not a substitute for proper diet. It is not an essential nutrient and it can be harmful if taken in excess. Some people find that they can never tolerate it without gas and discomfort.)

• Bran can be kept in a bowl or shaker on the table and sprinkled on cottage cheese, yoghurt, desserts, soups, and stews. Include it in baked dishes, cookies, muffins, and cakes.

• If it is difficult for the older person to keep up daily fiber requirements from food sources alone, or if plain bran is not tolerated, talk to the doctor about substituting a psyllium-seed preparation, such as Metamucil, Cillium, or Naturacil. Such products are sold in drugstores and can be taken three times a day in a glass of juice.

• New users of a psyllium fiber product should start by taking one dose a day. If minor gas or bloating occurs, cut down the quantity for several days, then gradually increase the dosage to three doses a day, if needed.

• Buy whole-grain breads and buns rather than highly refined white versions.

Approximate Fiber Content of Selected Foods
(grams of fiber in each 100-gram edible portion)

Grains and cereals		*Fruits*	
White bread	2.7	Prunes	7.7
Whole wheat bread	8.5	Banana	3.4
Pancake, waffle	0.9	Raisins	6.8
All Bran™	26.7	Apple (peel and flesh)	1.5
Corn flakes	11.0	Cherries	1.2
Rice Krispies™	4.5	Dried apricots	24.0
Special K™	5.5	Orange	2.0
Puffed wheat	15.4		
White rice	0.8	*Others*	
Oatmeal	7.0	Peanuts	8.1
		Peanut butter	7.6
Vegetables		French fries	3.2
Peas	12.0	Lentil soup	2.2
Spinach	6.3	Strawberry jam	1.1
Green beans	3.2		
Corn on cob	4.7	*Bulk laxatives*	
Cauliflower	1.8	Metamucil® (g/tsp)	3.5
Broccoli	4.1	Perdiem Plain® (g/tsp)	5.2
Baked potato	2.5	Fiber Med® (g/cookie)	5.0
Baked beans	7.3		
Lettuce	1.5		
Cucumber	0.4		
Onions	2.1		
Carrots	2.9		
Celery	1.8		

Source: *Handbook of Geriatrics*, Steven R. Gambert, ed., Plenum Press, New York, © 1987.

• Read labels when buying cakes and cookies and choose those containing fiber.
• Serve fruits and vegetables in their skins.
• Serve dried fruits; prunes are especially high in fiber.
• Top desserts and cereals with berries, nuts, and seeds rather than sugar and syrupy sauces.
• Include a salad with most meals.
• Keep a fruit bowl on the table. Fruits are laden with roughage and water.

• Keep a pitcher of water in the kitchen or other convenient spot and refill it daily with fresh water to ensure that plenty of fluid is consumed (unless the older person is on doctor-directed fluid restrictions).

• Instead of water, vary fluids with skim milk and clear liquids such as juice and broths.

Good Toileting Habits Help. Problems can result if defecation is frequently delayed. The longer the stool remains in the lower colon the harder and drier it becomes. Dry stool is one of the main causes of constipation. Also, neglecting the "urge to go" can eventually dull the rectal reflex. Anyone can avoid such difficulties by following these suggestions:

• When the rectal reflex is felt it is best to head for the nearest bathroom.

• Take advantage of the gastrocolic reflex that follows a meal or a hot drink within ten or twenty minutes.

• Try to routinely set aside a time in the day to go to the bathroom. This scheduling trains the bowel and gives a pattern to the digestive system.

• Early in the morning or after breakfast is usually the best time to establish as a "time to go." This timing often works because the largest meal of the day before will have had time to digest overnight.

• Do not strain. If nothing moves, leave the bathroom until the urge returns. Straining can cause hemorrhoids and strongly affect blood pressure and even the heartbeat in someone who is predisposed to heart attack or stroke. Straining can also aggravate hernias.

• Don't get obsessed with bowel habits and the notion that it is normal and desirable to have a bowel movement every day. The "normal" varies from individual to individual. For some people, normal can be twice a day, but for others twice a week is usual.

Exercise. Exercise can certainly help prevent constipation. The digestive tract functions best when the blood is actively circulating and the abdominal muscles are in a state of push and pull.

• Even a little exercise, every day, in the form of walking, does wonders for digestion.

• Complete bed rest is generally harmful, unless absolutely necessary. Anyone capable of getting out of bed should be helped to do so several times a day.

• An older person who is sedentary in a wheelchair or armchair will need a special program of exercises, introduced by the doctor, a nurse, or a physiotherapist.

• Rigorous exercise should not be done until two hours after a full meal.

What to Do If Constipation Occurs

An occasional short period of constipation is nothing to be alarmed about. Everyone gets constipated once in a while. Often the cause can be pinned down to a new medication that needs to be changed, a day without drinking enough, a few days of being ill in bed, or a period of nervousness or depression when good health habits are dropped.

One thing that does need to be brought to medical attention is a persistent change from the normal. Relentless episodes of constipation that cannot be helped with proper diet, bathroom habits, and exercise are signs of a disorder in the bowel that needs attention.

If the person you are looking after does become uncomfortably constipated with no relief in sight despite efforts to coerce a bowel movement, call the doctor and ask what laxative to buy and try. The doctor may recommend a laxative taken by mouth or a mild commercial enema preparation. Neglected constipation can eventually lead to stools so highly compacted that fecal or urinary incontinence occurs, or even the life-threatening emergency of a burst colon.

If a commercial preparation given at home does not move the bowels, such a miserable state of constipation has to be resolved under a doctor's care. A stronger enema can be given or the hard-compacted stool removed manually. Severe constipation is usually seen in those who are too ill to get out of bed. For someone not severely ill, and not on constipating medications, constipation like this should send out a loud alarm that the diet is much too low in fiber and fluid content.

Hemorrhoids

Almost everyone has had hemorrhoids sometimes, though usually not so uncomfortably that they merit medical attention. They are swollen veins in the anus or rectum. They can be *internal* beneath the soft folds of tissue in the rectum, or *external* at the outer edge of the anal opening. They can be painless — although sometimes prone to bleeding — or they can itch, burn, and hurt a lot. When they hurt it is usually because blood inside them has become thick and clotted, even infected. Sometimes they can drop down (prolapse) past the anal opening from an internal position, or balloon out from the external position of the anal opening. Prolapsed and ballooned-out internal hemorrhoids can become particularly painful when the anal sphincter muscles tighten and cut off their blood supply.

Hemorrhoids are primarily caused by the food we eat and the use we make of the bathroom. A low-fiber diet and straining to pass stool cause pressure on the anal-rectal veins. Other causes are heredity, pregnancy, heavy attacks of vomiting, sneezing and coughing, and standing or sitting for many hours. People who work at, or are retired from, jobs that involve physical strain are prime candidates for hemorrhoids, for it can put undue pressure on the veins and musculature in the rectal area.

When to Seek Medical Treatment

Hemorrhoid flareups can be dealt with by adding fiber to the diet and drinking plenty of fluids. Hemorrhoids usually settle down after two or three days of such treatment. Doctors often encourage those who have frequent hemorrhoid flareups to take daily dosages of a psyllium preparation. For someone who takes steps to prevent constipation, the areas of weakness and balloonings of skin remain, but typically are not a bother.

The bleeding that hemorrhoids cause is usually not a problem. It occurs at the time of bowel movements and shows up as bright red blood on the toilet paper or in the bowl. But new bleeding from the anus should always be checked with a doctor because bleeding can be a sign of cancer or other diseases of the digestive system.

Hemorrhoid Removal

A visit to the doctor's office is in order if hemorrhoids persist in being painful after dietary changes have been tried or if they are agonizingly painful in a flareup. The doctor can tell during an examination whether it might be a good idea to shrink them or to do away with the hemorrhoidal tissues altogether.

Hemorrhoid surgery has come a long way in recent years. Several techniques make the surgery a quick and easy office procedure done under local anesthesia. For ligation banding the doctor puts a tiny elastic band around the swollen veins. Cut off from blood circulation, the hemorrhoids just drop off in a few days, usually during a bowel movement. Cryosurgery destroys the cells of hemorrhoidal tissue with liquid nitrogen. Laser surgery is gaining in popularity with doctors; with infrared light, hemorrhoidal tissues are shrunk so that they reabsorb into the body.

Today few people need to undergo hemorrhoid surgery that is done under general or spinal anesthesia.

Hemorrhoid Relief

As every television watcher knows, we are offered innumerable over-the-counter preparations for temporary relief of pain and itching. Some are topical and others are in suppository form. Most experts do not recommend the latter because they are potentially more irritating. Many contain a short-acting anesthetic, and others have cortisone and other products to reduce inflammation. A preparation widely recommended by doctors and nurses is Anusol.

Beyond hemorrhoid preparations, we have other good self-help ways to ease discomfort.

A soak in the bathtub. Sitting in a tub of warm to hot water is called a sitz bath. The water helps to take away pain while drawing blood to the rectal area. Sitting isn't absolutely necessary; a long soak lying in the bathtub can also provide relief.

Witch hazel. The ancient preparation witch hazel has an astringent effect and may cause surface blood vessels to shrink and contract. Witch hazel can be bought in bottled form or on packaged soft-paper towelettes.

Ice packs. Cold can kill the pain and reduce swelling.

Cold witch hazel. Placing a cotton ball or cloth dabbed in witch hazel against the rectum can bring soothing relief. Keep a bottle of witch hazel chilled in the refrigerator.

Petroleum jelly. A dab of petroleum jelly placed about 1/2 inch into the rectum can make defecating less painful on hemorrhoids.

Pushing in protruding hemorrhoids. Hemorrhoids may easily slide in beyond the anal sphincter if the effort is made to do so. Moving them thus works best in the bathtub, because the water facilitates the job. Hemorrhoids left hanging are prime candidates for blood clots.

A doughnut. Sitting on a blown-up rubber or plastic ring can be a lot more comfortable than sitting on a hard surface. The cushions are available in pharmacies.

Rest. Lying down can take pressure off the veins that are struck by pain and discomfort.

Dampen toilet paper. It's important to keep the rectal area clean without irritating it. Purchase only nonperfumed, noncolored toilet paper and dampen it before use. Drugstore-bought witch-hazel pads, such as Tucks brand, are a good substitute.

Diverticular Disease

A Disease Caused by Diet

Diverticular disease is very common among the middle-aged and elderly in Western countries. Studies show that one third of Americans over forty-five and two thirds of those over sixty have the disease. Almost unheard of until 1900, today it is known to be a strong indictment of our highly refined diet, lacking in natural fiber. Africans, Asians, and the Indians of South America, who eat plenty of natural fiber or roughage, rarely get attacks of diverticulitis, which come about as a critical stage of the disease when the colon becomes infected and inflamed.

The basic condition, known as diverticulosis, is present if one has tiny pouches (diverticuli) pushed out from the inside lining of the intestine walls. Such ballooned-out pockets of the bowel can occur in the upper bowel, but usually they appear in the lower segment, the sigmoid (for S shaped) colon. Normally this part of the colon is narrow, muscular, and smooth.

It is thought that diet is the main cause of the disease, although aging and muscle shrinkage in the colon may weaken the walls, allowing pouches to form. After years of a low-bulk diet, which takes more pressure and sometimes straining to pass, the sigmoid colon becomes thicker and looks corrugated. Diverticuli form here along the corrugations.

Many people can have diverticuli without having symptoms. Often they are discovered by an x-ray or an intestinal examination done for an unrelated reason. On x-rays they look like clusters of grapes, varying in size from a fraction of an inch to slightly more than an inch in diameter.

Treatment of Severe Attacks

Although most people with diverticuli can sail along without severe repercussions, about 25 percent of those who have them suffer sudden attacks of diverticulitis, which recur in about 45 percent of cases. Diverticulosis becomes diverticulitis (*itis* means "inflammation") when digested material gets stuck in a pocket, therefore highly irritating to the surrounding tissues. Such inflammation can turn into a serious infection, just as dangerous as an attack of acute appendicitis.

Those who have a severe attack feel tenderness and pain, at times severe, in the left lower abdomen. Fever, constipation, perhaps diarrhea, and even rectal bleeding from blood vessels surrounding the inflamed diverticula can also be present. Anyone having such symptoms must consult a doctor immediately. An acute attack can cause complications, including inflammation of the surrounding bowel, rupture and leakage of fecal matter into the pelvic or abdominal cavity, or complete obstruction of the bowel.

The sufferer of a severe attack should be hospitalized for observation and put on intravenous antibiotics and fluids. This treatment is meant to knock out the infection while giving the bowel a temporary rest until a soft diet can be resumed.

Once the acute phase of the infection has been resolved, the doctor will make dietary recommendations gradually introducing fiber back into the diet. The current thinking is that a high-fiber diet, along with plenty of fluids, can prevent the likelihood of recurrent attacks. Most doctors advise a few restrictions: nuts, fruits (strawberries, grapes, raspberries) and vegetables containing seeds, and corn from the cob, although the proof for this recommendation is meager, at best.

Surgery

Usually an attack can be taken care of by prompt medical attention and dietary modifications. But when such measures don't work — and they don't in fewer than 10 percent of cases — surgery is the safest option.

Depending on the severity of the infection, a temporary colostomy, which involves bringing the bowel out to the abdominal wall for drainage, may be necessary. Most surgery for diverticulitis involves removing the infected area of bowel and sewing it back together without a colostomy. A colostomy is necessary only when the bowel is so severely infected that it can't be rejoined. The probability of recurrent attacks of diverticulitis becomes low after surgery.

Such surgery is usually successful in resolving the disease, and within a few months the bowel adapts well to the insult of surgery.

Following recovery, attention to proper diet is, of course, as important as ever.

Painful Diverticular Disease Without Inflammation

The presence of diverticuli in the bowel can cause discomforts that are not necessarily related to infection. Some people complain of gripping pain and tenderness, gas, and constipation, alternating with diarrhea when no inflammation of the bowel is present. Such episodes are called painful diverticular disease.

The person having the symptoms above needs to be seen by a gastroenterologist for a diagnosis of their cause. The doctor can run tests to determine whether or not diverticuli are indeed present. The tiny pouches can be seen through an endoscope or on a barium enema x-ray. If diverticuli are in the bowel, the doctor then has to determine how much they contribute to the symptoms. Painful diverticular disease usually occurs when one also has an "irritable bowel," otherwise known as a "spastic colon." People who have this condition express tension and fatigue through their bowels.

Painful diverticular disease often resolves itself after a few days. Getting rid of known stressors, or finding ways to cope with them effectively, can help. Attention to a high-fiber diet and plenty of fluid is vital. Medications that are designed to relax the spasmodic motions of the bowel are an option for those who find pain and other symptoms not clearing up spontaneously.

Surgery can help those who have relentless episodes of painful diverticular disease. It involves removing the area of bowel most heavily dotted with diverticuli.

Iron-Deficiency Anemia

After Mrs. Johnson's husband died, she became lonely and depressed. In happier times she had enjoyed shopping for the best fresh ingredients and cooking for him and for large groups at their house. She was always healthy, often gregarious, and well able to lead a full life at eighty-one. But in her depressed state she stopped having company and took to eating quick and easy meals out of cans and packages, along with cups of hot tea and an occasional scrambled egg. Six months after her husband's death her children worried not just about her mood, but about her thinner build, constant fatigue, and headaches. Finally, they got her to go to the doctor for a physi-

cal. A simple blood test showed she was anemic — her blood count was far below normal — and her anemia was related to lack of iron in her diet.

Mrs. Johnson was suffering from the condition that public-health nurses who visit the homebound elderly call the tea-and-toast disease, with tea blocking absorption of iron in the stomach and toast being an easy-to-prepare filler. Iron-deficiency anemia is the commonest anemia in the elderly and often causes older people to complain of feeling "old and tired," though their health is limited more by their poor diet than by their age.

Many elderly people, particularly those who are frail and living alone, give up preparing square meals with fresh vegetables and fruits, meat, poultry, and fish; instead they turn to nutritionally paltry convenience foods and snacks. These overly processed products contain little iron, among other essential nutrients. Iron deficiency can also be brought on as a side effect by aspirin and aspirin-containing drugs, which are often prescribed to those who have painful arthritis. Those taking arthritis medications need to be especially careful to eat an iron-rich diet.

Iron is vital in manufacturing red blood cells in the bone marrow, and it also acts as a carrier for oxygen on the red blood cells. When iron-deficiency anemia occurs, less-than-adequate supplies of oxygen circulate to every cell in the body, therefore explaining Mrs. Johnson's symptoms of overwhelming fatigue and headaches. When anemia grows particularly severe, the nails become brittle and streaked with ridges and the lips and skin tone are pale and ashen; also, fingers and toes may begin to feel tingly and numb. Many older people who are anemic also grow disoriented and confused. Anyone who is iron deficient will have a weakened immune system and will be easy prey to diseases of any kind.

Once anemia has occurred, no iron is left in the liver, where it is stored, and it is impossible to build up health-sustaining iron stores with diet alone. Older people who become anemic need to take iron supplements for a number of weeks, until a simple test on a finger-prick drop of blood indicates they can turn to iron-rich foods for the body's iron needs. No food in itself contains enough iron to "treat" iron-deficiency anemia; a person of average size would have to eat at least 10 pounds of steak daily to gain therapeutic amounts of iron.

A doctor will prescribe a schedule of iron-supplement injections for someone who is extremely anemic or unable to take pills; but usually over-the-counter pills are recommended. Often an anemic older person will feel better within a week or two after taking pills and improving the diet.

Iron pills do have mildly unpleasant side effects, such as gas, constipation, and tarry-looking stools, another reason for fending off anemia as well as constipation with plenty of fiber in the diet from fresh fruits and vegetables and bran cereals.

Older people often stop taking their iron pills as soon as they start to feel stronger and back to themselves. But stopping is a poor idea, because the purpose of iron-pill therapy is to bring them up to par and also build up iron storage in the liver. Timed-release capsules seem least disturbing to the intestinal tract. If the older person taking iron pills complains about a great deal of discomfort, do call the doctor and discuss alternative kinds of iron pills.

Milk and antacid medications interfere with iron absorption across the intestines. Anyone on iron pills should therefore drink or eat milk products three hours *after* taking iron pills. Because vitamin C helps the body absorb iron, a good practice is to drink a glass of orange juice, or to eat a fruit or vegetable rich in vitamin C along with the pill.

Pernicious Anemia or Vitamin B-12 Deficiency

Vitamin B-12 needs help from a substance called intrinsic factor so that it can be absorbed in the stomach. Although it is not considered a normal consequence of aging, many elderly people are deficient in vitamin B-12 because tiny glands in the stomach stop secreting intrinsic factor. The problem is especially prevalent among people of northern European extraction.

Older people who lack intrinsic factor develop pernicious anemia, or vitamin B-12 deficiency. If left untreated for years this condition can cause extremely serious symptoms. Vitamin B-12 is vital to a number of physiological processes, including the production of red blood cells, and for the growth of new cells, especially in the nervous system and digestive tract. Early symptoms of the disorder are severe fatigue, nervousness, and a sore tongue.

Pernicious anemia used to be fatal for those who lived long enough to be struck by it, but fortunately nowadays vitamin B-12 is easily given by injection so that it enters the blood stream without having to go through the stomach.

What Are Good Sources of Iron?

Food	Selected serving size	Percentage of U.S. RDA[1]
BREADS, CEREALS, AND OTHER GRAIN PRODUCTS[2]		
Bagel, plain, pumpernickel, or whole wheat	1 medium	+
Farina, regular or quick-cooked	⅔ cup	+ +
Muffin, bran	1 medium	+
Noodles, cooked	1 cup	+
Oatmeal, instant, fortified, prepared	⅔ cup	+ +
Pita bread, plain or whole wheat	1 small	+
Pretzel, soft	1	+
Rice, white, regular or converted, cooked	⅔ cup	+
Cereal, ready to eat, fortified	1 ounce	+ +
FRUITS		
Apricots, dried, cooked, unsweetened	½ cup	+
VEGETABLES		
Beans, lima, cooked	½ cup	+
Spinach, cooked	½ cup	+
MEAT, POULTRY, FISH, AND ALTERNATES		
MEAT AND POULTRY		
Beef		
Brisket, braised, lean only	3 ounces	+
Ground, extra lean, lean, or regular, baked or broiled	1 patty	+
Pot roast, braised, lean only	3 ounces	+
Roast, rib, roasted, lean only	3 ounces	+
Short ribs, braised, lean only	3 ounces	+
Steak, baked, broiled, or braised, lean only	3 ounces	+
Stew meat, simmered, lean only	3 ounces	+
Liver, braised		
Beef	3 ounces	+ +
Calf	3 ounces	+
Pork	3 ounces	+ + +
Chicken or turkey	½ cup diced	+ +

Food	Selected serving size	Percentage of U.S. RDA [1]
MEAT, POULTRY, FISH, AND ALTERNATES		
Liverwurst	1 ounce	+
Tongue, braised	3 ounces	+
Turkey, dark meat, roasted, without skin	3 ounces	+
FISH AND SEAFOOD		
Clams, steamed, boiled, or canned, drained	3 ounces	+ + +
Mackerel, canned, drained	3 ounces	+
Mussels, steamed, boiled, or poached	3 ounces	+
Oysters		
Baked, broiled, or steamed	3 ounces	+ +
Canned, undrained	3 ounces	+ +
Shrimp, broiled, steamed, boiled, or canned, drained	3 ounces	+
Trout, baked or broiled	3 ounces	+
DRY BEANS, PEAS, AND LENTILS		
Beans: black-eyed peas (cowpeas), chickpeas (garbanzo beans), red kidney, or white, cooked	½ cup	+
Lentils, cooked	½ cup	+
Soybeans, cooked	½ cup	+ +
NUTS AND SEEDS		
Pine nuts (pignolias)	2 tablespoons	+
Pumpkin or squash seeds, hulled, roasted	2 tablespoons	+

1. A selected serving size contains:
      + 10–24 percent of the U.S. RDA for adults and children over four years of age.
      + + 24–39 percent of the U.S. RDA for adults and children over four years of age.
   + + + 40 percent or more of the U.S. RDA for adults and children over four years of age.
2. Breads, pasta, and cereals listed are enriched.
This list of iron-rich foods was compiled by the U.S. Department of Agriculture in January 1990. The foods included are considered the best sources of iron in the standard North American diet, although other foods are also significant sources, such as chicken, iron-enriched whole grain breads, prunes, and raisins. Iron is lost in cooking some foods, so to retain iron, cook food in a minimal amount of water and for the shortest possible time.

Some medicines, by interfering with B-12 absorption through the stomach, create their own pernicious B-12 anemia, or make one that is already started worse. The medications to watch out for are those prescribed for Parkinson's disease, gout, and cholesterol reduction. Anyone taking these drugs needs to make sure the doctor is keeping tabs on blood levels of B-12 and the prospect of B-12 replacement therapy.

Any older person complaining of fatigue and nervousness should be checked for pernicious anemia. Diagnosing the disease is tricky, and so a doctor may have to run two or three blood tests, including the Schilling test, to find out if anemia is present.

Treatment is easy: giving injections of B-12 directly into the blood stream. For someone severely deficient in B-12 because of pernicious anemia it takes about a month to build it back up to normal levels, and so one injection of B-12 at the standard dose is given once a week for several weeks. After an initial series of injections the vitamin needs to be given by injection for a lifetime, but only three or four times a year. For the homebound, the doctor can arrange for a visiting nurse to come to the house to give the injections.

Unfortunately, a few charlatans prey on the pocketbooks of the elderly — unscrupulous doctors and nutritionists give B-12 injections to their patients every week for hefty fees. This racket is beyond control by the medical establishment because vitamin B-12 seems not to cause overload and toxicity problems in the body.

Peptic Ulcers

Ulcers created by stomach juices are called peptic ulcers. The gastric ulcer occurs in the stomach and the duodenal ulcer occurs in the duodenum.

The stomach's digestive juices — pepsin and hydrochloric acid — are supposed to digest food in the stomach and upper digestive tract. Most of the time they do so effectively. If we secrete too much of these juices or are hypersensitive to them, though, they eat away at the lining of the stomach and upper part of the intestine (the duodenum) and peptic ulcers form.

Approximately one in ten North Americans will have a peptic ulcer sometime during his or her lifetime. Duodenal ulcers are commoner in people in their twenties and thirties, but stomach (gastric) ulcers are more likely to erupt among people over forty.

The verdict is still not in on what causes peptic ulcers. Emotional conflict and stress are no longer thought to be primary causes, and diet seems a minor influence. Smoking, on the other hand, is a strong contributing cause. Studies show that people who smoke heavily get ulcers twice as often as those who don't smoke. Many medications, especially those used to relieve arthritis pain, can also cause ulcers (see Chapter 6, "Oh, My Aching Bones!").

Although peptic ulcers are *not* more frequent among older people, they are far more likely to become complicated and life-threatening in older age groups. Most people hospitalized for peptic-ulcer complications are over sixty-five. Complications include slow bleeding from the ulcer, sudden hemorrhage (gush of blood), obstruction of the stomach outlet, and perforation of the stomach or bowel.

Ulcer Symptoms

The classic warning sign of an ulcer is gnawing discomfort in the middle or upper abdomen. The pain can be so intense that it can be mistaken for a heart attack. Unlike the pain of a heart attack, though, it can be soothed quickly by food in the stomach or with an antacid preparation. The pain comes between meals or in the middle of the night.

Ulcer symptoms may be less specific and milder in older people. For this reason an ulcer can sit like a time bomb, while symptoms are dismissed as nothing much to worry about. Less-obvious signs of an ulcer include mild discomfort, gas, constipation, loss of appetite, and regurgitation in the mouth of a clear, tasteless fluid from the stomach.

An ulcer can even bleed without pain and other symptoms. Sometimes bleeding is slow enough that it is not seen in the stools. In time, anemia can develop. An ulcer should be suspected if you see signs of anemia, which include fatigue, faintness, pallor, and tingling sensations in the extremities.

Black or tarry stools indicate blood leakage, and merit immediate medical attention. A leak can turn into a hemorrhage if the ulcer crater expands into a major blood vessel. A hemorrhage is a medical emergency necessitating an *immediate* ambulance call.

Diagnosis

If your spouse, parent, or friend is having any of these changes in bowel habits or symptoms of an ulcer, then it's time for a doctor's consultation. Your general practitioner or internist may be qualified and equipped to run appropriate tests. If not, you will be referred to a gastroenterologist, specializing in disorders of the digestive tract.

Most gastroenterologists prefer to diagnose ulcers with a fiber-optic endoscope. Passing the instrument down the throat into the stomach and duodenum, they illuminate and examine the organs in magnification. The procedure usually takes about ten minutes, following a mild sedative to help the patient relax. An advantage of this procedure is that it also enables the doctor to take a biopsy of tissues so that they can be examined for cancer.

Although cancer is the exception rather than the rule, when someone has symptoms of an ulcer, it must be considered. Cancer of the duodenum is possible, despite its uncommonness. Certainly stomach cancer too must be looked for, because it is common among older people, especially those in the eighty to ninety age group.

Evidence is mounting that the bacterium campylobacter pylori is associated with ulcers. It is generally believed that this bug can colonize the stomach and duodenum and irritate its lining, joining with other factors that may cause an ulcer. Although the influence of campylobacter pylori in ulcer formation is controversial, many doctors are testing for it in people who have ulcer symptoms. The infection can be found in a biopsy sample, or even in a simple breath test.

Treatment

Peptic ulcer sufferers today are far better off than those of a generation ago. In the old days before antiulcer medications, having an ulcer meant a long siege in bed on a special diet, and surgery if this treatment didn't work. Today the chance that surgery will be necessary to treat ulcers is less than 1 in 18. Usually surgery is necessary only after complications have arisen.

The bestselling prescription drugs these days are the ulcer drugs called histamine$_2$ blockers. These are extremely effective at healing peptic ulcers and any other conditions related to stomach juices. These drugs reduce the quantity of acids that a billion or so cells churn out to digest food. Cimetidine (trade name Tagamet), famotidine (Pepcid), misoprostol, nizatidine (Axid), ranitidine (Zantac), and sucralfate (Carafate) are all commonly prescribed and approved for ulcer treatment.

Once a peptic ulcer has been diagnosed, drug treatment with an H_2 blocker starts immediately. If pain and other symptoms are felt, dramatic relief can come in a day or two. A small ulcer can heal in about four weeks, and healing a large ulcer takes six to eight weeks.

The doctor will encourage the patient to curtail any activities that appear to have brought on the ulcer, such as damaging medications. During the first two weeks of drug therapy, most doctors advise their patients to drink no alcohol and coffee and to eat a nonspicy, low-fat, low-residue diet. The loud, clear message to patients who smoke is to give up smoking.

If someone is known to have a campylobacter pylori infection, treatment may also include antibiotics and daily doses of a bismuth compound preparation (Pepto-Bismol, De-Nil).

Once healing from drug therapy has taken place, patients are told they can start to eat foods they customarily enjoy. Dairy foods, spicy foods, curries — any foods — as long as they are enjoyed and tolerated.

What about Recurrences of Ulcers?

Unfortunately for the majority of people (about 80 percent), ulcers can come and go after they have experienced a first one. The growing trend is to put ulcer patients on a low dose of an H_2 blocker for life. This treatment is known to be effective at preventing ulcers from recurring.

Most doctors agree that not everyone needs to take H_2 blockers indefinitely after an ulcer has healed. Instead, those with low risk factors for an ulcer and those who have a small ulcer are often carefully watched by their doctor.

If the person you are caring for is told to go on maintenance doses of an H_2 blocker, ask why continuation is necessary. You don't want another drug in the older person's drug regimen unless the benefit it contributes is essential. Not only are H_2 blockers expensive, they cause drowsiness in most people and confusion in some. Those who are put on maintenance doses of an H_2 blocker are told to take the drug before bedtime so that the drowsiness effect will be a benefit rather than a liability. The older person must also be told to watch out for unwanted side effects that are known to occur with the drug prescribed.

Heartburn

The name heartburn is appropriate because it describes a harsh, gnawing pain right in the middle of the chest near the heart. The pain is caused by backed-up stomach juices — the same ones that cause peptic ulcers — from the stomach into the esophagus. The irritation and subsequent pain these juices cause can be so intense that one can mistake heartburn for a heart attack, and vice versa. It is thought that the two conditions stimulate some of the same nerve pathways running through the chest.

As a rule, an attack of heartburn can be relieved as soon as the sufferer takes a liquid antacid, and even a glass of water can wash away stomach juices and provide relief. If heartburn cannot be quickly relieved, a heart attack must be suspected until disproved (see Chapter 10, "Meeting the Challenge of Heart Disease").

The medical label for heartburn is reflux esophagitis. Until quite recently, doctors blamed the problem on hiatus hernias, which are an extremely common anatomical change, hitting 50 to 70 percent of people over seventy. Hiatus hernias are protrusions of the stomach through the hole in the diaphragm where the stomach and esophagus join.

Although about half of those who have hiatus hernias do experience some esophageal reflux, it is now accepted medical opinion that most often hernias are *not* the cause of heartburn. Today it is known that most episodes of heartburn are caused simply by juices backing up out of the stomach, because the muscles at the entrance of the stomach become weak and flaccid.

Hiatal hernias, although common, are rarely dangerous. You can have one for years without noticing any symptoms. Occasionally, a hernia can become constricted (strangulated) so that surgical treatment becomes necessary.

Heartburn is most unpleasant. Anyone suffering it continuously needs to consult with a doctor, who can offer common-sense tips for managing the disorder as part of daily routine. If self-help measures don't work, then medications can be prescribed. Antacids can be helpful if taken cautiously, according to the doctor's directions. Then the histamine$_2$ blockers for peptic ulcers that we have described are a good choice. The decision to accept H$_2$ medications for heartburn should be made only as a last resort.

Treatment is important, not just for comfort, but to protect the esophagus. The constant backflow of gastric juices can damage and scar the delicate tissues of the esophagus. This irritation can lead to ulcers there and scarring and narrowing of the esophagus so that swallowing becomes increasingly difficult.

Ways to Prevent Heartburn
Fortunately, heartburn is one of the conditions that can usually be helped simply by doing things right, as opposed to wrong practices persistently followed. Some people are plagued by chronic heartburn unless they faithfully follow self-help measures as a matter of daily routine. Less seriously affected individuals need only pay attention during their occasional bouts with the problem.

Stop Smoking

- Ingredients in cigarette smoke quickly rush through the blood stream to relax the stomach sphincter, so irritating juices escape.

Meal Management

- Keep to a healthy weight. Obesity contributes to heartburn.
- Keep to a nonconstipating diet. Straining increases intra-abdominal pressure, and therefore reflux.
- Always eat sitting up.
- Stay sitting, or standing, at least an hour after meals.
- Avoid late-evening meals so that peak digestion is not carrying on at bedtime.
- Eat small to medium-sized meals several times a day, if necessary.
- Keep fat and excessive grease out of meals as much as possible.
- If necessary, avoid acidic fruit juices such as grapefruit and tomato. Also avoid coffee, both regular and decaffeinated, and strong tea.
- Avoid chocolate and peppermint, which can relax the stomach sphincter.
- Avoid excessively hot drinks.
- Stay away from carbonated drinks, which can cause belching.

Resting and Sleeping

- Don't rest or sleep propped up on a lot of pillows. This posture can add pressure to the problem area.
- Here is the best bed arrangement: elevate the head of the bed

---

During a Heartburn Attack

- Sit upright and drink a glass of cool water. It may help flush down acidic secretions.
- Don't try milk. Its fat content may relax the stomach sphincter and contribute to reflux. It also may stimulate production of stomach acid.
- Relax. Tension and stress can increase stomach secretion.
- If the urge to belch is present, let it happen naturally. Carbonated drinks or an over-the-counter effervescent will aggravate heartburn.
- Take an antacid as prescribed by the doctor. One such as Mylanta or Riopan may be helpful during attacks, or for prevention. A doctor or nurse practitioner's supervision is essential, for any antacid is a drug, capable of interacting with others or causing gastrointestinal complications.

---

by placing six-inch-high blocks under each of the two leg posts. Gravity will keep fluids flowing downward out of the stomach. A visiting nurse can help make the arrangements.
- Use one pillow only for head comfort.

Dressing

- While dressing, avoid bending at the waist.
- Wear loose clothing. Don't wear girdles, belts, and other garments that put pressure on the abdomen.

Gastrointestinal Cancer

The Annual Screening

We refer you to Chapter 14, on cancer, but we must emphasize early how important it is for older people to undergo regular screening tests for cancers of the digestive system. Two out of three patients hospitalized for colon and rectal cancer are more than fifty years old.

The key to cancer treatment is early detection. Cancer of the colon and rectum — if caught in time — can be treated successfully in many cases. Only lung cancer surpasses colon and rectal cancers as a cause of cancer deaths. Tragically, most of these deaths could be prevented by early detection.

The American Cancer Society currently recommends that once a year everyone over fifty have a test for hidden blood in the stool. The test can be quickly done by the doctor during a routine rectal examination. If stool is not present during the examination, the patient can perform the test at home; you simply smear a stool sample on paper sensitive to hidden blood. The home test is hygienic and very easy to perform, because the paper is attached to a thick envelope that closes tightly after use.

Besides the annual stool test, the American Cancer Society recommends that everyone beyond age fifty have a procto-sigmoidoscopy test every three to five years after two initial negative stool tests one year apart. For this exam, a thin, lighted instrument is inserted into the rectum. The procto-sigmoidoscope allows the doctor to see a good stretch of the lower colon. About 50 percent of colon and rectal cancers can be found with this "procto" or rectal exam.

Like it or not, rectal exams and tests are essential components of medical checkups. Be sure the older person you are caring for undergoes such tests every year. Far better to be safe than sorry.

Symptoms

Signs of cancer in the upper and lower digestive tract often resemble the signs of many other disorders, such as infection, diverticulitis, ulcers, and hemorrhoids. Any illness of the digestive tract should be brought to medical attention if symptoms last longer than a few days. A medical diagnosis can rule cancer out or provide the necessary information for appropriate treatment.

The symptoms listed here are possible warning signs of cancer, and also of more benign conditions:

- Diarrhea or constipation
- Blood in the stool (either bright red or very dark)
- Stools that are narrower than usual
- General stomach discomfort (bloating, fulness, cramps)
- Frequent gas pains
- A feeling that the bowel doesn't empty to completion
- Loss of weight for no discernible reason
- Constant fatigue

8

Managing Lung Disorders and Preventing Pneumonia

THE LUNGS are marvelous organs — they are able to inhale and exhale 25,000 gallons of air each day, even after losing a great deal of capacity with age. If we all lived in a perfectly clean atmosphere, free of smoke, germs, and many other irritants, they could serve us well for a hundred years. Of course we don't live in the best of all possible worlds, and older people's lungs reflect not only their age but also a lifetime of breathing a lot more than life-sustaining oxygen.

Older people are at high risk for developing pneumonia and other serious lung diseases. Their lungs are less efficient and less able to fend off disease, and many people have lungs ravaged by all that they have breathed in. Of all the body's organs (second only to the skin), the lungs are most exposed to the environment. When dirt lands on the skin it can be washed off; dirt that gets into the lungs can't be so easily gotten rid of.

Smoking and exposure to pollutants greatly accelerate the small normal decline in lung function that comes with age. People who have smoked throughout life inevitably have weak, damaged lungs, and are twice as likely to develop lung cancer as someone who has never smoked or who has stopped early enough. Likewise, anyone who has spent years in workplaces where the air was polluted will have lungs that are less than healthy and will be susceptible to respiratory diseases, especially emphysema and bronchitis.

Many millions of elderly people have pollutants' brands indelibly marked on their lungs, put there in years gone by when everyone was less aware of the poison in airborne pollutants. We now know that the danger list is long, beginning with automobile exhaust, asbestos, coal dust, plaster dust, formaldehyde, lead, hair spray, aerosol cleaning products, and, of course, cigarette smoke.

Older people can make the best of their lungs, no matter what the state of their health. Do stay with us, even if the person you are caring for has good, strong lungs, because there's plenty to know about how to keep them that way. If you're looking after someone who has a lung disorder, you should know not just how to seek good treatment, but how to help this person get the most out of every day despite the incapacitating difficulty in breathing.

RED ALERT: Colds and Flu Can Lead to Pneumonia

Medical professionals caring for the elderly take the subject of colds and flu very seriously. No trivial subject, colds and influenza can be deadly. These common illnesses can easily lead to pneumonia, an unpleasant, life-threatening infection of the lungs and the fourth leading killer of older people. Younger people who get pneumonia usually have powerful immune systems and strong lungs so that they can recover more easily. The threat of pneumonia to the elderly is all too evident: more than three quarters of those who die of it are men and women over sixty-five.

Older people usually take longer than those who are younger to get rid of a cold or the flu, and sometimes they don't feel back to normal for several weeks. The older person with a cold or the flu needs adequate rest, loving care, and perhaps medical attention to avoid the complication of severe pneumonia. For healthy children and adults, colds and influenza are typically a moderate to severe illness; they are usually back on their feet within a week.

Pneumonia sets in as either a bacterial or a viral infection of the lungs while the body is weakened by a cold or influenza. Both colds and flu are respiratory diseases, damaging the respiratory tract so that it is hospitable to other germs. A cold stays in the upper respiratory tract — the nose, sinuses, and throat, including the voice box — but influenza infects these areas as well as the lungs, which become swollen and inflamed.

Two prevalent kinds of pneumonia — bacterial and viral — are associated with colds and flu. The commonest form is bacterial pneumonia, caused by the pneumococcus germ. Normally, this germ lives in the throat without causing trouble. But when body defenses are weak the infectious organism multiplies in the throat and travels to the lungs, where it can do heavy damage. Viral pneumonia occurs when a particularly strong strain of influenza virus takes over in the lungs. Occasionally, a virus other than the flu virus is "caught" and enters the lungs. Viral pneumonia is considered more dangerous than bacterial pneumonia because viruses are usually harder to treat than bacteria, which can be knocked out by antibiotics.

Influenza and Pneumonia are Preventable with Vaccines

The news isn't all bad: influenza is mostly preventable. An older person can avoid the disease, which is highly contagious and abroad among us every winter. An excellent vaccine provides protection against prevalent strains of viral influenza. An antiviral medication can also be prescribed for those who have not been immunized. What's more, a vaccine can provide protection against bacterial pneumonia. Confused? Let's look at each vaccine and the antiviral drug. Inform yourself about these modern flu preventives, and keep this nasty disease out of your house this winter and every winter.

Influenza Vaccine
The American Lung Association and the Centers for Disease Control run an all-out campaign to spread the word that everyone over sixty-five should be immunized each year against influenza. Younger people who have heart, lung, or kidney disease, or diabetes, are also included in the high-risk groups who should be immunized. So too are doctors and nurses and people like you — caregivers.

The up-to-date kind of vaccine is designed to protect against each year's strains of viral invaders. Scientists can anticipate which ones to expect before they arrive early in December. The best time to get a shot is between October 15 and November 15, because it takes two weeks for full immunity to build up after vaccination.

Although the flu shot is very effective and extremely safe, far too few people are getting it. All kinds of myths deter people, mostly because of vaccines that made people feel rotten years ago. The old flu shot, prior to 1980, did sometimes cause bad reactions, including a mild dose of the flu and a big swelling where the shot was injected. Today's vaccine is pure and rarely has side effects (*very* occasionally, one may get a mild fever a day or so after taking the shot). Also, contrary to popular opinion, today's shot does not make other medications stop working or a current illness worse. If anything, people who are on medication, or ill, need the vaccine most; they are more susceptible to complications caused by influenza.

Countless studies show that 80 percent of those who have today's kind of vaccine will escape influenza. Furthermore, the 20 percent who do get some symptoms of flu after being immunized will have a modified, mild version. The only people who should not have flu shots are those who have severe allergies to eggs; also, no one should be vaccinated while ill with a fever.

Antiviral Medication: Amantadine

A new antiviral drug is now available for those who are not protected against influenza because they have neglected to get a flu shot or because they are allergic to eggs, which are used in manufacturing the vaccine. This drug, amantadine, can at best throw off the disease or, second best, modify the severity and duration of symptoms once they have started so that the disease is less dangerous. Even up to the third day of illness, amantadine will still modify the disease.

Although the drug is not a substitute for flu shots, it is far better than doing without protection. When influenza is raging through a community or household, many geriatricians and lung doctors recommend that unprotected older people — especially those who have lung disease, heart disease, or diabetes — hurry to get a flu shot and take amantadine to cover the two weeks that the vaccine takes to start protecting them. They recommend even more strongly that unprotected elderly take the drug if they come down with the disease. Those who are allergic to eggs are often advised to take the drug for the entire flu season.

Ask your doctor about this drug.

Antibacterial Pneumococcal Vaccine

According to the National Foundation for Infectious Diseases, about half of pneumonia cases are caused by bacteria, 60 to 90 percent of which belong to the pneumococcal bacteria family. These bacteria are extremely dangerous. If an older person comes down with pneumococcal bacterial pneumonia, he or she may require hospitalization, and it is known that if left untreated the fatality rate can reach 30 percent. Even among those who receive antibiotics, about 5 percent die.

Pneumococcal pneumonia is the only type for which a vaccine has been produced. This vaccine is underutilized, even though every major public-health group recommends it as safe and effective. Even Medicare provides coverage, as an incentive for people over sixty-five to get vaccinated. But the incentive has not worked. About 25,000 nonimmunized people die every year from pneumococcal pneumonia; three quarters of them are elderly.

The vaccine is recommended for *all* adults over sixty-five, not just people who are frail or ill. Until recently the vaccine was given only once to last a lifetime. Now, however, research shows that re-vaccination may be a good idea for some high-risk individuals. The vaccine takes effect about two weeks after injection. The side effects are minor — temporary soreness at the injection site. Check with your family member's doctor to find out about this vaccine.

Tender, Loving Treatments for Colds and Flu Are Best

Please believe us that vaccinations are important, so all the older people in your family can be spared most forms of the flu. Don't forget to talk to your doctor about getting a shot for yourself; as a caregiver you can't afford to come down with the disease. Left for you to catch are colds and flu strains not covered by immunization (20 percent of a season's flu cases are in this category).

Colds and flu are very easy to catch. What can you do to avoid the multitude of cold viruses floating around all winter? Not much, because people who are already infected are walking germ factories before they start to feel symptoms. Cold and flu viruses are usually picked up from surfaces that infected people have sneezed on or touched; the virus also floats in the air for a few seconds after someone has sneezed or talked. Certainly frail elderly people should stay away from sick members of the family, and if space allows they should be cared for in a sickroom away from household traffic.

Anyone around people who already have colds or the flu should practice common-sense strategies for protection, including frequent hand washing, especially before handling food or touching the mouth or eyes (the virus entry points); disposable handkerchiefs to be handled by the cold sufferer only; and separate dishwater for the sick person's dishes and utensils.

The Full-Fledged Cold and Cough

Sneezing, tearing, runny nose, scratchy throat, and cough are the common early signs of a cold. Mild muscle aches may accompany these symptoms later. Usually a cold will go away within a week if the sufferer takes it easy, gets plenty of rest, stays warm, and drinks ample fluids, including hot drinks. Homemade chicken soup and other nutritious warm drinks are good to provide; besides their food value, they are generally comforting and pleasantly steamy for a stuffed-up nose. Sitting in a steam-filled bathroom or near the gentle whoosh of a humidifier will also help to unclog nasal congestion.

Those older people who have malfunctioning lungs because of chronic bronchitis or emphysema may be given an antibiotic to prevent an overlying infection, but taking an antibiotic is pointless because a cold is a viral infection. A bacterial infection may be present if the sinuses start to hurt and produce a discharge of foul-smelling yellow or green pus into the nose, or if the ears feel painful. If these symptoms occur, the doctor should be consulted and antibiotic therapy considered.

Despite all kinds of claims to the contrary from over-the-counter drug manufacturers, no drug or other therapy can nip a cold in the bud or alter its course. All cold remedies do is mask symptoms. When a disease is as mild as a cold usually is, the body — young or old — is best served by taking the least medication possible. Most geriatricians urge older people to stay away from over-the-counter cold remedies. Instead, if necessary, they recommend using aspirin or a nonaspirin pain reliever to ease some of the aching discomfort.

Drugstore shelves proffer a kaleidoscopic feast of medications said to ease the miseries of a cold, but few of them do much good, and generally they are more harmful than therapeutic, especially to the elderly. So-called timed-release shotgun remedies for cold symptoms combine many drugs and are loaded with agents that the user probably does not need. Some remedies in liquid form contain as much as 25 percent alcohol, and a high concentration of sugar. Following is a rundown of common ingredients in cold remedies, with a quick analysis of their drawbacks, especially for older people. All these ingredients may be included in a shotgun product, or they can be packaged separately in different product formulations.

Expectorants. Many liquid cough medications include expectorants, which are intended to loosen up secretions in the lungs so that they can be coughed out more easily. No good studies demonstrate that expectorants loosen secretions beyond what steam and drinking plenty of fluids will do.

Cough Suppressants. Generally, elderly people should avoid cough suppressants because normal aging change already gives them a suppressed cough reflex. Besides, the objective of a cough is to bring up secretions so that they do not pool in the lungs. The doctor should be consulted for a dry, nonproductive, hacking cough that disturbs sleep and rest. The doctor may suggest a product to control the cough so that sleep is easier. Geriatricians recommend single-purpose cough-suppressant formulations containing dextromethorphan. Food and Drug Administration studies demonstrate this to be the only effective cough-suppressant drug on the market.

Decongestants. Most decongestants work by constricting the blood vessels and are found in both nose sprays and drops and oral medications. They should not be taken by persons with heart disease, glaucoma, high blood pressure, hyperthyroidism, and diabetes, all conditions aggravated by constricted blood vessels.

Antihistamines. Taking antihistamines for a cold is essentially an exercise in futility. Antihistamines do relieve sneezing, runny nose, and tearing eyes if you have allergies such as hay fever, but not the symptoms of a viral cold. Besides, they cause drowsiness, dry mouth, dizziness, and constipation, and should not be combined with other sedative or painkilling medications. People with glaucoma should never take antihistamines, for they raise fluid pressure within the eye.

Anticholinergics. Included in some cold medicines to help dry the nasal secretions, anticholinergic agents are only mildly effective at doing this job. They do little good while giving you a dry mouth and sometimes a feeling of general nervousness and drowsiness; they have also been known to cause confusion in the elderly. Anyone suffering from asthma, glaucoma, enlarged prostate, or incontinence should not take anticholinergics.

Treating Flu at Home

Is It the Flu?
Know how to tell a cold from the flu — the distinction is vital. A doctor should be consulted if you suspect that symptoms are indeed caused by influenza. No older person should fight flu alone or under the family's care. The situation is too risky. Pneumonia is one loom-

ing threat for the older flu victim, but other risks loom too, such as dangerous dehydration and pulse irregularities.

Influenza is a much more serious illness than a cold, although at first it can be difficult to tell them apart, for both are strictly respiratory infections sharing some symptoms. The influenza virus can cause plenty of coldlike symptoms — runny nose, sore throat, burning eyes, and a *dry* cough — but it is a very different illness. Although classic influenza always infects the lungs, the whole body suffers. The respiratory symptoms the virus produces are usually slight compared to symptoms such as chills, loss of appetite, weakness, and the misery of an aching head, back, arms, and legs. Older victims are generally ill longer than younger victims.

Flu behaves differently from year to year, from person to person, and from age group to age group, and so no one symptom distinguishes it from a cold. Although very old people frequently do not register the same kinds of symptoms as those who are younger and heartier, usually signs are pretty obvious that an illness is more than a cold. If flu is around in your community, watch your older friends and be alert to any signs of illness. An older person can have the flu and not run a high fever or a runny nose, but may instead express the illness with obvious weakness and malaise, and disoriented behavior (see Chapter 1).

For most of us, flu onset is usually abrupt and severe, unlike the slow buildup of a cold. The flu almost always starts with a fever of at least 100 degrees F (38 degrees C), whereas only children usually have a fever with colds. Flu symptoms are much nastier than those of a cold, such as headache, weakness, chills, and miserable muscle aches, and those usually overshadow its coldlike symptoms. Flu victims usually have a *dry* hacking cough, but colds are less often accompanied by a cough, and if they are, the cough comes from fluid dripping into the throat.

The flu symptoms usually subside after three days; if they do not subside, the doctor must certainly be told. The fever goes down each day, and temperature should be normal by the fourth. It can last longer, though. Once the fever has gone, the aches and pains lighten and fade away. The runny nose and sore throat continue after the fever, sometimes for days, and the cough can go on even longer as the lining of the lung heals. After these symptoms have abated, the flu victim is left feeling profoundly tired, because the body has been thrown off course.

Now for Flu Treatment

How can you help the flu victim elude complications and get better as soon as possible? Above all, do not think you can hurry full recovery. Treatment for flu begins with complete bed rest — except for trips to the bathroom — allowing all available energies to go toward fighting the infection. If the elder's other medications and state of health allow it, the doctor will recommend aspirin or an aspirin substitute to ease discomfort and bring down the fever. The temperature should be checked three times a day — morning, noon, and evening — each at the same time of day.

Keep a written record of the illness so that you will have accurate information to present to the doctor. Call the doctor if the temperature reverts to nearly normal and then soars later; a high or prolonged fever could indicate a secondary pneumonia. Call the doctor too if your patient is not drinking enough, or not urinating every three hours. Dehydration is very dangerous to the elderly; their body chemistry can easily go out of whack with slight changes in fluid intake. Provide lots of fluids — eight ounces of hot or warm fluids every two hours. Coldlike symptoms should be treated as for a full-fledged cold and cough.

How to Recognize Pneumonia

As pneumonia progresses, the tiny air sacs that give the lungs their spongelike texture fill with pus, mucus, and other liquids so that breathing becomes difficult. Pneumonia is considered dangerous because it causes oxygen deprivation; the bacterial kind, if it gets from the lungs into the blood stream, can also cause serious infections of other organs, as well as blood poisoning or shock.

If the older person you are taking care of has influenza, you must watch for signs of pneumonia so that you can call the doctor well before the disease has caused extreme difficulty in breathing and harm to the entire body.

Now for the classic signs of bacterial pneumonia. The cough is much more productive than a flu cough, and the small amount of thin watery mucus that accompanies the dry hacking cough of flu turns to profuse mucus, usually of thick yellow or greenish material, sometimes rust colored by blood. When bacterial pneumonia comes on the tails of the flu, it usually makes itself known by a sudden rebound in temperature that rapidly rises, together with shakes, chills, and chest pain. As the victim's need for air becomes apparent, the patient's lips will become blue and breathing will be rapid.

Viral pneumonia has a less obvious onset. The fever usually stays low, with a persistent hacking cough and moderate to profuse mucus, often blood-tinged.

Remember that a very old person may not show the classic signs of pneumonia described here. The only clues you may have that pneumonia has set in are confused behavior, drowsiness, quicker-than-usual breathing, and breathlessness. Left to carry on, these not-so-obvious symptoms can lead to labored, panicky breathing, which is a medical emergency necessitating an ambulance call. Any of these clues should be brought to the attention of the older person's doctor well before the critical "air hunger" starts.

If you do come upon someone suffering air hunger, while waiting for the ambulance sit the older person up in bed against pillows and calm and reassure him or her with your presence. Air hunger is frightening; no one should be left to experience it alone.

Pneumonia Treatment
The treatment for pneumonia involves a course of strong antibiotics. The drugs are given at home in pill form if the illness is not critical and, if it is, in the hospital through an intravenous line with support fluids. Even those who are found to have viral pneumonia are put on antibiotics to prevent an added bacterial infection.

Convalescence from pneumonia can be a long haul. Even after the infection has left the body the sufferer may be weakened by days, even weeks, in bed. While taking care of someone who has pneumonia, follow the same kinds of nursing measures that we recommend for treatment of flu, and consult Chapter 14, on "Caring for the Convalescent at Home."

Two points to remember: Offer plenty of fluids and nourishing soups and light meals designed to coax back the older person's appetite. The antibiotics as well as the illness and time spent in bed will probably dull the appetite. Also, encourage the older person to cough up secretions several times a day, either in response to the cough reflex or as an exercise in controlled coughing (described at the end of this chapter). To promote coughing, and possibly breathing comfort, the patient should be propped up on pillows while in bed.

If you arc having difficulty in planning what to do, ask the doctor if it makes sense to arrange for a visiting nurse to come to the house and support you with caregiving.

Chronic Obstructive Lung Diseases: Emphysema and Bronchitis

COPD — A Serious Disease

Older people should notice no more difficulty in walking at a normal pace on level ground that they did in their twenties, although if they exert themselves they may notice more huffing and puffing, and may need more rest time than when they were younger. Generally the lungs, with their tremendous margin of extra tissue, will serve them well.

Older people who look weak and tired, breathing with obvious difficulty as they walk around, are most probably suffering the earlier stages of a condition called chronic obstructive pulmonary disease (COPD). That is the blanket name for the closely related and coexisting conditions of emphysema and bronchitis, both of which permanently damage the lungs so that they are incapable of functioning properly, and can no longer take in oxygen and exhale carbon dioxide easily.

In emphysema, the lung tissue breaks down and fills up with dead spaces, where stale air is trapped and little oxygen is exchanged. In bronchitis, the airway tubes of the bronchial tree — the bronchi — are damaged, with scarring inflammation and thickened structure. The person who has chronic bronchitis coughs and wheezes frequently because the bronchi are unnaturally quick to produce excessive secretions of mucus. The bronchi may also be especially sensitive to stressful circumstances — exertion, anxiety, and irritants — so that they go into a state of spasm that can cause panicky, labored breathing.

Although millions of people have COPD, few healthy people know how crippling and how serious it is. Those who are in the advanced stages are rarely seen out of their homes because they are extremely weak, barely able to breathe. As a major cause of death, COPD is right up with heart disease, and deaths from it have increased about 900 percent since 1960.

COPD Prevention

Although COPD is primarily a disease of smokers, years of breathing in badly polluted air can also cause it. The combination of smoking and air pollution is especially destructive. People who have been exposed to frequent lung infections — influenza and pneumonia — and those who have severe chronic asthma can also have COPD as a consequence of these illnesses.

We can prevent COPD by not smoking and by staying out of polluted places. Flu shots and early treatment for respiratory infections and asthma are another good way to ward off the damage these diseases cause in the lungs.

Most sufferers of COPD caused by smoking and polluted air are over sixty-five, because it takes about twenty years for disabling symptoms to appear. Once COPD damage has been done to the lungs they cannot be repaired. We can prevent further damage, though, by curtailing cigarette smoking and exposure to pollutants, once and for all.

Why Early Detection Matters So Much

The outlook for someone with COPD is much brighter than it was just a few years ago. As more older people get the disease, more is learned about how to manage it. Thanks to much-improved drug therapies and better understanding of lung rehabilitation, and things that aggravate the disease, people can live into their eighties with COPD. But they can do so if, and only if, they take steps early enough to arrest it, including immediate cessation of smoking.

Realize that COPD must be treated under a doctor's care as soon as signs of lung damage become apparent. The disease has no cure, but a lot can be done to treat its symptoms so that they do not quickly get worse and totally disabling.

Unfortunately, the signs that bring many people to the doctor mean that much has already been lost in the fight against the disease. In very severe cases the individual may have to stop all normal activity, give up work completely, and concentrate on just staying alive with every labored breath.

Very often if the disease is far along, the heart may have been affected. If one is constantly laboring to breathe, the heart as pump has to toil relentlessly to keep up with the body's need for oxygen. Patients who seek help too late have a condition called cor pulmonale: the heart becomes enlarged and stretched and so is less efficient. The condition leads to chest pains and swollen legs and ankles. All this trouble goes on top of desperately difficult breathing, weakness, headaches, insomnia, irritability, and impaired mental acuity.

If anyone in your family or any friend is still smoking or breathing in obvious pollutants, speak up and tell them for love of life to stop. One way may be to show them pictures of what lungs ravaged by COPD look like, and ask them to read literature about the disease. Write or call the organizations listed under lung diseases in the Appendix for brochures and information you may need.

Symptoms You Can Watch Out For

For symptoms of chronic lung disease to be obvious and easily felt, 50 to 70 percent of the lung surfaces have to be damaged. The signs that finally move most individuals to seek help are: breathlessness combined with colds that hang on too long, perhaps all winter, repeating year after year; and a cough that is steady, persistent, and racking and brings up large quantities of mucus. But even in periods free of colds and coughing, unmistakable and continuous signs reveal chronic breathlessness. Whether exercising or just sitting around, the sufferer pants for air. Instead of the usual fifteen breaths a minute, victims may find themselves panting twenty times a minute, even thirty in extreme cases — and still they are hungry for air, though exhausted by their battle to breathe.

Beyond the obvious symptoms that the lungs are damaged, watch for telltale warnings that they are losing their capacity. After a run of only a few steps to catch up with her husband, a woman may notice she gasps for breath while coughing loudly and says, "Been smoking too much lately, I guess." Or a grandfather, giving up after a few minutes of backyard romping with his grandchildren, may say, "I can't take getting winded any more. I'm too old for this sort of thing." Both of these people probably have COPD, and they need treatment.

But how does one draw the line between normal shortness of breath — we all experience it sometimes — and breathlessness that is not normal? It is not easy. Generally any change in breathing means things are not right; no one should be breathless while performing routine tasks and just walking about. If a woman can barely make it from her car to the house with a bag of groceries, the breathlessness is not normal. But walking up a hill for the first time in months may leave her breathless at the top, just because of unaccustomed activity.

If you notice that an older person in your family is breathless a lot or coughing often, especially in the morning, talk to your doctor. The doctor will need to do a complete physical examination for

COPD. A spirometry test is also needed, to measure lung efficiency in exhaling, along with a blood-gas analysis, judging oxygen–carbon dioxide exchange in the lungs and how much air is left in the lungs after each outward breath.

How Do Doctors and Respiratory Therapists Treat COPD?

For milder cases, medical supervision combined with good health habits and regular checkups will keep symptoms from interfering with most activities. Remember, however, that any treatment can only keep the condition stable, and away from becoming worse, it will *not* restore damaged tissues.

We do not intend to tell you all about the various in-home emphysema and bronchitis treatments that help make breathing easier and coughing less exhausting. Below we simply present the kinds of treatments available so that you can seek them out, preferably with a doctor who is expert in managing emphysema and bronchitis. Most treatments can be taught as self-help measures, for someone to apply at home, and some require medication. After prescribing treatments the doctor will steer you to health professionals — visiting nurses and respiratory and physical therapists — in your community, who teach people management techniques especially designed for everyday application in the home.

The person who has COPD may need treatment that includes:

Bronchodilators. These drugs relax and widen the bronchial tubes to increase airflow. They are inhaled through a small handheld plastic device placed in the mouth.

Antibiotics. Lung infection can be devastating and very dangerous. As soon as an infection — a cold, the flu, pneumonia — is suspected, antibiotics are prescribed.

Steam Treatments. Breathing air saturated with water vapor can help loosen phlegm. Medications are often administered in mist form on a schedule through specially adapted steam nebulizers (available in drugstores).

Oxygen Therapy. Some people need carefully prescribed doses of oxygen to keep going. A portable oxygen carrier may be suitable.

Only the prescribed amount of oxygen should be provided — never adjust the flow without the doctor's consent.

Breathing Exercises. Special breathing techniques can help a sufferer breathe with diaphragm and abdominal muscles instead of weakened chest muscles. Pursed-lip breathing techniques allow gentle expiration of stale air trapped in the depths of the lungs.

Positioning to Drain Secretions. Gravity can be used to make built-up secretions move out of the lungs, just as we can turn a ketchup bottle upside down to move its contents out. Different positions can be worked out for the individual on the back or sides, and a schedule is planned for taking each posture several minutes each day before controlled coughing.

Chest Percussion. Gentle but forceful pounding on the back and chest can help break mucus away from the bronchi so that it can be expelled by coughing and positioning for drainage.

Graduated Exercise. Small strides; small goals leading to larger strides; and larger goals — this is the sequence followed in graduated exercise. Many COPD sufferers may have been sedentary for years, and they need to work on muscle fitness. Muscles in good shape need less oxygen. Exercise is also good for the heart problems that can accompany COPD.

How You Can Help Make Breathing Easier
You can do much to make the air safe to breathe and daily living easier. The biggest problem for emphysema and bronchitis sufferers is their fatigue, for everyday activities that the rest of us take for granted can quickly exhaust them. You can help the person you are caring for find economical ways of doing things, tricky ways to go about tasks more simply so that they are less taxing. Edit out activities that will not be missed. *Simplify, simplify* should be your daily motto.

Patients with COPD have good days and bad days. Try to figure out what makes for a good day so that you can do your best to repeat its circumstances. When bad days happen you can learn how to feel out ways of helping make the best of things. You may need to be sympathetic to the older person's need to just loaf, or encourage

Controlled Coughing Is Important

Elderly people — especially those who are sedentary — need to do "controlled coughing" at least twice a day. Coughing clears the lungs of secretions, so that the chest is more comfortable and less vulnerable to infections. Good times are before breakfast, to clear mucus that has built up during the night, and in the evening, at least an hour before bedtime.

Those who have lung disease may need to do controlled coughing many more times throughout the day, according to the doctor's directions.

The elderly have a less sensitive cough reflex and weakened respiratory muscles and lungs. Often they are not aware that "stuff" has built up in the depths of their lungs until it has reached levels that are tiresome to cough up and out. Understand that mucus breeds mucus: while any is there, more will be produced. Another problem is that many people simply do not know how to cough effectively; they go red in the face, feel giddy, and forget to breathe.

Coughing is a lot easier if lung secretions are liquefied as much as possible — with water. Water is the best expectorant, just as good as over-the-counter remedies, and it is completely safe and beneficial to the body. Be sure those eight glasses of water are downed each day, and humidify the air so that secretions move in the lungs. Again, humidifiers and any source of light steam will help.

Always remind the person you are caring for to cough up secretions during times of illness. The COPD sufferer also needs to be on a schedule of special times set aside to concentrate on clearing the lungs. Here are the words you can use to teach controlled coughing:

1. Take a deep breath in — think of filling the bottom of your lungs; push the stomach area out as you draw air in.
2. Hold that breath for a few seconds.
3. Cough twice — first time to loosen mucus, second time to bring it up.
4. Breathe in by sniffing gently.
5. Wait a few minutes before trying again if necessary. Avoid exhaustion.
6. Sit down for coughing, leaning slightly forward with feet on the floor.
7. If mucus is still present but the cough is not productive enough, try lying down for ten minutes on each side. Cough, then repeat on the other side.
8. Use disposable tissues. Never swallow mucus — it upsets the stomach.

the opposite — an outing to lift flagging spirits. Damaged lungs are temperamental; sometimes they are clearer of mucus than at other times, and better able to take in oxygen.

COPD does not have to be an isolating and depressing disease. Many COPD sufferers give up on going out and getting together with friends, embarrassed about needing to do things slowly, anxious and obsessive about respiratory therapy at home. Yet a social life and suitable hobbies can be worked out with careful planning. The American Lung Association has local chapters in all major and medium-sized cities. Contact a nearby office — its staff should be able to steer you to support groups for COPD sufferers, called respiratory or breathing clubs, as well as social, recreational, and sports programs. When you inquire, ask for a copy of the excellent booklet *Around the Clock with Chronic Obstructive Pulmonary Disease*. It is loaded with suggestions that will help ease living with the disease.

Above all, anyone with the disease will benefit from loving support from family members and friends, kind people willing to be there as good company, to chip in and help with strenuous tasks as well as with any self-help therapy techniques that require a partner. If everyone in the family organizes, the person with breathing difficulties should be able to lead a pleasant enough life, with modifications in the manner and pace of doing things.

Helpful Hints for Organizing Home Life
Offer these tips, some of which you may have thought of already; choose among the others.

Dust Busting

• Dust is a real enemy and can cause relapses. All dust-collecting objects should be removed unless someone is willing to dust and vacuum everything in the entire house every day. Loosely woven and shag rugs, pillows, curtains, clutter, and items under the bed all gather dust.

• Enclose dust collectors in clothing bags, behind closet doors. Pillows, mattress, and box springs can be zipped into allergy-proof covers. Use pillows and comforters made of synthetics rather than down or feathers.

• A COPD sufferer should wear a mask when doing dusty jobs.

The vacuum-cleaner bag should be changed by someone with healthy lungs.

• Sweeping with a broom and dusting with a feather duster are out (they spread dust). Use a lightweight electric broom, a rechargeable electric handheld vacuum, a lambswool duster with an 18 to 24 inch handle, and wet cloths for surfaces.

• Use no aerosol or powder and make no excuses: any product for the home is available in liquid form. But also, avoid using anything harmful that can vaporize, such as mothballs, kerosene, perfume — anything volatile.

Air Quality and Temperature Control

• Stay home on days that are smoggy or otherwise likely to be high in pollution. Find out where to get a daily air-quality report for your area. Smog and air pollution can cause wheezing and airway injury. Also, avoid walking around near heavy traffic.

• Don't stay in the room with anyone who is smoking. Put up no-smoking signs at home and throw out any ashtrays.

• Don't use woodburning fires or kerosene stoves.

• Fans stir up dust; use an air conditioner instead to cool a room.

• Controlling temperature and humidity is important. The house should be kept at around 70 degrees F (21 degrees C); the ideal humidity is between 40 and 60 percent. Be aware that COPD sufferers are extra sensitive to extremes of hot and cold.

• Don't go out for any length of time if the temperature is below 25 degrees F (− 6 degrees C). Cold air can cause bronchospasm. In cold weather wear a scarf or soft cold-weather mask over the mouth.

• Humidify the air with a humidifier or bowls of water placed near radiators.

• If steam and humidity become too oppressive in the bathroom, buy an exhaust fan or leave the door ajar.

Eating Properly

• Six small meals are usually better than three larger ones. A full stomach squeezes the lungs, and prolonged digestion draws blood and oxygen to the stomach and away from other parts of the body.

• To encourage drinking (fluids liquefy lung secretions) keep plenty of nourishing fruit juices in the refrigerator.

- On "bad days," make every effort to eat soups and light, flavorful meals. Bronchodilators can be nauseating, and overall lack of energy and feeling ill can dull the desire to eat.
- Do avoid gas-forming food. Common culprits can be cabbage, melon, grapes, carbonated beverages, onions, radishes, and of course beans and other legumes.
- Do talk to the doctor about antinausea medication if nausea is frequently oppressive.
- Buy a microwave oven, which can be extremely helpful. The older person has to be convinced and taught that the appliance is easy to use, safe, and effective. Already-prepared food that is frozen or straight from the refrigerator or cupboard can go into the oven and onto the table in the same dish. Food cooks quickly, too, and no heat leaves the oven to heat up the kitchen. Even paper plates can be used in the microwave for days when doing dishes is too exhausting.
- Buy a Crockpot. Stews and soups can be easily prepared in it.
- On good days, make double or triple servings of a meal and freeze the extra portions.
- Do reset the table after each meal and leave pots and pans on the stove after they have been washed.
- Find out if nearby grocery stores have delivery service.
- Do investigate meals-on-wheels food programs, if preparing meals is too great an exertion.
- When friends ask what they can do to help, answer, "Bring me a one-course meal."

Medical Self-Help for Respiratory Health

- Dental hygiene can keep germs from spreading to infect the lungs. With a rechargeable electric toothbrush (soft bristles), you can brush teeth three times a day using little effort.
- For medication and steam treatments, set up a table with drawers in a pleasant corner of the house, preferably close to a sink and near a window with a pleasing view, if possible.
- Store small items in a plastic box so that parts can be soaked and sterilized — as directed — in the container.
- Any motor-driven equipment will hum more quietly with a pad under it.
- Do keep telephone numbers of equipment suppliers, doctors, and respiratory therapist next to the phone, just in case you have problems or questions.

• Play relaxing music while doing treatments. Keep a tape deck handy.

• Buy the Medi-Alert bracelet service. In an emergency, medical personnel can call the service number on the bracelet to find your normal blood-gas needs.

• Keep normal blood-gas levels in your wallet and on the refrigerator door. Medical personnel must understand your oxygen needs in an emergency.

Making Light of Clothes and Bedding

• Any clothing that is uncomfortable or that restricts breathing is out. Tight belts and constricting bras should not be worn. Girdles are not a good idea.

• Suspenders are more comfortable than a belt for holding up pants.

• Slacks do away with elastic-waisted pantyhose that are difficult to put on and constricting.

• Sweat clothes are very comfortable, easy to wash, and need no ironing.

• Shoes should be slip-ons. Do use a 12- to 18-inch-long shoehorn, if reaching down is too troublesome.

• A heavy coat can wear you out — down is much lighter and is warmer, too. Many older people need to be converted to down's advantages.

• A lightweight shawl is a must for shivers. As the temperature goes down a bit, you don't need to put on another sweater. Both men and women should wear shawls.

• An electric blanket is ideal for the winter. It is light in weight and does away with heavy blankets; making the bed is easier, too.

Relaxation Is Indispensable

• Never rush — unless the house is on fire. Set things up so that you don't have to rush anything.

• Take a nap or a rest after lunch.

• Sleep propped up by pillows to facilitate breathing.

• Learn how to do relaxation exercises, and do them routinely.

• Practice how to do "panic training," using exercises when you find yourself breathing fast with rising fear. You need a secret word to tell yourself to be calm, and special slow, even breathing techniques (talk to the respiratory therapist about these).

• Join an American Lung Association support group for company and relaxation.

When to Call the Doctor

Call if:
• You suspect influenza.
• Classic signs of pneumonia appear.
• The cough is dry and hacking, as if the lungs were slightly irritated. (Could be a symptom of congestive heart failure, because lung tissue swells slightly. See Chapter 10, "Meeting the Challenge of Heart Disease".)
• You notice signs of oxygen deprivation to the brain: unusual drowsiness, disorientation, or confusion.
• You need more pillows to sleep. (Visiting nurses ask, from visit to visit, how many pillows their COPD patients use.)
• You see air hunger and breathing panic.

9

Getting Treatment
for Adult-Onset Diabetes

"DON'T WORRY, *I just have a touch of sugar," said seventy-eight-year-old Mrs. Smith to her daughter Susan. "The doctor said I don't need to take insulin, I just need to lose a little weight."*

Susan did worry and went to the local library's medical section to find out what "high sugar" means for an older person's health outlook. Surprised, Susan discovered that high blood sugar — at any age — is a form of diabetes.

Susan read on to find that untreated diabetics are generally ten years older than their chronological age. The disease can make one feel fatigued and "not right," but beyond discomfort it can shorten the life span by wreaking havoc on the body's tissues, especially the eyes, the blood vessels, and the nervous system. Recent research confirms too that high sugar levels weaken the immune system.

Not satisfied with her mother's or her doctor's relaxed attitude toward the problem, Susan encouraged her mother to see a diabetologist. He diagnosed Mrs. Smith as having adult-onset diabetes and put her on a treatment plan, including daily blood self-monitoring to know her blood sugar, or glucose, and a specially tailored diet and exercise program. Each week Mrs. Smith returned to the doctor's office to meet with a nurse certified in diabetes counseling, who reviewed what Mrs. Smith had eaten and how it had affected her blood glucose level. Although two months after starting the program, Mrs. Smith no longer had excess glucose in her blood, she was told to continue her special treatment program as a lifetime commitment, under medical supervision.

Besides the relief of knowing her body was functioning more

normally and was no longer prey to body-damaging high blood-glu-cose levels, Mrs. Smith felt better than she had in a long time. Gone were the constant fatigue and nagging infections she had experi-enced in the past few years, which the doctor said were related to the disease.

Diabetes: A Widespread, Underrecognized Disease

Mrs. Smith was fortunate in getting appropriate medical help for diabetes. Large numbers of older people are walking time bombs for diabetes-related complications, because they do not know they have high blood sugar. The American Diabetes Association (ADA) claims that of the 11 million people who have maturity-onset diabetes, only 6.5 million have been properly diagnosed and treated. Also, of those who are diagnosed, only one in four gets suitable treatment.

An appalling state of affairs, especially because diabetes compli-cations — which show up after years of high sugar — can be grisly. Diabetes is the seventh highest cause of death, besides doubling the risk for heart disease and stroke, and the leading cause of blindness in those middle-aged and beyond. Uncontrolled diabetes can also cause a form of gangrene in the extremities, especially the legs. At least half of the limb amputations performed in the industrialized world are done on people who have severe diabetes, most of them over sixty-five.

Why Is Diabetes an Undertreated Disorder?

Most of us, including plenty of doctors, have an outmoded view of what the disease is about. Not so long ago, adult-onset diabetes was poorly understood, and it was broadly thought of as "mild" or "just the other kind of diabetes." Unlike the insulin-dependent kind, which typically appears in childhood — the majority of cases start between the ages of twelve and seventeen — and requires daily insulin injec-tions for survival, maturity-onset diabetes usually creeps up slowly, with vague physical symptoms, or none at all. Symptoms often are ignored because they can easily be obscured by other medical prob-lems of the elderly, or they are blunted because of changes brought on by aging.

A recent American Diabetes Association survey showed that the public has a long way to go in awareness of how serious adult-onset diabetes is. The survey found people were aware of and being tested for high blood pressure and cholesterol far more than for high blood sugar. According to the study, 50 percent of Americans knew their blood-pressure numbers and 34 percent knew their cholesterol count. But only 10 percent know their blood-sugar number, which is the best indicator of diabetes.

Many people are astonished to find that they have the disease. Typically the doctor calls to say "your blood test came back from the lab with a reading of high glucose." As part of a routine physical, doctors draw a small vial of blood to be tested for glucose, as well as cholesterol and many other blood products.

The next step depends on the doctor's knowledge about and interest in diabetes. Proper diabetes management takes effort, time, and patience, and many doctors find the job frustrating, especially with patients who are elderly and need to change a lifetime of eating habits, among other problems that may have contributed to the disease.

Busy doctors often take the easy and quick route of care for their older diabetic patients by alerting them to their high blood glucose and simply handing out a printed diet plan. Often such patients have little idea of how serious their diabetes is, and so at best they become frustrated by the diet, or they ignore it altogether. Usually patients handled in this way come back a few months later with even higher, *not* lower, blood-glucose levels. And they quickly end up relying on medications to control their blood glucose.

The Up-to-date Attitude

The current attitude, based on years of hard research, is that maturity-onset diabetes is just as serious as its more dramatic counterpart, insulin-dependent, juvenile-onset diabetes. The maturity-onset variety is a different disease, but it nevertheless causes the same kind of high blood-sugar levels that can damage the body.

To make a dent in the problem of untreated diabetes, the ADA has set in motion a wave of programs to educate doctors and other health professionals on how to help older diabetics control their problem. The emphasis is on glucose self-monitoring with state-of-the-art home blood-testing meters (urine testing for glucose is now a medical dinosaur), dietary restrictions, and exercise; and medications only if other approaches have not worked. Getting people to recognize and prevent complications of the disease is also a big area of concentration. Risk factors for adult diabetes are also emphasized so that people understand their need for diabetes testing and how to do away with risks within their control.

The Basics: What Is Adult-Onset Diabetes?

If you are offering support to someone managing diabetes, you need a basic understanding of the intricacies of the disease. Read on.

What is insulin? Insulin is made by the pancreas, a small gland behind the stomach. Normally, insulin hormone constantly trickles into the blood stream, with larger amounts secreted during eating. Insulin's job is to move glucose or sugar, and also fats and proteins, from digested food into the body's cells so that they can thrive. In a sense, insulin can unlock the doors of cells so that digested food can enter.

What is the difference between juvenile diabetes and adult-onset diabetes? In juvenile diabetes, also called type I, the pancreas goes awry and produces too little insulin to properly manage the body's glucose supplies. Type I diabetics need daily injections of insulin; without them they can lapse into a life-threatening coma.

In adult-onset diabetes, also called type II, the problem is a contrasting one. Often type II diabetics have normal or high levels of the hormone, but for some reason the body is unable to put it to good use.

Why is someone's own insulin not used effectively in type II diabetes? The causes of type II diabetes are not fully understood, although researchers are finding out more about who is at risk and how the disease involves insulin's not working to move digested food into cells.

Diabetes is on the rise in industrialized societies such as ours, in which plentiful food and sedentary lifestyles are a norm for many. It is clear to researchers that as overweight people become older, the cells in their tissues change so that their own insulin is resisted. Ninety percent of adult-onset diabetics are overweight.

Other investigators are seeking to explain why thin people also can get adult-onset diabetes. One theory looks at how insulin resistance may also have to do with a deficit in the body's immune system, whereby it perceives its own insulin as foreign and attacks and renders it no longer useful.

How does uncontrolled diabetes harm the body? Uncontrolled, the disease gluts the body with glucose and harms it in two ways. First, it "starves" the body's cells, depriving them of needed glucose, and badly affects their ability to function and reproduce. Second, it causes glucose to build up in the blood stream, irritating and damaging the cardiovascular system's sensitive walls, eventually causing hardening of the arteries, and also causing damage to the retina of the eye, deterioration of the nervous system, and skin disorders, among other problems. In this way it can be compared to a drug given in such high doses that harmful side effects occur.

Who Gets the Disease?

These are the four main risk factors for adult-onset diabetes:

- Being overweight
- Having the disease in one's family history
- Being over forty
- Having diabetes in pregnancy

Although the disease does run in families and comes on more easily as people age, being overweight is the strongest influence that sets it off. More than 90 percent of adult diabetics are overweight at their initial diagnosis. In fact, "diabesity" is used of those who have diabetes and are overweight.

For reasons not clearly understood, women are likely to develop diabetes more easily than men. One contributing factor is well understood: women who have temporary diabetes during pregnancy are at high risk of contracting it later in life, particularly if they remain overweight. Women who have had pregnancy diabetes can improve their chances of avoiding diabetes if they keep their weight down.

What You Should Know about Diagnosis in Older People

Symptoms May Not Be Noticed
As we have said, most people over sixty-five may have the classic symptoms of diabetes, but may not recognize them. On the American Diabetes Association list of symptoms, the first three — frequent urination, excessive thirst, and extreme hunger — arc the stand-

out symptoms for diabetes in young people. Ironically, though, these are the symptoms least likely to be paid attention to or "felt" by those who are old and frail.

Changes with aging can cause stand-out symptoms to get lost. The older person may not think it unusual to urinate frequently as the body tries to rid itself of excess sugar by losing water. The resulting thirst may not be noticed, for the elderly often have a dulled sensation of thirst. And hunger — the cells are starved for glucose — may not be sensed because of age-related changes in perception of physiologic messages.

Nevertheless, if you recognize that your mother or father is showing *any* of these symptoms, take action and call the doctor for an appointment so that diabetes can be ruled in — or out — of the picture:

> frequent urination
> excessive thirst
> extreme hunger
> drowsiness
> dramatic weight loss
> irritability and mood swings
> weakness and tiredness
> sore gums
> frequent bladder infections
> frequent vaginal infections
> blurred vision
> tingling in hands or feet
> itching
> frequent skin infections

Blood Testing Is In, Urine Testing Is Out

The doctor who suspects that one's symptoms may point to diabetes should get a test reading for glucose on the spot. In an up-to-date office the doctor will be able to make a quick and accurate reading of the patient's blood from a finger droplet of blood put in a small metered machine. Some meters work almost as fast as electric thermometers, and the patient and doctor can quickly see the patient's glucose level on a tiny screen at the sound of a beep.

Any medical person involved with diabetes would agree that the blood-glucose monitoring meter is the second-best advance in diabetes, next to the injectable insulin developed by Banting and Best in the 1920s. The machines are a lifesaver, not only because they allow doctors to more accurately check on a patient's blood-glucose level in the office or at the bedside but also because they have made it possible for diabetic individuals to easily pinpoint how food, exercise, and other behaviors affect their glucose level. With the machine, doctors and patients and caregivers can check glucose at any time, anywhere, and in any situation in a most efficient way. A definite diagnosis of diabetes is *not,* however, made from meter readings. It is made by analyzing, in a laboratory, two or more samples of a patient's blood.

Urine testing has its place for some medical diagnoses, but as a way of testing glucose levels it is heading toward extinction, although not fast enough. When it was the only easy test around, urine testing for glucose was used despite its imperfections. Now that blood-monitoring machines are readily available, the urine test is totally inappropriate.

Some physicians not up on diabetes management, and even some hospitals, are still hanging on to urine testing, but no health practitioner these days has any acceptable excuse for using urine testing to check glucose levels.

Besides being messy compared to modern blood testing, urine tests are highly inaccurate. Patients undergoing urine tests miss out on being told that their blood glucose is beginning to go high — or too low, which can happen if they are on medications. Urine tests pick up positive readings for high glucose only when blood levels have zoomed to *twice* their normal level; by then, diabetes is harder to control. Because of aging changes in the kidneys, older people can also have an overload of glucose in the blood stream, and no sign will appear in a urine test. (Another reason for inaccuracy is that a urine test reading depends very much on one's state of hydration, activity, and blood pressure on that day, all of which constantly fluctuate.)

Blood-monitoring machines are relatively inexpensive and compact — easily carried in a pocket or purse. When machines came on the market in 1980 they were extremely expensive. Today a savvy shopper can buy one for well under $50, using a manufacturer's rebate or refund policy. In some states Medicare will reimburse the cost.

If a doctor diagnoses diabetes by urine testing alone, or recommends that your mother or father buy a urine-testing kit to use at home, go elsewhere for diabetes treatment.

The Correct Way to Test for the Abnormal Number

Everyone should find out the number that comes up on a blood-glucose test and what diabetologists consider an unacceptably high or abnormal number. If your parent is not interested or is befuddled by talk of numbers, call the doctor and find it out yourself.

The American Diabetes Association now says someone has true diagnosed diabetes if the reading is 200 milligrams per deciliter (mg/dl) within two hours of a meal, and 140 mg/dl after not eating for ten hours but no more than fourteen hours (beyond fourteen hours the reading would be based on starvation conditions). Anyone showing a reading higher than these numbers should be put on treatment to bring the sugar level down. Generally, 140 to 180 mg/dl, with 200 mg/dl as borderline acceptable, within two hours of a meal is thought of as a good range to head toward — as an ideal goal.

Do make sure testing has been done correctly, for often it isn't. Many people fall through the cracks of glucose testing because they have a basic glucose screening test when their last meal (which converts to glucose in the body) was hours back and is already digested. The very best time to test for the basic screening is within an hour after a full meal, although two hours is acceptable.

Be wary of results from a general blood test, the kind done for the annual physical that measures all sorts of blood products. Some doctors and testing-center employees ask people *not* to eat breakfast before a general blood test. Some blood products — though not glucose — produce a better reading if the patient hasn't eaten for hours.

Although a fasting glucose test is an excellent test for doctors to use in testing for diabetes, the fasting approach is wrong for a basic glucose screening. A basic screening test can easily show glucose to be far below the reading considered indicative of diabetes if it is done on someone who has not eaten for several hours. Mrs. Jones may go home and eat a big dinner after a visit to the doctor, happily thinking her sugar has tested just fine. Yet as she eats her meal and later snacks, her sugar shoots up to harmful diabetic levels. Ideally, a basic screening for blood-glucose level should be done within two hours of a meal.

What Is Normal Glucose for Older People?

The goal of keeping blood-glucose readings under 200 mg/dl is an ideal — and it is certainly reached by plenty of people — but as time goes on that goal may have to be changed. Diabetes is a long-term disorder that stays with someone for life. It is likely to get progressively worse, but usually does so very slowly if the person is put on a good treatment program. The course of the disease and the response to treatment are highly individual.

As people get older their readings will usually be naturally higher, whether they are diabetic or not. In subtle ways the aging body does put out less and less insulin, and for many complicated reasons sugar metabolism becomes less efficient. As a rule of thumb, diabetologists take into account that blood glucose normally reads about 10 mg/dl higher with every decade after we reach age sixty-five.

Today the drift in diabetes is for doctors to take into account, not discount, this factor. In other words, 10 mg/dl or 20 mg/dl, or 30 mg/dl above the number of 200 mg/dl is still too high for comfort and safety at any age and should be brought down. The aim is not just to prevent the serious complications of constant high sugar in the blood, which take about fifteen years to fully develop, but to prevent the subtler symptoms.

Elevations from the normal can make older people feel irritable and tired and in need of more trips to the bathroom. Even slight modifications in diet and activity can make a difference in how they feel.

What Is Proper Treatment?

Now we are ready to move on to treatment. Our job here is *not* to give you a how-to lesson so that you and the older person you are caring for can go it alone. You need professional help and guidance, specially worked out to suit the person you are caring for, and the best you can get. We will tell you how you can find treatment and what it should be.

Start with a Good Specialist

Diabetes treatment amounts to very little unless the diabetic individual is in the hands of a doctor who is well up on things. The doctor your relative or friend uses must be willing to take the time to teach patients how to lower blood-sugar levels, or delegate the job to a specially trained nurse or nutritionist.

The trend these days is for a diabetic — at any level of the disease — to be under the care of a specialist who will provide and supervise an individualized program of diabetes control, built around blood self-monitoring. Here is some advice about finding such a specialist.

The doctor who diagnosed diabetes in the first place may be just the one your mother or father needs. If so, the task should be easy from the beginning. Or the doctor may recommend a colleague who is excellent at managing diabetes. The two might collaborate on your parent's case, and together find solutions to problems as they arise. Your doctor may also choose to send your parent to a diabetes clinic at a local hospital. Most major teaching hospitals and many community hospitals have such clinics, and with the population aging more of these are opening across the country.

If you have trouble finding a diabetes specialist, call the local chapter of the American Diabetes Association. The organization has 800 chapters in major cities in 46 states. Each chapter has a list of carefully screened local diabetes specialists and clinics. Most ADA chapters also have a telephone information service for the public to call with questions about diabetes.

Another option is for you to call the Association of Diabetes Educators for the names of diabetes counselors in your area. Call 1-800-338-DMED. These are health professionals, nurses, and dieticians, all well trained and certified to offer diabetes counseling. Some are in private practice, but most work in joint practice with a doctor so that an attempt to get public and private insurance reimbursement for their patients can be done, as part of general prescribed diabetes care.

Five Mainstays of Treatment

The five-pronged approach to treatment taught by those who do diabetic counseling includes: (1) blood-glucose self-monitoring, (2) weight loss, for the overweight, (3) healthy food in appropriate amounts, (4) exercise, and (5) medications. Go with your parent to teaching sessions so that you will understand how to help at home. Expect to go to one start-up teaching session and to follow-up sessions every two to three weeks for several months. Most insurance companies will cover such visits if they are prescribed by the doctor.

1. *Blood Self-Monitoring.* The first lesson the newly diagnosed diabetic needs to learn from the doctor or counselor is how to use a self-monitoring blood-sugar meter as a surveillance tool. Accuracy depends on using the monitoring device correctly. Because scores of meter machines are on the market, rely on the counselor's recommendation of a model. An experienced counselor will help you order a meter directly from a catalog or a company at low cost, and advise you if Medicare will cover the cost in your state.

Learning how to use the device should not be difficult, and if done correctly pricking the finger to draw a drop of blood is gentle. The drop is carefully expressed on a special test strip inserted into the machine with each use. The chemical reaction that takes place on the paper is read by the meter and shown as one number value on a screen.

The person with vision problems can decide whether it is easier to read numbers on the screen, or to remove the paper strip and match its color against a color chart, which is divided into several color ranges, varied according to how much glucose is in the blood. The higher the blood glucose, the darker the strip. Someone who finds reading both strips or numbers confusing can store strips selected for their chemical stability in a container and take them to sessions with the diabetic counselor.

In the first few weeks of treatment your counselor will ask your parent, and you if need be, to keep a daily diary of blood-glucose values, food consumed, activity, and any medications taken over several days. She will ask that meals be "bracketed," which means taking a blood reading before and after all meals, and perhaps she will ask for blood values taken in the morning and late evening before bedtime.

The diary allows counselor and patient to sit down at appointments and review how food and activity affect the patient's blood glucose so that a diet and exercise plan can be worked out. If glucose levels spike up any day, the events of that day are analyzed against those of other days. For example, what caused Mrs. Jones to have an unusual spike in glucose on day six? Was it the cake eaten after lunch, or the canceled daily walk that afternoon? Answer: the canceled daily walk, rather than the cake, because she ate a similar lunch on day three, also followed by the same kind and quantity of cake.

2. *Weight Loss and Dieting.* The weight-loss approach should be tried on those of any age who are heavier than normal, and of course

under the doctor's supervision. Amazingly, as an overweight person's weight drops, blood glucose shows a remarkable tendency to move toward the normal. Rarely, someone will not respond to weight loss and proper diet as a treatment. Simple weight loss can improve and invigorate insulin production and the body's sensitivity to the hormone.

As motivation to lose weight, your parent needs to understand that weight loss does indeed work. Often, blood sugar will go down after as little as five to ten pounds have been shed. Losing weight is not an easy task for anyone, though, especially the older person who may like to eat more than he should to compensate for loneliness, boredom, and depression. Typically, older people resist the idea of going on a special diet and losing weight. "At my age, why bother?" is a common response to the mere idea of dieting.

If a calorie-counting weight-loss program is kept simple and as close as possible to one's usual diet, it can be easy to follow. Most counselors look at a diabetic individual's typical eating habits, with an eye to keeping as much of them as possible within the plan. The idea is to cut down on sugar, shrink portions, and emphasize nutrient-dense food over food containing empty calories. Sometimes just giving someone a list of foods to avoid, such as sweets and table sugar, will make compliance with a diet easier.

3. Healthy Foods in the Diet. The thinking behind what diabetics can and cannot eat has changed in recent years. Carbohydrate restriction and rigid meal patterns are no longer the rule. Your parent may well remember the days when diabetics had to put a skull and crossbones on spaghetti, potatoes, and bread, but protein foods and fruits and vegetables were considered safe.

New ways of looking at diabetes and how body cells process and use food nutrients have allowed researchers to see that the old diet caused harm. It was actually starving body cells of energy-providing nutrients, while overloading the body with harmful side products of excess protein.

Nutritional guidelines have recently been revised by the ADA. The new kind of diet may look complicated at first, but it actually isn't. Nothing is mysterious about it — it is simply a generally healthy diet, almost identical to the one recommended by the American Heart Association. These guidelines now call for the following.

Lower protein and fat intake. About 15 percent of the diet should be made up of protein. Fat intake should be limited to 30 percent or less of calories. Although some fat is essential in the diet, saturated fat should be limited (it is found in animal meats and high-fat dairy products and coconut and palm oils). High-cholesterol sources of protein should also be limited (found along with saturated fats as well as in egg yolks and organ meats, even though these are actually low in fat). Half the battle can be won if fried foods are nixed, and dishes broiled, boiled, baked, or grilled without added fat.

Higher carbohydrate intake. Up to 60 percent of daily calories can come from carbohydrates. Higher carbohydrates improve the body's ability to maintain normal glucose levels. Of the two types of carbohydrates (starches and sugars), starches should be increased, but sugars such as table sugar, honey, corn syrup, and maple syrup should be limited, for they quickly raise blood sugar. Starches include whole-grain breads and cereals, pasta, rice, dried beans, and peas. Blood monitoring and weekly record keeping allow the diabetic to find out how particular starches affect glucose levels.

Stress some fiber-containing foods. Fiber is the indigestible part of plants, found in dried peas and beans, vegetables, and whole-grain cereals and breads. Fiber in the diet slows digestion and allows glucose from all food sources to enter the blood stream gradually.

Limit fruits. Notice that fruits are not included as a source of carbohydrate or fiber. Most fruits are high in sugar content and should be eaten in moderation. Also, concentrated fruit juices are high in sugar. Vegetables are a better source of vitamins and minerals, and contain little sugar. Broccoli, cauliflower, and carrots are great choices.

Limit alcohol. It's best to leave alcohol out of the diet. But if someone really wants to have an occasional drink, it can be worked into an overall meal plan.

Limit salt. Salt is known to raise blood pressure, or aggravate high blood pressure, which can make diabetes control more difficult.

Although the counselor will work with your parent on a custom-designed approach to eating, she may provide an exchange list of foods for meal planning that have been put into food-group categories (starch and bread, meat and protein substitutes, vegetables, fruit, milk, and fat). The exchange-group approach allows you to trade food within each list category for other foods on the same list and so keep calorie, carbohydrate, fat, and protein intake fairly constant. The ADA publishes the booklet, "Exchange Lists for Meal Planning," available from any of their chapters.

The exchange list is very helpful because it simplifies the entire picture of what to eat. But no one should turn to a list without proper counseling. Self-monitoring shows that each diabetic individual has a unique response to food and how it converts to sugar, and all diabetics need to be taught how to work around this limitation.

4. *Exercise.* Exercise is just as important as proper diet in the program. In the short term, it lowers blood glucose, because muscles put to use draw glucose instantly from the blood stream. In the long term, a regular program makes the body more sensitive to insulin so that wide swings in blood glucose are prevented.

Although many elderly people are limited in their ability to exercise, some form of it should be undertaken every day. Walking and swimming are excellent for the able-bodied who can easily get out of the house. If an older person really can't do much because of disability, he or she should at least do something and work at not being constantly sedentary. The counselor will be able to recommend a program for anyone who is wheelchair or bedbound, or able to do only simple exercises indoors. Even exercise that is not at all rigorous will influence glucose levels.

To keep glucose levels even every day, it is a good idea to do some form of exercise on a schedule. In the beginning of a glucose-control program, scheduling is needed so that the daily diary can be easily understood.

5. *Medications.* For some people with type II diabetes, diet and exercise just aren't enough to control the glucose. Medication — hypoglycemic pills — is needed to boost insulin production and help glucose enter body cells. The pills are not a form of insulin, and anyone taking pills needs to understand that they work best within a program of diet and exercise.

Most older people with type II diabetes can keep taking their pills without having to rely on insulin injections. If the diabetic lives long enough, however, the disease may eventually deplete the body's natural insulin, so that a pharmacological version will need to be injected. If injectable insulin is needed, as a lifetime replacement for the body's own, the older person's doctor will enlist a visiting nurse or a diabetic counselor to teach him or her and any caregivers how to manage daily injections.

Those who work hard at diet and exercise should not think of having to go on pills as a failure of character, or proof that they didn't try hard enough. They must be reassured that their need for medication is a natural consequence of the disease as it affects them. As we have said, the disease can get progressively worse, although usually very slowly if someone is put on a good treatment program with counseling.

The need for medication is highly individual. Fortunately, most adult diabetics can go without it, and some people are advised to use it after a three-month trial of exercise and diet. Others can go for years before diet and exercise no longer keep their blood sugar in line.

Another highly individual variable is how well diabetes control pills work for those who need them. For some individuals, especially those already thin, the pills do not work at all. Or they may work initially, but then give out. In fact, only one in seven individuals will continue to respond to pills after taking them for ten years. If they do not work, injectable insulin is needed.

Pills Involve Precautions
Pills are a good choice for those who must have them, but they do have the potential to cause problems, especially for very old people. For this reason, hypoglycemic pills are held off until diet and exercise are absolutely not working. Also, once pills are taken regularly, the doctor should keep a check on the patient to see if they have jump-started insulin production so that it can carry on without continued use of the pills; they sometimes do so. Too many people take pills indefinitely, when they need them only for a short time.

Because old people are often on other medications and may have sluggish kidneys, the hypoglycemic medication should be started with a low dose and gradually increased. Self-monitoring of blood glucose helps the patient and doctor make necessary adjustments so that the medication does not back up in the blood stream to such high levels that too much sugar is broken down.

The most serious potential problem with the medication is that it can cause a dangerous state of hypoglycemia or low blood sugar. This state can happen if the diabetic individual eats less food than usual, skips a meal, exercises too much, becomes ill, or takes a new medication. To prevent sugar from going too low, scheduling of meals and exercise must *be consistent every day*. Also, no drugs should be taken that haven't already been approved by the doctor caring for the older person's diabetes, because some medications can contribute to hypoglycemia.

Oral hypoglycemics are very sensitive to many drugs commonly prescribed for older people. Some drugs increase the glucose-lowering action, especially large quantities of aspirin taken to relieve arthritis pain, other arthritis drugs, and several drugs commonly prescribed for lowering high blood pressure. Some drugs have the opposite effect, pushing blood sugar too high, including some diuretic agents, the cortisone drugs, estrogen, niacin, adrenalin, decongestants that contain ephedrine or epinephrine, nasal sprays that contain phenylephrine, and many cough remedies. Caffeine, which is an ingredient in many over-the-counter preparations, may also raise blood sugar.

Alcohol does not mix well with oral hypoglycemics, especially diabinese. Those who are taking pills are advised to cut out drinking alcohol, for even a moderate amount, such as a glass of wine with dinner, can bring on lightheadedness, dizziness, and red flushed skin. Some doctors, however, will allow occasional drinking, depending on the patient's condition and medication regimen.

Insults to the body such as fever, infection, periods of stress, or trauma, as from a fall or car accident, can also cause blood sugar to shoot up dangerously so that hypoglycemic pills are no longer effective as prescribed. Thus contributing double trouble, the ill person may not be able to prepare or eat proper meals on the usual strict schedule.

The doctor should always be called when a person who is on diabetes medication becomes ill with the flu or anything else. The doctor may decide to arrange for a nurse to visit the home, to provide the sick person with insulin injections, or to teach the family how to give them. Usually after an illness has resolved, insulin is discontinued and pills are started again.

The Hypoglycemic Emergency

Although low-blood-sugar emergencies are much more frequent for people who use insulin, they can happen to people who use oral hypoglycemics. If your parent is on oral medication, know that signs of hypoglycemia mean the body is not getting enough sugar to maintain itself. Symptoms of hypoglycemia can come on so rapidly that within minutes or almost immediately they can progress to unconsciousness or an altered mental state.

Your doctor or counselor may advise you to fill a prescription for a glucagon emergency kit and teach you how to use it to treat the emergency before the ambulance arrives. The glucagon in the kit is for use when a diabetic individual becomes unconscious or is too groggy to swallow milk, juice, or soda. A neighbor should learn how to use the kit if the diabetic individual is living alone, or is alone during the day. The kit includes injectable glucagon. Glucagon is a hormone — a chemical messenger — that moves sugar out of storage in the liver to the blood.

You need to talk with the doctor or counselor about how to recognize and prevent the early signs of dangerously low blood sugar, so that you can take action to prevent unconsciousness. Unfortunately, old people sometimes don't have the usual warning signs, and it can be quite difficult to tell if an attack is going on. The older person may simply appear and act confused, or weak and drowsy.

Those who have had awareness of their attacks often report that initially their mouths become tingly and dry, as in an anxiety attack, and that they have a profound and frightening nervous sensation of "losing control." Typical obvious symptoms include feeling cold, clammy, shaky, weak, or very hungry. Some people become pale, get headaches, or act irrationally.

When you have any doubt about whether or not the older person is having a hypoglycemic attack, a finger-stick blood test can quickly provide a clear answer. If you are sure an attack is going on, react quickly:

1. Begin treatment IMMEDIATELY. Delay allows the reaction to become more severe and harder to treat, and unconsciousness will result.
2. Offer a glass (8 ounces) of milk. If unavailable, offer orange juice, or any other fruit juice, or *non*dietetic soda pop. Or offer several hard candies, sugar lumps, spoonfuls of honey or jam (special glucose tablets can also be used for this purpose).
3. After twenty minutes, check blood glucose to see if it is within safe limits.
4. If blood sugar is still too low, repeat the snack, or move on to the next scheduled meal if it is ordinarily within the next hour.
5. If symptoms persist after the first snack, CALL YOUR DOCTOR OR COUNSELOR promptly. You will need extra help.
6. CALL THE DOCTOR, if attacks occur frequently over several

days, or more than once in twenty-four hours. It may be time to change the dosage of oral hypoglycemics.

7. If the diabetic individual is unconscious, or too groggy to swallow, use the glucagon kit as you have been taught by a doctor or diabetes counselor.

8. After administering the glucagon, call the doctor. If no immediate response is available, call for an ambulance. Hypoglycemia can kill, and a dangerous possibility is that it will rebound from thirty minutes to two hours after the initial attack. A doctor also needs to determine what caused the initial attack.

Medical Complications

Severe medical problems, or complications, are caused by high sugar levels and take many years — about fifteen beyond the start of the disease — to develop. Years of high sugar work in the same way as years of cigarette smoking: the damage is progressive and cumulative. The doctor, the older person with diabetes, and the family, all must be on the lookout for early signs of such complications, which stem from damage to blood vessels and nerves. Prompt treatment is necessary to keep them from getting worse.

Control of sugar levels is the best way to prevent or postpone complications. But even if a type II diabetic older person is on an effective control program, checkups for complications are essential. Many older type II diabetics are at high risk for these complications, because often their disease was "hidden" for a long time before being diagnosed. If someone already has a diabetes complication, keeping very good control may prevent it from getting worse or slow it down.

Here are especially worrisome problems:

Vision loss. Although about 5,000 new cases of blindness related to diabetes are reported each year, untold numbers of diabetics suffer severe, irreversible visual impairment. The typical cause is diabetic retinopathy, a condition of quick-to-bleed blood vessels growing over the inner surface of the retina, at the back of the eye. Retinopathy originally forms without symptoms, and so the only way to catch it early is with regular checkups — done by an eye specialist — at least once a year.

Heart disease, hypertension, and stroke. These problems are twice as common for diabetics, and even more frequent for diabetics who smoke. Turn to Chapter 10 to read how these disorders can be prevented, recognized, and safely treated.

Nerve damage. Known as diabetic neuropathy, the signs of nerve damage are repeated burning, pain or numbness, and tingling in the legs or feet. If nerve damage causes loss of feeling, minor foot injuries may go unfelt and can become badly infected. Sometimes nerve damage can interfere with the functioning of the digestive system and cause diarrhea that may come and go, bloating, and frequent nausea.

Poor circulation in the feet and legs. Legs and feet can feel cold, crampy, with shiny dry skin because of poor circulation. Even slight injury on the feet or legs can be dangerously slow to heal, for immune cells have a hard time getting to the area to fight infection. When combined with loss of feeling from nerve damage, undiscovered injuries can fester unnoticed and become so severely infected that amputation is necessary to save the rest of the foot or leg. On a bright note, amputations have been far fewer in recent years, as a consequence of better antibiotics, improved treatment for poor circulation, and awareness among diabetics and their families that feet have to be well taken care of.

Good Foot Care Is Essential

The feet should be checked twice daily, when shoes are put on in the morning and when they are taken off at night. If anything looks suspicious — a cut, a bruise, a hangnail — the doctor should be alerted. The description of the injury will determine whether or not an appointment should be set up for an examination before a difficult-to-treat infection sets in.

If the person you are caring for finds looking at the soles of the feet difficult to manage, someone else should do the checking. Second best is for the older person who can see well to use a mirror to examine the undersides of the feet.

Those who have a tendency to diabetes-related foot problems should know about some very definite do's and don'ts for foot care. We know these precautions sound strict to the point of obsession, but obsessive or not, they are essential for the diabetic individual to follow.

Don'ts!
- Don't use hot-water bottles or heating pads.
- Avoid extremes of temperature; test bath water before bathing.
- Don't walk barefooted.
- Don't wear tight shoes.
- Don't cut toenails, corns, or calluses (leave the job to the doctor or a podiatrist recommended by the doctor).
- Don't use chemical agents for removing corns and calluses.
- Don't wear socks or stockings with seams, or tight elastic.
- Don't break blisters — unbroken skin is the best defense against infection.

Do's
- Do bathe feet daily in warm water. Dry them thoroughly with a patting, not a rubbing, motion.
- Do use mild soap (avoid deodorant soaps and soaps containing fragrance).
- Do massage feet once or twice a day with a lanolin-base cream or lotion to prevent scaling or cracking. (See Chapter 5 for advice on preventing dry skin.)
- Do not leave cream between the toes; it may promote an infection.
- Do put talcum powder between the toes to create comfort and to maintain dryness.
- Do insert lambswool padding between toes, to separate them, but only if necessary.
- Do wear cotton socks at night if feet are cold.
- Do visit a podiatrist, *at least every two months.*

10

Meeting the Challenge of Heart and Blood-Vessel Disorders

FIRST THE PRAISEWORTHY NEWS. In the past two decades or so, people in the industrialized countries have learned to control blood pressure; they've also made changes in their eating, smoking, and exercise habits. Good habits have shown rewards: death rates from heart attack and stroke have *declined dramatically*. Lifesaving advances in medical treatment have also contributed to a much happier picture for heart and blood-vessel disease. One of the main reasons people are living longer than ever before has to do with these positive trends.

The news isn't all so good. Heart and blood-vessel disease, known as cardiovascular disease, is still the number-one killer of people over sixty-five, as it is for middle-aged people. It causes almost as many deaths as cancer, accidents, influenza-pneumonia, and all other causes of death combined. Many deaths could be prevented if people would lower blood pressure, stop smoking, reduce the cholesterol in their diet, and recognize the warning signs of heart disease, particularly heart attacks.

To be complacent about cardiovascular disease is folly indeed. We all need to educate ourselves about how to prevent it. Four fifths of the cardiovascular deaths are in people over sixty-five. It can be found in 50 percent of those aged sixty-five to seventy-four, and 60 percent of those seventy-five and over, with percentages growing.

In this chapter we take a two-pronged approach to the subject. In one direction we inform you about how older people can avoid disorders, because strong, clear evidence indicates it's never too late to start. In the other direction we identify the most common disorders, and show how they can be successfully diagnosed and then treated through the medical system, and with established recommendations to apply in daily life at home.

Here are the disorders we cover:

- High blood pressure
- Coronary heart disease
- Peripheral vascular disease
- Congestive heart failure
- Slow heartbeats
- Stroke

How Do the Heart and Blood Vessels Normally Age?

Now for more good news.

As recently as ten years ago, the prevailing attitude toward older people was that they were more susceptible to heart attack, stroke, congestive heart failure, and high blood pressure simply because the cardiovascular system wears out and clogs with plaque as a consequence of normal aging. This attitude has been turned around, now that current research indicates that disease and disuse, rather than age itself, account for most of the changes seen in the cardiovascular system of elderly people. It seems that those risk factors — which can be modified — cause far more heart disease than aging does.

A number of changes are more or less inevitable with aging, but they are subtle alterations in a system that is designed to last a long lifetime. The research keeps showing that there is no such entity as "an old heart that gives out." We have only to look at those healthy people up into their nineties who have healthy hearts — slightly different from younger hearts but completely free of disease. Likewise, medical studies of elderly people in cultures with relatively fat-free and cholesterol-free diets show that significant numbers of people have clear, well-functioning heart and blood vessels, wherein changes were the common ones of aging, such as some thickening and loss of elasticity in blood vessels and a thickened heart muscle.

The best evidence to date on the aging heart and blood vessels — with the largest number of subjects, the widest range of ages, and the most extensive testing — comes from the Baltimore Longitudinal Study on Aging, carried on for twenty-five years at the National Institute of Health. Older volunteers from the study who showed no

---

Cardiovascular Risk Factors

Uncontrollable Risk Factors

Age   Family history

Controllable Risk Factors

Cigarette smoking   Obesity
High blood pressure   Diabetes
High blood cholestcrol   Stress
                                     Lack of exercise

---

evidence of heart disease on various tests were compared to younger volunteers who also seemed to be free of heart disease.

The investigators found interesting details about young versus old hearts, and two main discoveries. The first showed that older subjects had slight increases in blood pressure relative to their age, whether they were at rest or actively exercising. This discovery was not unexpected, but the second was a surprise. It showed that the ability of the older subjects to effectively pump blood through the heart remained about the same as that of the younger people's.

The Challenge of Risk Factors

Unless you have been living on another planet for years, you probably know the risk factors for heart disease and stroke. But it is worth reviewing them because many older people, and even those working with them on their health, share the belief that only younger people need to make changes in lifestyle. This impression is false: living a healthy lifestyle and diligently taking care of medical problems makes a difference in anyone's cardiovascular health at any age.

Some risk factors are considered *uncontrollable*. For older men and women, thesc include heredity and advancing age.

Heredity is a risk factor for those who have parents, aunts, uncles, or siblings who were victims of angina and heart attacks at relatively early ages. Such a pattern means the family blood lines may harbor genetic susceptibility to heart attacks. Although heart disease is not directly caused by aging, age is deemed a risk factor, because heart disease is so common among older people. Those who have heredity as a risk factor need to be especially conscientious about tackling controllable risk factors so that they can stack the odds in their favor for a longer life and a comfortable old age free of heart disease.

Everyone has the power to modify the controllable risk factors. Cigarette smoking can be cut out entirely. Smoking has immediate as well as long-term damaging effects on the entire cardiovascular system, and it is the most preventable cause of disability and death from cardiovascular disease.

Smoking, obesity, diabetes, lack of exercise, and stress are controllable risks that interact with the two most important physical risk factors — high blood pressure and high blood cholesterol. We move ahead to what you need to know about how these conditions can be prevented and treated in older people.

CONTROLLING HIGH BLOOD PRESSURE

A Powerful Risk Factor

We should all make sure to keep our blood pressure within normal limits. The reasons are very compelling. High blood pressure is known as one of the most powerful predictors that someone will have a heart attack or a stroke; more than half of those who have heart attacks, and three quarters of those who have strokes also have high blood pressure. It is also a major factor underlying other unpleasant problems, such as congestive heart failure, poor circulation in the leg (peripheral vascular disease), and kidney failure.

The problem of high blood pressure is very common in industrialized societies. In the United States alone at least 30 million people have it. The association between increasing blood pressure and advancing age is strong: 55 percent of people over fifty-five have abnormally high blood pressure.

Both men and women are highly susceptible. In fact, contrary to the popular misconception that high blood pressure is primarily a man's affliction, older women are slightly more susceptible to it, and more than 50 percent of women over fifty-five are affected. Also, studies show that high blood pressure is generally more dangerous to women; for unknown reasons, women do not survive heart attack and stroke as easily as men. Untreated high blood pressure in a man doubles his risk of cardiovascular disease, but a woman's risk is increased by two and one-half times.

Luckily, most everyone can respond to treatment for high blood pressure either with practical changes in lifestyle, or, if these don't work, with medication. It matters less that someone has the disease than that he or she follows through on proper treatment so that blood pressure goes down. By bringing blood pressure down to safe levels, one can prevent some of its serious consequences, such as stroke and heart attacks.

Because no one can feel high blood pressure unless it has reached nearly fatal levels, it should be checked at least once a year and whenever a medical examination is performed. Make sure that the older people in your family and circle of friends are having this checkup done; and also, don't neglect to find out if your own blood pressure is within safe limits.

What Is Blood Pressure?

Blood pressure is the force that moves blood through the blood-vessel tree, every branch of it, from the trunklike tubes feeding in and out of the heart and down through the center of the body, to the minute vessels transporting nutrients to and from cells.

The heart's forceful, rhythmic pumping action is the main mover of blood throughout the system, but a complex network of nerve signals, hormones, and other elements regulate the blood flow to each organ by widening or constricting small muscular blood vessels called arterioles, much as a faucet controls the flow of water. The walls of the arterial system are elastic, constantly stretching and contracting to take the ups and downs of blood pressure as it changes from moment to moment, depending on the body's needs.

The medical name hypertension describes the abnormal condition of too much tension in the walls of the arterioles. In someone who has hypertension, the regulatory system controlling blood flow goes awry: arterioles throughout the body stay tense and constricted, driving up the pressure in the larger blood vessels.

Hypertension, with its constant rush of high-pressure blood flow, gradually strains and weakens the blood-vessel walls, as well as the heart itself. Even mild hypertension can make blood vessels more likely to tear, leak, and gather deposits of fat, cholesterol, and cellular debris. Over the years the heart has to work harder at pumping, with the result that it alters structurally.

The precise cause of high blood pressure isn't known, although researchers do know of factors that increase the chance that one will develop it. They include heredity, age, smoking, obesity, and sensitivity to salt. Heavy alcohol consumption also has a bearing on high blood pressure. Although the reasons are not definitely known, race is also a strong factor; black Americans are especially prone to high blood pressure.

Many people incorrectly think hypertension is caused primarily by mental and emotional tension. Although stress can raise blood pressure in all of us, it is not by itself a cause of hypertension. Very calm people can get it as well as high-strung types, who are often physically tense. Furthermore, not all high-strung people have it.

What Do Blood-Pressure Numbers Signify?

Blood pressure is expressed as two numbers, such as 130/80, and is measured in millimeters of mercury. The top number is the systolic blood pressure, the force exerted by blood pressing against the artery in the arm being tested, while the heart is pumping. The bottom number, or diastolic blood pressure, is the pressure that remains in the arteries when the heart is relaxed.

Most people have their blood pressure taken without much understanding of what the numbers mean. We suggest you encourage the older individual you are helping to learn about the meaning of numbers for blood pressure, and other basic tests, such as cholesterol and blood glucose, and to keep a notebook of medical information. Such a record will help keep the older person, and all involved with his or her care, better informed at home and when visiting doctors. Also, a record will provide you with some basic understanding of what's going on, so that you can weigh the older person's response to the high blood-pressure treatment. Progress that shows in the record can also become a powerful reinforcer to the idea that treatment is well worth undergoing.

Safe Numbers: Are They Different for the Elderly?

Until the mid-1970s it was commonly believed that elderly people had high blood pressure as part of normal aging, to compensate for their hardened arteries and weaker heart. Most doctors left high blood pressure alone in the elderly, thinking that it was best to do so. Even today there is controversy about what levels of high blood pressure should be treated in older people, especially those who are very old (eighty-five plus).

Some doctors still hold to thinking that high blood pressure should be left alone in very old people. Such doctors don't see the sense in asking them to change their lifestyle to lower their blood pressure. These doctors also may argue that it is right to be supercautious about treating blood pressure with medications because the job is too tricky and complicated to do in the elderly body, especially if the person is suffering from other chronic conditions that require medication.

Because of such doctors, older people and their families really must "know the numbers" — what's normal and what's not — and must be fully aware that the National High Blood Pressure Education Program published a report in 1988 to impress on doctors that treatment should be sought by people of all ages. A range of treatments work very well for most patients, even those who are old and frail.

Here is a summary of some of the main guidelines in this report.

• High blood pressure is not "normal" in the elderly and should be lowered to established safe ranges.

• Treatment should be started if the blood pressure reading is higher than 160/90 on three consecutive visits, on different days.

• If the diastolic number stays lower than 90, and the systolic number goes up higher than 160, a condition called borderline isolated hypertension is present. "Isolated" means that only the systolic is elevated. It should be cautiously treated so that the systolic reading comes down to 140–160, without lowering the diastolic number so far that dizziness and falls occur.

• Blood pressure should be read in both sitting and standing positions at every visit.

• Follow-up visits in a doctor's office or clinic should be scheduled every two to four weeks until antihypertensive therapy has stabilized the pressure.

• Diuretics are the preferred first drug to try in elderly patients with diastolic hypertension or isolated hypertension.

• The initial dose of a drug for elderly patients should be one-half that prescribed for young and middle-aged adults.

Treatment for Older People

The Nondrug Measures
When blood pressure is not drastically above normal, nondrug measures are tried first to lower it, usually for up to three months. Often adopting just one or two of the measures will lower blood pressure so that pills are unnecessary.

The measures listed here are recommended for all people with hypertension, whether or not they are candidates for drug treatment.

Lowering Salt. Everyone differs in sensitivity to salt, and many older people seem very sensitive to salt's effect on their blood pressure. At least half of those who try cutting down on salt intake can reduce their blood pressure, many of them to safe levels.

Most people consume far too much salt, probably about two teaspoons a day if they add salt to their food and if they eat canned soups, canned vegetables, fast-food meals, salty snacks, and processed meats such as hot dogs, salami, and ham. This total is about twenty times more than the body actually needs. The general recommendation is that anyone trying to lower blood pressure consume no more than a teaspoon or so a day, or 2,000 to 3,000 milligrams. Your parent's doctor should make an appropriate recommendation.

Many elderly become so used to easy-to-prepare processed foods that it can be quite difficult for them to switch to basic foods that they can salt themselves. Although favorite salty foods don't have to be cut out entirely, they certainly should be limited, and supplanted by appetizing substitutes. Encourage your parent to follow these five steps to lowering salt in the diet, or follow them yourself while planning meals.

1. Don't add salt at the table; leave the shaker near the stove just for cooking.
2. Avoid obviously salty foods. These include the ones mentioned above and also potato chips, pretzels, crackers, and other salted snacks; pickles and pickled foods; and salted nuts.
3. Read labels carefully to find "hidden" sodium. When you see the word *sodium* with another word attached to it, the num-

ber listed applies to the sodium content. It can be shocking to read labels and find out how much salt is in commercially prepared or packaged foods. Many of these foods that don't taste salty can be loaded with it — even some dessert products.

4. In cooking try using alternatives to salt and salty condiments. Herbs and spices can perk up home-cooked meals, as can a little lemon juice and anything from the onion family. Limit ketchup, soy sauce, mayonnaise, and packaged salad dressings and dips.

5. Go easy on processed cheeses and buttermilk. Low-sodium cheeses and low-fat milk are better substitutes.

Weight Control. Those who are overweight have more fluid in their system and a tendency to develop high blood pressure because the heart has to pump harder to make up for the extra fluid load. Often when people lose even a small amount of weight — as little as five pounds — their blood pressure can go down.

No older person should go on a weight-loss program without a doctor's supervision. Also, careful attention must be given to the nutritional content of any weight-loss diet; older people often have specific nutritional needs and it is becoming more and more evident that they need essential nutrients at least as much as younger people do. Exercise is a vital adjunct to a weight-loss plan.

Exercise. Some people become afraid to exercise after a diagnosis of high blood pressure, not realizing that regular exercise is considered a promising way to improve general health, lose weight, and lower blood pressure. Moderate exercise — walking, swimming, bicycling — should be done for at least 20 minutes several times a week, if possible, for full conditioning effect. Those with chronic ailments who can't move easily should try to do some form of exercise so that they are not sedentary. The doctor should always be consulted before the start of an exercise program, especially if the older person has heart disease.

Most older people who are able to get out and about prefer walking because it's easy and pleasant. The trouble with most North American cities, however, is that they depend so heavily on automobiles and are so crime-ridden that pleasant walks aren't always right outside the door. Many cities now have senior citizens' walking clubs, which find ways for people to walk in parks, malls, school tracks, and gymnasiums.

Stress Management. Stressful situations can raise blood pressure, especially in people who are stress sensitive. Older people are buffeted by multiple stresses and frustrations from failing health, death of people significant in their lives, loss of income, or inability to continue activities they had enjoyed. Family members need to do all they can to help the older person cope with stressful situations. When a crisis occurs, be there to listen, help with details that need handling, and above all, show that you care.

If your parent seems overwhelmed by events and depressed, talk to the doctor about strategies to make things easier, such as consulting a mental-health expert who understands the problems of the elderly. Be wary, though, of the doctor who is quick to prescribe tranquilizers.

Drug Treatments
Although a few old-standby medications are still appropriate, many new medications available today are extremely effective against high blood pressure and have fewer side effects than those used just a decade or so ago. Your mother or father, and anyone else you care about, should be fully aware that drug side effects previously taken for granted, such as drowsiness, dizziness, nervousness, depression, and sexual impotence, need not be suffered silently and rarely need to be tolerated. Your parent may well have recollections of friends or older family members "zonked" and depressed by blood-pressure medications. He or she may fear taking medications, or if taking them, may assume that side effects are the price for lowering blood pressure.

These days, the blood-pressure drug regimen is tailored to the individual. Doctors have so many good drugs to choose from that they can fine-tune treatment to the patient's specific health needs and to the cost the patient can afford. There may be some false starts along the way, and it can take up to three months for a program to show beneficial change without significant side effects, but eventually a doctor who knows how to manage blood pressure should be able to find a drug, or combination of drugs, useful for the patient and well tolerated.

Drugs are given in much lower doses than they used to be, and often in mix-and-match combinations. If a combination is prescribed, ask the doctor if it can be given in one pill, to simplify things. People with heart disease, for example, can sometimes be given one medication to take care of both their angina and high blood pressure. Such combinations may also be cheaper.

The cost factor should not be overlooked. Though unfair, it is a well-known fact of life that many older people, if their prescribed blood-pressure medications are prohibitively expensive, will not take them. The newer drugs, though often very effective and with fewer side effects, can be extremely expensive, running up to $200 a month. In selecting a medication the doctor must pay heed to the patient's budget limitations.

If cost is troubling, the doctor may decide to carefully prescribe one of the less-expensive medications in a dose that creates tolerable side effects that the patient can learn to live with. Many of the diuretics, which are old standbys, can cost as little as $2 a month (see Chapter 13). Although diuretics can cause potassium depletion, this problem can be taken care of safely and inexpensively with potassium supplements. For a drug that causes dry mouth, the patient can learn to abate this side effect by chewing gum and hard candies, and by drinking enough fluids.

More and more doctors are helping patients cut costs of high blood-pressure medication by combining effective but new, expensive drugs with cheaper old standbys. The doctor might give an expensive drug in a dose smaller than recommended when the drug is used alone, in very effective combination with a low-cost diuretic. We list here categories of drugs prescribed to lower blood pressure.

Diuretics. Known as water pills, diuretics eliminate salt and water into the urine so that less fluid is in circulation. Usually a diuretic is the first drug tried, but for someone who is on heart medications, sometimes in just a small amount. A major side effect to contend with is loss of potassium, which can if severe lead to leg cramps, fatigue, and palpitations. The doctor should test blood levels of potassium regularly, and if need be prescribe potassium supplements. Many older people, particularly women, also, find they have urge incontinence within an hour of taking pills. This side effect is most common during the initial days of therapy and will reappear if daily pills are skipped.

Beta Blockers (timolol, atenolol, propranalol). Also used for heart disease, these beta blockers blunt the force of the heart's pumping

Blood-Pressure Medication Tips

• If the older person has complaints that could be side effects, call the doctor. Watch out for fatigue, dizziness, confusion, tiredness, depression, leg cramps, constipation, nausea.

• Be especially observant during the beginning of drug treatment, or after a dose has been increased, or a new drug added. Elderly people can be exquisitely sensitive to the medications, and sometimes pressure drops too low, which can cause confusion and dizziness, sometimes so severe that the person doesn't have the wits to call the doctor.

• If a known potassium-lowering diuretic is prescribed, make sure plenty of potassium-rich foods are eaten daily. They include potatoes with the skins left on, bananas, orange juice, and raisins.

• Potassium supplements have such a nasty, bitter taste that many people refuse to take them. Ask for the pill form and take it with fruit juices, apple sauce, and other sweetish foods.

• Diuretics can cause urge incontinence, especially in older women. Usually the urge to "go" comes about half an hour after taking a pill. Incontinent episodes can of course be highly embarrassing and create fear of "accidents." Ask the doctor to schedule the time to take a daily pill when your family member will be at home, or close to a bathroom.

• Ask if a diuretic can be taken only once a day and in the morning after getting up from sleep.

• Keep to the prescribed schedule: very important. If a dose is missed, tell the older person to get back on the prescribed schedule. Don't allow him or her to take several pills at once to make up for the missed ones.

• If the older person is making a concerted effort to change — cut down on salt, lose weight, relax, and give up smoking — ask the doctor to assess how these changes have affected blood pressure. Perhaps medications can be reduced or cut out entirely.

• Periodically, encourage your family member to take a brown bag with all current medications to the doctor, who can then see what drugs are being taken along with those for high blood pressure.

• Never take a new drug without consulting the doctor. Watch for side effects caused by the interactions with the new drug.

action, also causing the arteries to dilate. A beta blocker is either prescribed alone to treat high blood pressure, or in combination with a small dose of a diuretic. Besides the most common side effect of pervasive fatigue, other possibilities include constipation, depression, sleep disturbances, and a slow pulse.

Calcium Channel Blockers (nifedipine, diltiazem, verapamil). Among the expensive choices, these blockers lower blood pressure by relaxing the muscular aspect of arteries, thus causing them to dilate. Originally used for coronary heart disease, these drugs can be ideal for those who have angina and high blood pressure. Each calcium channel blocker has unique side effects. For example, constipation can accompany verapamil, but it can be managed with a high-fiber diet and plenty of fluids. Stomach and intestinal disturbance can occur with nifedipine. Diltiazem rarely causes side effects, but it is not as potent as the others and so is not the best choice for some patients.

ACE Inhibitors (captopril, enalapril). Also expensive, these inhibitors lower blood pressure by blocking the action of angiotensin, a hormone secreted by the kidneys, which modulates blood pressure as well as levels of salt in the body. Some evidence suggests that ACE inhibitors may have a protective effect on the kidneys of those who have diabetes as well as hypertension. On the other hand, they are used with caution in those who have kidney disease. People who are on ACE inhibitors need to have their blood count and potassium levels checked periodically at the doctor's discretion.

LOWERING CHOLESTEROL

Why Lowering Cholesterol Is Important

Cholesterol is a fatlike substance normally produced by the liver, but also found in animal-food products, meats, poultry, fish, dairy products, eggs, and some oils. A surplus of cholesterol in the blood stream has a tendency to stick to the inside of the blood vessels so that they become narrower and narrower, much as water pipes build up scaly mineral deposits.

This clogging up of blood vessels is known as atherosclerosis.

Too much cholesterol in the blood is a culprit, but other factors contribute, too: smoking, high blood pressure, diabetes, being overweight, and a sedentary lifestyle.

Although cholesterol buildup can begin early in life, it can take decades for clogging to get so bad that blood has difficulty getting through blood vessels. Excess cholesterol accumulates either because one has an inherited tendency to produce much more of the stuff than the body needs, or because the diet is overloaded with cholesterol-rich foods.

The condition is usually not noticed until a major illness occurs. Either discomfort is noticed in and around the chest because the arteries around the heart are blocked (ischemia), or blood is completely blocked so that the catastrophe of either a heart attack or a stroke occurs. When a complete blockage happens in one of the arteries surrounding the heart (the coronary arteries) the result is a heart attack. When blockage occurs in one of the arteries leading to the brain, or a vessel within the brain, the result is a stroke. Another illness usually caused by high cholesterol is peripheral vascular disease in the legs (see page 227).

The research resoundingly states that people of any age who have high cholesterol in their blood have an increased risk of having heart attacks and strokes. Studies on people under sixty also show that for those with high cholesterol, just a 1 percent reduction in cholesterol translates to a 2 percent reduction in heart-attack risk. Similar studies still need to be done on people in their seventies, and beyond. But until the verdict is in it seems to make sense for older people to consider adopting at least a modified healthy diet. Healthy habits can probably keep atherosclerotic blockage from getting worse.

What Do the Numbers Mean?

Cholesterol readings taken from a simple blood test are now a routine part of physical exams. The test is done so that doctors can inform patients about whether or not their cholesterol is within safe limits.

Just as there is a report by the National High Blood Pressure Education Program to clarify questions about blood-pressure treatment, so too a National Cholesterol Education Program is designed to give doctors the information they need to correctly treat high blood cholesterol. No solid research has been done on the effects of low-

Total blood cholesterol		
DESIRABLE	BORDERLINE HIGH	HIGH
200 mg/dl	200–239 mg/dl	240 mg/dl and above

LDL levels (the harmful kind)		
DESIRABLE	BORDERLINE HIGH	HIGH
Less than 130 mg/dl	130–159 mg/dl	160 mg/dl

ering cholesterol in people over sixty, and so the information in the report is based primarily on research done on younger people. Older people who are interested in the cholesterol factor, however, can certainly benefit by discussing with the doctor the meaning of their tested cholesterol numbers, compared with those generally considered safe. Most elderly people test at the low end of the range considered high cholesterol, at least in countries where diets prevail that are high in cholesterol, high in salt, and depleted in fiber.

The doctor will check the total cholesterol number first, and if it is not good, will test for the two basic cholesterol types — one is beneficial to the body, and the other can lead to cardiovascular disease. Both are transported in the blood by protein packages called lipoproteins. The protective kind, which is good to have at high levels, is called high-density lipoprotein (HDL) and is processed by the liver and removed from the blood stream. The harmful kind, known as low-density lipoprotein (LDL) stays in the blood stream and deposits itself on artery walls. A high LDL number greatly affects one's chances of having a heart attack.

The table shows the categories of cholesterol numbers and how they should be managed, according to information in the report.

If cholesterol is at the desirable level:

- Plan to repeat the test in five years.
- Evaluate other risk factors (smoking, high blood pressure, diabetes, obesity) with the doctor and consider steps to control them.

If cholesterol is "borderline high":

- Plan to repeat the test annually if at low risk (no history of heart disease and fewer than two risk factors).
- Consider asking for an analysis of LDL and HDL levels.

- Take steps to modify heart-disease risk factors.
- Reduce cholesterol in the diet.

If cholesterol is "high":

- Consider asking for an analysis of LDL and HDL levels.
- Take steps to modify heart-disease risk factors.
- Reduce cholesterol in the diet.
- If diet, conscientiously adhered to for six months, fails to reduce cholesterol sufficiently, then drug therapy for lowering cholesterol can be considered (although the research evidence is scant on the efficacy of cholesterol-lowering medications for patients over sixty-five).

Should Elderly People Lower Their Cholesterol?

Being really aggressive about lowering high cholesterol usually is highly practical for younger people, if they want to live out a long life span. But the choice is not as clear for elderly people. Cholesterol may not necessarily be the most important risk factor for their age group; more significantly, getting compulsive about lowering cholesterol may be just too confounding for some.

As a family member wanting the best for your relative, you must be careful not to go overboard on the cholesterol issue. Likewise you should be supportive if your relative wants to make cholesterol-lowering changes in diet and to keep up healthy habits, or if he or she has already had a heart attack and wants to prevent another.

We have heard plenty of stories about young family members badgering their elders into feeling guilty about eating food they have enjoyed for a lifetime. The idea is for all of us — most of the time — to eat a sensible diet, not obviously overloaded with high-fat and high-cholesterol foods. No harm should come of eating ice cream, eggs, favorite cheeses, and so on once in a while, and certainly if one has a hard time eating and preparing meals at all, foods one is used to and likes should not be abandoned.

Older people have very different responses to finding out that they have high cholesterol. After a lifetime of cooking and enjoying food, an eighty-year-old woman may find out her cholesterol is 300 milligrams and say, "No way will I stop using butter, cream, and eggs in my cooking. I feel fine; I must have done something right!"

Or a recently widowed man, frail and eighty-six years old, told by his daughter he has to cut out scrambled eggs and bacon for breakfast every day, says, "Leave me alone. I look forward to my breakfast, and besides it's the only easy-to-fix, wholesome meal of the day." It seems both of these people probably will be happier living out the rest of their years enjoying their usual way of eating.

On the other hand, some older people take on lowering cholesterol with a sense of great purpose. Doing so makes them feel in control of their longevity, and, eventually research may well prove their way to be right.

Know Which Foods Cause Atherosclerosis

The very best way to lower cholesterol is to reduce the amount of saturated fat in all meals and snacks. The main atherosclerosis builders are saturated fats. Reducing cholesterol-rich foods is important, but saturated fats raise blood cholesterol more than anything else in the diet.

Currently, about 35 to 40 percent of the calories in the average diet are derived from fats — about 16 percent from saturated fat and 24 percent from mono- and polyunsaturated fats. To reduce the risk of cardiovascular disease, the experts recommend that people reduce total fat intake to about 30 percent of total calories, with saturated fat making up less than 10 percent of fat intake, no more than 10 percent from polyunsaturated fat, and 10 percent or more from monounsaturated fat.

Dietary cholesterol should be reduced to less than 300 milligrams per day. To give you an idea of what this number means, consider that one egg yolk contains about 213 milligrams of cholesterol.

But which fats belong in which category? And what foods contain cholesterol? Here's how to tell.

• Cholesterol is found only in animal products (meat, poultry, seafood, organ meats, eggs, and dairy products such as butter and cheese).

• Vegetables, fruits, cereal grains, and foods such as rice or pasta are good sources of starch and fiber, and generally contain no cholesterol and little or no saturated fat.

• Saturated fats tend to be hard at room temperature. They can come from animal sources, butter, high-fat cheeses, whole milk, ice cream, and cream. A few vegetable fats are also high in saturated fats: coconut oil, cocoa butter (found in chocolate), palm kernel, and palm oil.

• Polyunsaturated fats should be substituted for saturated fats whenever possible; they actually help lower cholesterol. These fats are found primarily in liquid vegetable oils, such as safflower, corn, soybean, sesame, and sunflower oils. Another type of polyunsaturated fat is found in the oils of seafood, and these are referred to as fish oil or omega-3 fatty acids.

• Monounsaturated fats are said to lower cholesterol. They can be found in high amounts in olive oil, canola oil (rapeseed oil), and peanut oil.

Tips for Preparing Meals

• Choose fish, poultry, and lean cuts of meat, and remove fat from meats and skin from chicken before cooking. Keep portions moderate.

• Avoid organ meats such as liver, kidney, and brains; also cut down on sausage, bacon, and processed luncheon meats.

• Substitute skim or low-fat milk for whole milk or cream. Use low-fat cheeses and yoghurt.

• Instead of butter, use margarine high in polyunsaturated fats.

• Remember, egg yolks are high in fat, and especially cholesterol. Limit whole eggs to three a week on the plate, as well as in cooking. Egg Beaters, containing no cholesterol, are an excellent substitute in cooking, and often egg whites alone can be used in place of whole eggs.

• Always use vegetable oils for sautéing vegetables, cooking rice, popping corn, and for making baked goods, pancakes, and waffles.

• Read labels carefully on commercially baked goods, crackers, prepared foods, and snacks. Although consumer pressure has forced some food companies to turn away from using lard, coconut oil, palm oil, or shortening, many products still contain them.

CORONARY ARTERY DISEASE

In this section, we describe how coronary artery disease presents itself, and how it is diagnosed and treated.

If someone in your family develops coronary artery disease, you will become involved in arranging how to get it treated medically, or if necessary, surgically. Your support will make a big difference in how the person you are helping lives with the disease and all its contingencies. It will allow him or her to carry on activities as comfortably as possible without undue symptoms and anxiety.

The stage is set for coronary artery disease when the coronary arteries surrounding the heart are progressively narrowed by fatty buildup (atherosclerosis), severe enough to slow blood to the heart, and "starving" the heart muscle for oxygen, in a condition called ischemia. The coronary arteries encircle the heart like a crown, hence their name, from the Latin word for crown, *corona*. These vessels, no wider than a drinking straw, are so prone to blockage because of their narrow diameter.

Mild blockage doesn't usually create significant, noticeable problems because enough blood passes to the heart. But when deposits take up 75 percent or more of the artery's diameter, temporary chest discomfort and breathlessness can occur, among other symptoms. When these symptoms strike, the victim is said to be having angina.

An anginal episode is not the same as a heart attack. The life-threatening emergency of a heart attack comes when blockage bars oxygen to an area of heart muscle so that it dies, thus stymieing the heart's ability to pump effectively.

The person with angina has a greater risk of having a heart attack than someone with no angina. For this reason you and your relative need to fully understand how to recognize angina when it first comes on, and how to determine if anginal symptoms are severe enough to warn of an impending heart attack or an attack in progress. See page 220 on the Heart-Attack Emergency so that you will know when to call the doctor or when to punch 911 on the telephone for an ambulance.

Be glad to know that not everyone who has angina is about to have a heart attack; plenty of people with angina — if it is well managed — live out long lives and die of causes other than those related to heart disease. The aim of treatment is to stabilize the disease so that one can carry on activities as normally as possible, and to forestall a heart attack.

What Does Angina Feel Like?

Typically, a person has no problem with angina while resting or doing slow activities. It comes on when extra demands are placed on the heart — climbing a flight of stairs, mowing the grass, doing a large load of ironing, vacuuming the house, eating an especially heavy meal, or experiencing an emotional upset.

Because angina comes and goes with activity, many older people dismiss their anginal symptoms as trivial. Classic angina symptoms include chest pains, or an ache that starts in or spreads to the neck, jaw, throat, shoulder, back, or arms, or complaints of indigestion, belching, muscle cramps, or shortness of breath during times of moderate to strenuous activity. If the older person you are with has any of these symptoms accompanying activity, do call the doctor to explain the symptoms and to make an appointment. Chest pains, breathlessness, and any quirky feelings or pain in and around and above the chest are not normal — no matter what your spouse, parent, or older friend may think. You must get them analyzed by a doctor to see if coronary artery disease is in or out of the picture.

Certainly, anginal episodes during activity are a serious warning sign that the heart is temporarily not getting enough blood and oxygen. The anginal condition needs to be treated medically and with modifications in the way activities are performed. If this warning is ignored, the heart muscle suffers ischemia and can be damaged. The damage can be subtle, or it can be dramatic if the angina becomes "unstable," on its way to spiraling into a heart attack.

How Is Angina Diagnosed?

Usually if someone comes to a doctor's office complaining of classic anginal symptoms that last from three to fifteen minutes before going away, the doctor will strongly suspect that the cause is coronary heart disease.

But not all chest pain or discomfort during exertion is angina. Pain that mimics angina can arise from a lung disorder, or trouble in the esophagus and stomach (for example, a hiatus hernia — see page 142), or a musculoskeletal problem. It can also arise from a different kind of heart problem, perhaps a disorder in one or more of the heart valves, which can sometimes show up with symptoms similar to those of coronary-artery disease. The doctor will need to do an examination and run tests, perhaps with a cardiologist, to check such possibilities.

The history and physical, including an electrocardiagram (EKG), count for a lot, and provide useful information for a diagnosis of angina. But an EKG is generally not helpful for angina, for the reading can be normal in more than half the patients with chronic angina, whose angina would show up only in a stress test. Although the EKG needs to be done when someone shows heart-disease symptoms because it can provide information about the state of the heart, it will not provide positive proof of angina. It's a common misconception among patients that a normal EKG means their heart is functioning normally. An x-ray will highlight enlargement of the heart and large blood vessels, and signs of fluid backed up in the lung, as a consequence of heart failure. It will not, though, visualize disease within these structures, or confirm that anginalike symptoms are caused by blocked coronary arteries.

If a doctor wants to start treatment for your relative or friend, based on a history, physical, an EKG, and perhaps a chest x-ray, you may want to insist that arrangements be made for further diagnostic tests. Only cardiac tests can give a definite rather than a presumed diagnosis of angina. Check your family member's insurance status first: some cardiac tests can be expensive, and cost may have to enter into the decision you make with the doctor. Such tests will confirm the diagnosis more precisely, and put the severity of the underlying coronary artery disease in perspective, so that decisions on treatment can be carefully reached.

Most doctors will go ahead and make arrangements for a cardiologist to do the testing as a matter of course. If you feel you need to make your own arrangements, though, find the name of a nearby cardiologist either through a local hospital's referral service or the service at the nearest chapter of the American Heart Association.

Once you have connected with a cardiologist, you and your relative can decide whether this doctor should be in continuing charge of heart-related problems. You may feel most comfortable having the older person's usual doctor handle the case, once testing has been done. In making this decision, however, take into account that if the older person is hospitalized for a heart-disease-related condition, a cardiologist will probably be in charge, as a matter of hospital policy. Recognize that it will be comforting and helpful to have a cardiologist already lined up whom everyone trusts and likes.

Noninvasive Tests for Coronary Artery Disease

The Electrocardiogram (EKG) Exercise Stress Test
This test is the one most often done on presumed angina patients, and it is relatively inexpensive (around $400). It's an EKG done while the patient walks on a motor-driven treadmill, or pedals a stationary

bicycle. The idea is to stress the heart under controlled conditions while an EKG is reading out to the cardiologist in charge. If the person being exercised experiences an inadequate flow of blood to the heart, the EKG will usually (but not always) display an abnormal reading, showing how degrees of activity affect the heart muscle and how much activity it can handle.

The stress test is, more often than not, very helpful in evaluating pain and other symptoms in and around the chest. It is particularly valuable in diagnosing the severity of coronary-artery disease in older people who do not have typical angina symptoms. The test will often point out symptoms far more severe than the older person may "feel." If the EKG shows changes suggesting that the heart is ischemic, the test is considered "positive" for coronary-artery disease.

Properly performed, the stress test is accurate about 80 percent of the time. If the test is inconclusive, the cardiologist may next do a nuclear scan.

The Nuclear Scan
Also called myocardial imaging, the nuclear test gets pictures of the blood supply within the heart. It is usually done as a stress test, while the subject is on a treadmill or bicycle; however, it can be done with the patient at rest. If the old person is particularly frail, ill, or so arthritic that active leg movement presents a difficulty, it is substituted for the standard EKG exercise stress test.

A radioactive thallium dye is injected into the patient's arm, either on the treadmill or bicycle, or at rest. The thallium diffuses into the heart muscle, mostly into areas well supplied with blood, less in areas inadequately perfused with blood.

Following exercise — if it is part of the test — the patient is asked to lie under a computerized imaging machine. The cardiologist can read the film for "cold spots," where blood supply is inadequate, and get a good idea of how coronary artery disease is affecting the heart.

The Two-Dimensional Echocardiogram
The echocardiogram uses safe, painless ultrasound waves to form an image of the heart on a television screen. The images are two-dimensional, in a way representing slices of the heart, and they can visualize the heart in motion. The cardiologist can read them while the test

is being run, or later by viewing a videotape, which can be put on file for future reference.

An extremely useful test for various forms of heart disease, the echocardiogram is usually ordered for those suspected of having enlargement of one or more heart chambers, or valvular problems. The film can record the internal structures of the heart, and can also measure the thickness and size of the heart walls, including those four chambers. The opening and closing motion of the valves can be recorded too, and in a newer version of the test, the Doppler echocardiogram, blood flow through the valves can be assessed for abnormal, turbulent flow patterns.

Stable versus Unstable Angina

Stable Angina and Subtle Changes

In its commonest form angina has a "stable" pattern. Symptoms feel about the same over months and years and occur during the same kind of activity. Most people learn to adapt to their angina by doing slowly or differently the activities that provoke it, and by taking special anti-angina medications.

Consider these examples of adaptive behavior. A woman notices that she starts feeling pain in her chest after ironing eight shirts, and so stops to rest for half an hour before moving on to do more ironing. A man whose apartment is up four steep flights of stairs finds he has to stop at each landing for a minute or two. Another man, reluctant to give up his weekly golf game, is able to keep this pleasure; he takes nitroglycerin before starting his game and rents a golf cart instead of walking.

A "stable" pattern of angina can gradually get worse. If the person you are caring for has angina that starts to change in subtle ways from its typical pattern, the doctor needs to be notified. Don't allow this person to wait until pains and other discomforts grow more and more severe. Remember that every time symptoms are felt the heart is deprived of oxygen and put into a state of imbalance. Pain means ischemia. Look for these situations: an increase in the frequency or severity of pain with the same activity, angina at a lower level of exercise, or decreased responsiveness to nitroglycerin medications.

When changes are reported, the doctor will consider changing angina treatment medications, and may order further cardiac tests to assess progression of the coronary artery disease and how it has affected the heart. No doubt the older person will already have modified any activities that bring on angina.

"Unstable" Angina

The unstable variety of angina is a lot more noticeable than a subtle change in symptoms. It merits an immediate call to the doctor's office and for an ambulance first if you have any suspicion that a heart attack is in progress (see "The Heart-Attack Emergency" on page 220). This kind of angina indicates that one or more of the coronary arteries has become so severely narrowed that a heart attack is certain to happen within hours, days, or a few months.

The person with unstable angina needs to be hospitalized, preferably in a coronary-care unit, where he or she can be watched and medically managed until symptoms have "cooled off." After the cooling-off period, the patient, doctor, and patient's family need to make some hard decisions about whether to continue treating angina with medications or to choose angioplasty (see page 216) or surgery to unclog the heart vessels that are causing the trouble.

How then do you recognize if your parent, spouse, or friend is having unstable angina? First, and foremost, you and your relative need to discuss with the doctor how to recognize medical emergencies related to the older person's heart condition. Get some good, solid answers about how you can analyze changes in symptoms, so that you will know exactly when to call the doctor, and when to waste no time but call an ambulance first. Write out a list of such symptoms for each situation and make sure the family, neighbors, friends, and caregivers understand them.

The doctor will give you specific symptoms to look out for, but generally it is said that angina has turned unstable — and the doctor should be notified immediately — if the following conditions appear.

• If there is a sudden change in the typical pattern of angina during exertion. For example, your parent may feel angina after walking one block instead of eight, all of a sudden for the first time while washing hair in the shower, when sweeping one room instead of two, or while ironing three shirts instead of eight.

• If nitroglycerin does not relieve symptoms, after three tablets have been taken, at intervals, over a fifteen-minute period.

• If chest pain, sudden breathlessness, belching, indigestion, and other symptoms start for no apparent reason when the older person is at rest — lying in bed, sitting in a chair, standing up, or lying in the bathtub.

Angina Medication

Nitroglycerin is a proven and generally safe, low-cost drug given to everyone suffering from angina. It remains the most effective drug for promptly relieving an angina attack, and for those with severe angina to take at the same time each day to prevent attacks. The drug is non–habit-forming and short-acting, and does not accumulate in the body to toxic levels. No one need be afraid to take it, and several tablets can be taken in a day.

Nitroglycerin works by relaxing the blood vessels surrounding the heart and throughout the body. When this relaxation takes over, blood flow to the heart muscle is increased and at the same time the blood pressure goes down so that the heart has less hard work to perform. For prompt relief, people are given pills to put under the tongue. For long-acting results, a skin patch can be applied, to be replaced after twelve or twenty-four hours. Many angina patients wear skin patches and keep pills handy to use when they feel chest pains or other discomfort related to their disease.

Angina patients are told to first stop doing the activity that brought on the angina, and take it easy for a minute or two. If the symptoms persist, a pill needs to be put under the tongue and allowed to dissolve. Patients are warned to take the pills sitting or lying down, because they can cause a lowering of blood pressure that can bring on dizziness. Relief should come quickly. If pain hangs on after a few minutes, then another pill can be taken, and still another if necessary. Usually rest and a pill or two will do the trick; however, if after fifteen minutes medication gives no relief, the doctor *must* be called.

Beta blockers (such as propranolol, atenolol, and timolol), and calcium channel blockers (including nifedipine, verapamil, diltiazem) are two kinds of drugs commonly taken regularly by angina patients. Beta blockers help the heart beat slower and pump with less force. The heart therefore needs less oxygen during physical activity or at times of emotional stress. Calcium channel blockers are helpful because they relax the arteries all over the body, reducing the workload on the heart. They also prevent the coronary arteries from going into a state of spasm, which becomes part of an angina attack for some people. (We have discussed common side effects of these drugs in the preceding section on drug treatment for high blood pressure.)

Helpful Tips for Good Angina Control

The techniques in these four categories will help reduce anginal episodes. They will also give your parent a sense of control over the disease, as well as a feeling of security.

1. Slowing Down

The pace at which we do things has a lot to do with angina. The heart needs more oxygen when one is very active, in a hurry, or upset. You need to help your parent, other relative, or friend be well organized so that tasks and necessary everyday activities can get done at a slow pace without bringing on an angina attack.

• The person prone to angina may have good days and bad days. On the bad days it is sensible to stay close to home and completely edit out activities that bring on angina.

• Many activities can still be carried on, if just done slowly. Some people can walk a mile or more without distress if they pace themselves, but might have an attack walking rapidly for half a block.

• Brief, intensive physical effort will very quickly result in anginal discomfort. Such hard upper-arm activities as raking leaves, lifting heavy objects, and straining to open windows should be avoided.

• Remind the older person to take it easy in hot or cold weather, and to dress appropriately. What your parent can do in mild weather may bring on angina in the cold and wind, or on a hot or humid day. Make sure the indoor heating system is adequate and rooms air-conditioned in hot weather.

• Look into the same kinds of assistive devices recommended for people with arthritis. Select items in a catalogue or a surgical supply store. You can find those for food preparation, lifting, grabbing, and transporting things indoors and out (see Appendix).

• Arrange for strenuous household and garden tasks to be done by someone else in the family, a volunteer, or paid help. Sit down with your parent and list such tasks and a schedule to get them done.

• Encourage the older person to talk to the doctor about a program of moderate exercise. Your local chapter of the American Heart

Association may have an exercise program for angina patients, or may know about programs in your community. Many people experience reduced anginal symptoms with a progressive exercise-training program.

2. Rest and Relaxation

Tiredness can trigger angina, and so can frustration, outbursts of anger, and distress over bad news.

• Encourage the older person to have rest periods throughout the day, and if necessary a nap in the afternoon on a schedule that will keep it from interfering with adequate sleep at night.

• If at all possible, avoid any kind of situation that is emotionally and physically fatiguing.

• Keep communication open: talk to the older person about everyday situations that cause feelings of pressure and frustration. Think about ways to control such situations or keep them out of his or her life completely.

• Be there in person if you have to break bad news to your spouse, parent, or older friend about a death or other distressing loss. Make sure he or she is sitting down at home, or in familiar surroundings, with nitroglycerin on hand. Be on the alert for angina to turn "unstable."

• Seek help from a mental-health professional or clergyman if continuing tensions seem to be aggravating your parent's angina. Talk to the doctor or visiting nurse about this option.

• Encourage the older person to do relaxation exercises, and do them routinely.

• Urge your parent, spouse, or friend to join an American Heart Association support group, for company and relaxation.

3. Eating Properly

Like physical activity, digestion causes the heart to work harder and to require more blood. Encourage the person who is prone to angina to:

• Eat a sensible low-fat and low-cholesterol diet, in an attempt to abate the atherosclerosis blocking the coronary blood vessels.

• Avoid hard-to-digest, large meals and rich foods.

• Rest for a while after meals.

• Eat slowly, sitting down in a comfortable atmosphere. Never eat on the run.

- Use nitroglycerin before eating, if it brings on angina.
- If three normal-sized meals incite angina, try six small meals instead.
- Drink plenty of fluids. Dehydration will thicken the blood stream and contribute to angina. Fluids will also prevent strain from constipation.
- Avoid gas-forming food in quantity. Common culprits can be cabbage, melon, grapes, carbonated beverages, onions, radishes, and of course dried beans and legumes.
- Find out if local restaurants and food stores deliver, for the bad days.
- Avoid alcohol, especially if nitroglycerin is part of the angina-control program. Any alcohol in the blood stream will combine with the drug and cause a drop in blood pressure.

4. Nitroglycerin

The drug nitroglycerin is not "just for emergencies," it is for routine daily use. Nitroglycerin must be used whenever pain and other anginal symptoms act up. Remember, anginal pain means ischemia, and that can damage the heart. Give the older person the following information.

- Never keep going with an activity despite the pain. Stoicism is not a virtue in angina control, it's complete folly.
- Sit down while taking pills, and stay sitting down for a few minutes after the angina has gone away. The medication causes a drop in blood pressure, and older people are especially prone to lightheadedness if they get up too soon after taking the medication.
- Nitroglycerin causes headaches in some people, especially when they first take it. Call the doctor if headaches become pronounced. The doctor can lower the dosage and offer suggestions for headache relief.
- Wet the tablet with saliva before putting it under the tongue; it will dissolve faster.
- Nitroglycerin causes a tingly sensation under the tongue. If the tingling is not there, the pill may have become stale and weak.
- Ask the doctor how often each refilling of the prescription can last before tablets lose their strength. An opened bottle — stored and handled correctly — should last six months at most.
- Tablets must be kept in the dark-tinted bottle in a dry place. They're very sensitive to heat, light, and air. Do not carry in a pocket next to the body, or in the car.

• Do not keep cotton in an opened bottle; it will absorb the nitroglycerin.

• Take a tablet just before starting an activity that you know is going to cause angina. For example, before tumbling with grandchildren, before climbing steps or an incline in the road, before clipping bushes, or before a meal.

• Call the doctor, if pain does not subside as easily as it did before. The dosage may need to be upped, or the pills may have lost their potency.

• If a skin rash from using patches necessitates a return to pills, ask the doctor for only a small supply at the start.

• Ask the doctor if a patch can be worn twelve hours a day instead of twenty-four. The twelve-hour rest period will reestablish sensitivity to the next day's nitroglycerin.

• Follow these hints for wearing patches: put the patch on a different part of the skin each time; make sure the skin is free of hair, rash, cuts, scars, or calluses; avoid skin folds, such as the elbow or under the breast; and put the patch on at the same time each day.

• Ask the doctor about prescribing nitroglycerin ointment instead of patches. Considerably cheaper than patches, ointment is a good choice for those on a tight budget. Cream may also be easier to use for those with arthritis who have difficulty dealing with the layers of packaging. Squeeze the prescribed amount of ointment onto the piece of special paper marked in inches. Apply the paper to the skin and tape it on.

• Anyone helping your parent apply ointment must be careful not to get it on his or her own skin. It must also be kept out of the way of small children, who might mistake it for hand cream or toothpaste.

The Angioplasty and Surgery Options

Two options are available for those who have coronary arteries plugged up with plaque to the *n*th degree. Angioplasty is a newer treatment that involves inserting a tiny inflatable balloon into one or more coronary arteries to squash the plaque. The coronary-bypass operation has been around since the early 1970s. Segments of a healthy blood vessel, usually a vein from the leg, are grafted onto the heart's surface to bypass the clogged areas of the coronary arteries.

Both these options are offered to elderly people who are deemed healthy enough to make it through surgery, and able to benefit from the results. The angioplasty or bypass surgery does not cure under-lying coronary artery disease, but in most people who have them, angina symptoms either go away completely or are relieved enough that the operation is worthwhile.

The decision to have angioplasty or surgery may be thrust upon your parent in the days, or sometimes hours, following a heart attack. The decision comes up less abruptly if anginal symptoms become obviously painful and difficult to live with, and if the doctor feels they may lead to a heart attack.

The Cardiac Catheterization Test

This procedure can give the cardiologist a very clear look at the heart and all points of blockage within the coronary arteries. But because the procedure is invasive, slightly risky, expensive (more than $5,000, including a night in the hospital), it is generally reserved for people who are surgical candidates, willing to have surgery if the test confirms they need it.

During the procedure, a thin and flexible plastic tube is inserted into a vein or artery in the groin or arm and threaded to the heart. The progression of the tube is followed by special x-ray equipment and shown on a television screen. A contrast die is injected through the catheter directly into the coronary arteries so that they can be picked up on film. During the cardiac catheterization, each artery is examined from two to five separate camera angles to completely evaluate all the coronary arteries, as well as their smallest visible branches. The plaque within can be visualized and measured on the film with calipers, or simply looked at by the experienced eye of the cardiologist doing the procedure. The course of blood flow can also be determined during the procedure.

Cardiac catheterization usually involves one to two hours for the procedure in a catheter laboratory, usually on the day of admission to the hospital. The procedure is not painful, although a small incision does have to be made at the catheter entry point in the skin. Most people report the worst part is thinking about the procedure before it starts, and having to lie still for a long time.

Angioplasty

This procedure, which squashes plaque against the walls of an artery with a tiny balloon, has several advantages over coronary-artery bypass surgery: it doesn't require opening the chest or general anesthesia. The recovery period is short, usually a day and an overnight stay in the hospital and two days of taking it easy at home. The cost is quite a bit less than for heart surgery.

The results of angioplasty are a dream come true for those who have special kinds of blockages amenable to it. These people are a testament to the miracle of modern medicine. They can go from experiencing the rigors of painful, persistent angina, to complete loss of symptoms as soon as the procedure is finished.

If you are not familiar with angioplasty you must be wondering why everyone with angina can't have it done early in the game. Why too does open-heart surgery ever have to be done? Certainly, angioplasty sounds like an ideal way out of coronary-artery disease, especially for an elderly person, who, simply by being elderly, may not be an ideal candidate for the rigors of surgery.

The answer to the first question is that angioplasty is not done on those who can manage their angina with medications, because it does carry some risk, as well as the possibility that the procedure will not work. Only when angina becomes difficult to manage with medications or really dangerous does the prospect of benefit from angioplasty outweigh its risk. Then most cardiologists will say, "Go ahead and try it. It may work, so that surgery can be avoided." Here's a rundown of the risks and benefits, based on studies done through the National Heart Blood and Lung Institute, for you to use in reaching a decision with the cardiologist:

- The chance of successfully passing the balloon through a blockage is higher than 80 percent.
- There is a 30 percent chance that the vessel will slowly close down on itself within six months, in which case symptoms will return.
- Even for the most experienced cardiologists, 5 percent of the angioplasty patients wind up having coronary-artery bypass surgery anyway, because the vessel being angioplastied closes off completely during the procedure. A surgical team is always on standby, just in case.

But beyond this emergency reason for coronary-bypass surgery, the operation is done — around 200,000 times in the United States each year — because not everyone with clogged arteries is a candidate for angioplasty.

The technique is neither technically feasible nor safe unless the lesions are soft enough (noncalcified) and in easy-to-reach places. The lesion (or lesions) to be angioplastied need to be on a reasonably straight part of a coronary artery, away from where it forks into another branch of itself, and it needs to be small enough to take pressure from the balloon. Angioplasty is rarely considered if a lesion is on the left main descending artery, which nourishes a large area of heart muscle. This major vessel is considered too important to put in jeopardy during the procedure, and those who have severe blockage here are encouraged to have surgery if they are fit enough to be candidates.

Bypass Surgery

For older people who want to enjoy more years of relatively healthy living, but who are dangerously set back by severely clogged coronary arteries — not amenable to angioplasty — the decision to choose or forgo coronary-bypass surgery is a tough one. The operation is open-heart surgery under general anesthesia, followed by a long recovery period. The decision is loaded with contingencies: What if I do? What if I don't?

The surgery is a big-time, high-risk procedure, especially for older people. The operation lasts from three to eight hours, depending on the patient's condition and how many vessels are grafted. While the most delicate part of the operation is performed, the heart is temporarily stopped and the circulation is maintained with a heart-lung pump machine. Once off the operating table and into the recovery room, there is still the danger of postoperative complications, including lung disorders, vein blockages, and even a heart attack. The person undergoing such a procedure will be far better off from the start with healthy blood vessels and lungs.

Middle-aged people who have the surgery usually stay in the hospital ten days, stay in the house about three weeks before they can carry on moderate activities, and need about three months before they can get back into the groove of full-time work and normal life. Older people usually have a longer recovery.

Older patients who might benefit from the surgery are not denied it because of age alone. At major medical centers across the country plenty of people in the seventies, eighties, and (rarely) nineties are operated on with successful results. But such people are selected carefully, depending on their state of health, and told that for them surgery is riskier than for younger people.

In discussing the risks to older people and their families, heart surgeons quote statistics from surveys of "all comers" to the surgery. For all comers the chance that they might die from the surgery is 1 to 2 percent and the chance of complications that would mean a longer hospital stay is 3 percent.

A recent study done through the Mayo Clinic in Rochester, Minnesota, now gives surgeons a good look at how a group of those over eighty do with the surgery. In the study, 159 people over eighty had bypass surgery after being selected because they did not have other diseases that made the risk of surgery unacceptable, such as severe cerebrovascular, lung, or kidney disease. Most of the octogenarians had excellent relief of their symptoms and went on to a "good" survival capability from future heart attacks. But 12 percent of the people in the study died probably as a result of the surgery, which is no surprise, considering their advanced age.

If your parent is a candidate for bypass surgery, make the decision very carefully, with a realistic understanding of what the surgery involves. You will find the surgeon quite clear in his or her opinions about whether surgery is a wise decision, and forthcoming about the risks. Bypass surgery is a very costly operation and the heart surgeons doing it are under close scrutiny from within their profession, as well as from the insurance groups footing the bills. Heart surgeons are an extremely well-trained group, perfectionists by nature, and not interested in taking on patients who might be likely to die as a result of surgery. Death statistics are a matter of public record in hospitals, and no good surgeon wants to take on patients who will up his operative mortality record.

In considering surgery, you need to meet with the cardiologist and discuss what medical management can offer, in place of surgery. Next, meet with the surgeon and go over the benefits of the surgery as opposed to the extensive risks. If you feel confounded by the whole business, or uncomfortable with either doctor's opinions, seek out second opinions. A cardiologist who is familiar with your parent's history and tests should be in charge of the case. The surgeon will be involved only for the operation and postoperative period.

The Heart-Attack Emergency

Minutes Count

When a heart attack occurs, the ability to recognize that one is oc-curring (see next section) and time are the most critical factors. Min-utes, even seconds, count. Most victims of heart attacks who die, do so within two hours of the onset. But life itself is not the only issue: when a vessel becomes completely blocked, its related heart muscle dies gradually over several hours, usually in four to six hours. Once in the hospital, prompt emergency care can dramatically reduce damage to the heart, so that the person may not only survive the attack but recover more easily.

Besides getting treatment to prevent sudden death from an ab-normal heart rhythm, another vital reason for a heart-attack victim to get to emergency room care *fast* is for thrombolytic therapy, sometimes called clot busting. It is now known that over 95 percent of heart attacks are caused by a clot that forms around a coronary artery, where an atherosclerotic piece of plaque has ruptured. Clot busting involves administering medication intravenously (i.v.), which can thwart and dissolve a clot.

The procedure began widespread use in the mid-1980s, and, as a revolutionary development, it has contributed significantly to the lowering of deaths from heart attacks, especially among people over seventy-five, the age group in which heart attacks are most prevalent and lethal. In a few communities where ambulance care is superbly organized, clot busting is even started in the ambulance during the rush to the hospital.

Although it is well known that a speedy trip toward treatment is essential, studies show that most people procrastinate, on the aver-age, two to three hours after the onset of symptoms before calling for an ambulance. It's very common for victims alone, or in concert with their family, to sit around waiting for their doctor to call back so that they can get the go-ahead to move to the hospital. People also stall while determining whether the heart attack-like symptoms are getting better or worse. Another delay that is just about standard is the heart-attack victim's denying that what's going on is really as serious as a heart attack. Add denial to the list of heart-attack warn-ing signs. If your strong-willed parent, spouse, or friend doesn't want you to call an ambulance, call one anyway.

Heart Attack Signs

To be safe, not sorry, you must know the usual warning signs of a heart attack, and also the "typically atypical" signs that older people sometimes experience. Doctors familiar with the very old (eighty-five plus) say about half of them do not experience heart attacks with classic symptoms.

"Typically atypical" symptoms in the elderly usually occur as isolated symptoms, with no chest pain at all. Sudden breathlessness, passing out completely and coming to, sudden confusion, and for a diabetic individual a sudden, high rise in blood sugar, may all be signs of a heart attack in progress.

The classic symptoms most commonly associated with a heart attack may or may not occur in an elderly individual. They include: an uncomfortable pressure, tightness, heaviness, squeezing, burning feeling or pain (often extreme, but not always), usually felt in the center of the chest, upper part of the stomach, arms, throat, neck, jaw, or middle of the back between the shoulder blades. Other symptoms include sweating, nausea, vomiting, shortness of breath, feeling weak, and feeling faint.

Those who have had typical angina for some time usually can tell the difference in degree between anginal pains and those of a heart attack in progress. Usually their pain is more intense, and, as you know, it is not relieved by nitroglycerin. One man we interviewed for this book told us, "Of course I was having a heart attack, I felt like an elephant was stepping on my chest. My angina was different, like a balloon swelling up inside me."

Know What to Do Before the Emergency

If a heart attack does occur, you don't want to waste time deciding which ambulance service to call, or which hospital to direct it to. Be prepared by taking these steps:

- Ask your doctor which nearby hospital to go to. It should have twenty-four-hour emergency cardiac care.
- Find the telephone number of the best ambulance service(s) that goes to this hospital. Ask the doctor for this information.
- Keep a list of emergency rescue services next to the telephone, or stuck to the phone, and in your parent's pocket, wallet, or purse.
- Consider taking a cardiopulmonary resuscitation (CPR) life-

saving course in mouth-to-mouth breathing and chest compression.

RED ALERT: What to Do Before the Ambulance Comes
- Call the ambulance first.
- Make sure the person suffering the heart attack is kept calm and still. Activity and excitement will put the stress of increased oxygen demand on the heart.
- Loosen clothing and let the person choose the best position for breathing — usually sitting up.
- If the victim accepts it, apply a wet cloth to the head.
- Be kind and reassuring. Advise the person that medical help is on the way.

CONGESTIVE HEART FAILURE

Heart failure means the heart isn't pumping blood through the circulation as well as it should, because the heart muscle is damaged. The damage can come from a heart attack, atherosclerosis, lung disease, untreated high blood pressure, or valvular problems. With blood flow slowed in the damaged heart, blood flow either backs up into the lungs, or is slowed down and backed up in the veins, causing fluid congestion in the tissues.

In the days before much was known about the condition, it was called "dropsy." Back then, people would suffer terrible fatigue and the weighty discomfort of swelling throughout the body. The disease is referred to in literature and paintings dating back to ancient times, with old people often shown propped up in bed with pillows so that they could breathe more easily. Today, early recognition of symptoms, prompt treatment with medications, and appropriate changes in lifestyle can give the person with heart failure a more nearly normal life.

People who have underlying heart or lung disease usually are carefully watched by their doctors, who look for signs of heart failure at every checkup. If high blood pressure or a heart condition is under treatment, prevention of heart failure becomes part of the plan. The earlier congestive heart failure is diagnosed, the better the outlook.

Symptoms to Watch For

Heart failure usually comes on gradually, although sometimes it can strike out of the blue as a sign that the heart is undergoing drastic changes. It can develop during illnesses with fever — as the heart pumps harder to cool the body down — in anemia, during overexertion, and if someone susceptible to heart failure has a particularly rough day with anginal symptoms.

Symptoms generally depend on which side of the heart is damaged, unless both sides are damaged, as they often are if the disease progresses. Left-sided heart failure is more common at the start of the disease as residual blood backs up in the left chamber of the heart, rather than shooting forcefully forward into the aorta, the main blood vessel carrying newly oxygenated blood from the lungs to the tissues. Right-sided heart failure occurs when the heart is not well able to receive blood coming into it, on its way to the lungs for oxygenation. The veins then first expand to hold the extra fluid backed up in the circulation. Soon, however, the legs swell, and swelling may appear in and around the liver.

If the person you are caring for has heart disease, be on the lookout for these symptoms so that you can alert the doctor. Your parent, spouse, or friend may notice:

- Fatigue.
- Shortness of breath, all the time or with exertion, as a sign of fluid in the lungs.
- A dry, hacking cough, also a sign of fluid in the lungs. Wheezing may be present, too.
- Trouble sleeping unless propped up on two or more pillows.
- Waking up at night suddenly with feelings of suffocation.
- A sudden weight gain (two to four pounds in one to four days).
- Tenderness over the abdomen and clothes not fitting properly at the waist.
- Swelling in the legs or ankles or arms.
- Rapid heartbeat.

Drug Treatment

The doctor will do a physical assessment to determine what heart problems are causing the circulatory difficulties. Most cardiologists order an echocardiogram to look for evidence of such causes and to find out how the heart has been changed under the strain of circulatory overload and the backing up of blood.

Medications, the mainstay of treatment, need to be selected according to an individual's heart condition. They are designed to complement each other and to reverse the body's tendency to compensate for fluid overload. Four types of medications are usually prescribed to treat congestive heart failure:

- Digitalis is a time-honored drug for the condition; it strengthens the heartbeat so that more blood is pumped with each beat.
- Diuretics, or water pills, help the kidneys rid the body of excess fluid. As salt and water are taken from the blood stream with diuretic usage, less excess blood remains for the heart to pump.
- Potassium supplements are usually prescribed as an adjunct to diuretics, which leach potassium from the body. If the individual develops low potassium, the danger arises that digitalis will cause heartbeat arrhythmias.
- Vasodilators, usually prescribed for high blood pressure, help relax the blood vessels. Relaxed vessels help the heart pump blood more easily and gently. Usually an ACE inhibitor, which blocks a hormone that raises blood pressure, is prescribed. This medication lowers blood pressure and also controls salt and fluid accumulation in the blood stream. Recent studies show that the combination of digitalis, diuretics, and ACE inhibitors prolong the lifespan of those who have severe congestive heart failure.

Helpful Tips for Controlling Congestive Heart Failure

Taking medications correctly is essential in controlling fluid buildup. But plenty of other self-help measures will also reduce demands on the heart. First we cover such measures for your relative or friend to follow, then provide tips on taking medication.

Ways of Improving Heart Function
- Talk to the doctor about an appropriate activity schedule. The extent of physical activity allowed must be adjusted to the older person's symptoms and level of heart failure.

• Ask the doctor to recommend a daily program of walking.

• Plan rest periods throughout the day.

• Plan a nap after lunch, short enough so that it does not interfere with sleep at night.

• If swelling starts, put the feet up for a few minutes while sitting upright in a chair.

• If chest congestion is chronic, sleep upright in bed against pillows. Of course, the congestion must already have been reported to the doctor and must be under medical treatment.

• Avoid extremes of temperature. The heart works harder in a heated or chilled body.

• Avoid garters, kneehighs, or tightwaisted hose: they slow the flow of blood.

• Ask the doctor to recommend special elastic stockings to keep blood moving rapidly in the legs.

• If heaviness is a problem, ask the doctor to recommend a weight-loss program. The heart beats less hard to send blood through a thinner body.

• Limit high-sodium foods. Very important. Excess sodium makes the body hold on to fluid.

• Ask the doctor to recommend a level of sodium restriction.

Medications

• Be sure to talk to the doctor about how to recognize signs of digitalis toxicity. The difference between an effective dose and a toxic dose is very narrow. Toxic effects can cause life-threatening heart arrhythmias and lowered heartbeat.

• Meet all appointments with the doctor during the first few weeks after digitalis has been started. Blood tests on digitalis and potassium levels in the blood stream need to be done within a week, then two weeks, a month, and every six months thereafter.

• Feeling better or free of symptoms is no excuse for missing these appointments.

• Be alert for signs of digitalis toxicity. They include loss of appetite, bad taste in the mouth, nausea or vomiting, seeing green or yellow halos around objects, confusion, skipped heartbeats, palpitations, and rapid breathing.

• If toxicity is obvious, hold back on the next dose of digitalis, and call the doctor immediately.

• Take digitalis at the same time every day.

• Take a wrist pulse every time before taking digitalis. If it is under 60 beats per minute, or greater than 110 beats per minute, withhold the next dose and call the doctor. If the pulse is hard to find, unsteady, or changed from its typical pattern, call the doctor.

• If a dose is forgotten and skipped, take digitalis within twelve hours of its usual time, and take the next dose next day at the usual time. *Never* double a dose.

• Call the doctor if a dose is forgotten for two or more days in a row.

• If digitalis is given after an acute episode of congestive heart failure, ask the doctor if the dosage can be lowered or discontinued once the congestive heart failure has been dramatically reduced.

• Never discontinue the drug without the doctor's recommendation. Doing so can be extremely dangerous.

• Never take other medications — over-the-counter or prescription — without consulting the doctor. Digitalis is highly sensitive to the effects of other medications.

• Store digitalis safely. It is the drug that most often causes accidental poisoning, because the pills are white and easily confused with other medications such as aspirin and vitamin pills. A good idea is to put a bright-red heart sticker on the bottle (buy a pack of stickers at a stationery store or drugstore).

• One unusual side effect of ACE inhibitors is their ability to cause a dry, hacking cough. This symptom needs to be distinguished from a cough caused by heart failure.

• Keep digitalis completely out of small children's reach. Do not keep it in a purse, in drawers, or in accessible medicine cabinets when kids are around. The drug is a major cause of accidental poisoning in children, some of whom die of heart arrhythmias.

• Increase potassium-rich foods in the diet to replace potassium leached from the body by diuretics. Some people are able to keep potassium levels high enough from food sources.

• Call the doctor if a diarrhea-producing illness occurs. It can cause a large loss of potassium and the potential for digitalis toxicity, because the body needs potassium for digitalis to work correctly.

• If an ACE inhibitor is prescribed, meet *all* appointments with the doctor. Within a month, or other interval designated by the doctor, tests need to be done to check the blood count and potassium levels.

PERIPHERAL VASCULAR DISEASE

Atherosclerosis is a systemic disease that rarely manifests itself in just one part of the body. Many people who have heart disease caused by atherosclerosis also develop peripheral vascular disease, a condition in which the arteries of the lower abdomen and legs become blocked with plaque.

Such blockage is not always felt. Some people can have blockage in several large vessels, but reasonably good circulation in surrounding vessels, which take over the job of perfusing the legs with a sufficient blood supply. It is not unusual for a doctor to feel an absence of pulse in the lower legs — a sure sign that blood is not flowing through with force — of someone who doesn't complain of painful symptoms in the calves or anywhere else in the legs.

But plenty of older people do have noticeable symptoms of peripheral vascular disease, and left untreated at this stage it can become debilitating. Those who have it severely find that just walking a few steps across the room is excruciatingly painful, for in a sense angina is occurring in the legs. Usually symptoms come on gradually, and come and go with activity. In the early stages of the disease it is easy for people to dismiss their symptoms.

The hallmark symptoms of peripheral vascular disease are aching or tiredness in the muscles of a leg, or cramping when walking, both of which are relieved completely with rest. The medical name for this affliction is intermittent claudication, and it is an almost certain sign of blocked arteries in the legs. Older people often call it the stop-and-go disease. You and the older person you are looking after need to recognize that foot fatigue and tired hips, as well as cold feet on warm days, may all be signs of peripheral vascular disease.

Walking Is the Best Treatment

If your parent goes to the doctor complaining of the symptoms of intermittent claudication, you may be surprised at the simplicity of the treatment — provided that the doctor determines the disease is not dangerously compromising the circulation. The treatment is a program of walking to develop the blood-vessel pathways around the blocked vessels. Studies show that most people who go on a regular program of walking can significantly improve their circulation.

Many who go to the doctor able to walk only half a block return several months later after a program of walking, well able to walk three blocks without having to stop and rest.

Most people with the problem expect they will need to go on some form of medication. Walking just seems too easy a treatment. But in fact a walking program usually works, though medications don't. Any good vascular specialist will tell you that despite the drug-company claims, the vessels in the legs are not usually amenable to medications, at least when it comes to treating intermittent claudication. The vessels in the leg become very rigid in atherosclerosis, and no nitroglycerinlike drug is available.

When your relative or friend is put on an exercise program, do all you can to encourage it. Symptoms of peripheral vascular disease are more likely to become progressively worse if a walking program is not earnestly tackled.

Most people are told to take a simple walk at least three times a day, and to build up their tolerance gradually. Walking should be done at a steady pace until pain starts to really get distressing. It is not a good idea to walk in spite of excruciating pain, but experts say it is all right to walk through the beginnings of pain waves. Increased pain or excruciating discomfort should be reported to the doctor. Help the older person keep a daily log of progress. The information it provides will show progress, and it will be helpful to take it to the doctor at every visit.

Signs of Worsening Disease

Peripheral vascular disease can sometimes get worse, so that the tissues of the limbs are in danger of eventually being completely cut off from their blood supply, followed by gangrene. Usually the progression is gradual. Here are the signs of a limb heading toward gangrene; learn them and call the doctor if they occur.

- Pain occurs at rest, not just with walking.
- The limb feels particularly painful at night while flat on the bed.
- Pain seems to be relieved while the limb is dependent, with the foot pointing toward the floor. People with severe peripheral vascular disease often report that they have spent several nights sleeping in an armchair.

- The limb looks pale when elevated, and looks deeply red, almost purplish, when pointed toward the floor.

If surgery is indicated, your doctor will want your parent to have special tests from a vascular specialist, who may or may not be a surgeon. If surgery is recommended, the surgeon you select should have specialized training in vascular surgery.

RED ALERT: The Gangrene Emergency

Occasionally a small percentage of those who have peripheral vascular disease find their condition worsens because of sudden blockage in a leg artery — in a sense a heart attack of the legs. Just as for a heart attack, early treatment is needed to avert severe damage. A blockage takes from eight to twenty-four hours to create complete gangrene, which is tissue death. Those who ignore the early warning signs of a limb becoming gangrenous often end up having their affected limb amputated. If the problem is caught soon enough, surgery can be attempted to save the limb, either angioplasty or bypass graft surgery on the leg. Some lesions in easy-to-reach arteries can be treated with laser surgery.

Call for the doctor immediately if a sudden excruciating pain in the leg persists, or if the leg suddenly becomes cold and very pale and blue. If you can't reach the doctor within a few minutes, call an ambulance. While awaiting medical help, keep the leg pointing toward the floor, and do not apply heat or ice.

Tissue-Preserving Measures

Those who have circulatory problems in the legs need to follow the same kind of scrupulous foot care as diabetics (see Chapter 9). The feet need to be kept clean and dry and should be checked morning and night for signs of sores, cuts, and abrasions. A podiatrist or visiting registered nurse should cut the tocnails and examine the feet once a month. Pants are good to wear because they can protect the skin from injury. Report any signs of an open wound — no matter how small — to the doctor immediately. The doctor may want to start a course of antibiotics to help healing along if arterial blood flow is inadequate. Left untreated, a small wound can easily progress to one that is extremely slow and difficult to heal.

SLOW HEARTBEATS

Under normal conditions of rest, the heart beats 60 to 100 times a minute, carrying essential oxygen and nutrients throughout the body. The heart beats at a steady pace thanks to special kinds of heart cells that produce tiny electrical currents. If the cells become damaged, though, they can't do their job properly and an abnormally slow heartbeat, or a telltale rhythm of fast followed by slow beats can develop. Then the brain and the entire body receive insufficient blood supply, and one can experience symptoms such as fatigue, dizziness, and loss of consciousness.

Luckily for those who have unsteady or slow heartbeat, an extremely effective, lightweight device, the pacemaker, can be implanted in the chest. Pacemakers have saved hundreds of thousands of lives since their invention in the late 1960s, and have allowed people to resume their normal activities. Before pacemakers, many people with slow or irregular heartbeat were "cardiac cripples." Prone to fatigue and fainting spells, they had to give up driving, climbing stairs, and just about all strenuous activities.

Many elderly people benefit from pacemakers — the average age is seventy. Here is what you need to know so that the pacemaker can be worn safely and comfortably in the weeks after surgery, and in the years ahead.

Pacemaker Implantation

Pacemaker surgery is not considered a high-risk procedure, and the recovery is generally not at all unpleasant. The idea of having a device put inside the body and connected to the heart sounds much worse to most people than the reality proves to be. The surgery is usually done by a cardiologist or chest surgeon, using local anesthesia in an operating room, and takes from one to two hours. Most patients are asked to stay in the hospital for two days postoperatively so that medical personnel can check the incision as it heals, and verify that the pacemaker is effective.

To implant the pacemaker the surgeon makes a small incision underneath the collarbone. Through the incision tiny wires are slowly slid into a vein until they reach the heart, where they are directed and attached to the inner surface. The opposite ends of the wires are then connected to the pacemaker's electronic command center and power source, a small (about 2-ounce) rounded box, which is set in a pocket underneath the incision and close to the skin.

Compared to earlier models, today's pacemakers are well designed, extremely effective, and much smaller. The technology is now so sophisticated and sensitive that pacemakers can be programmed to "kick in" only when one's heart rate goes below a specified minimum. They can also be checked and reprogrammed from outside the body. In the past, pacemakers had to be readjusted or replaced in a surgical procedure.

Surgical Recuperation

Most people can resume their normal activities within four to six weeks after pacemaker surgery. But during the first month they must abide by definite restrictions in activities to ensure that the incision will heal properly, settling the pacemaker wires into their place within the heart. Strong fibrous tissue must build up around the wires where they are attached to the heart so that they cannot be dislodged.

If you're bringing a patient home after a pacemaker implantation, make sure before you leave the hospital that the person is given easily understood directions for general care of the incision. Specific advice an caring for the wound must come from the surgeon or nurse. We list here general advice that patients should be given before leaving the hospital.

• Call the doctor if signs of infection appear: the incision will be red or draining, hot to the touch or very tender, or if there is fever.

• Permit no lifting of anything heavy or arm exercises on the pacemaker side of the body, and no extreme stretching or bending of the upper body.

• A loose sling worn around the shoulder and arm on the pacemaker side of the body can serve as a reminder not to do any strenuous arm lifting or stretching. At the Johns Hopkins Hospital in Baltimore, patients are told to wear an arm sling on the operated side of the body for four weeks in daytime. The sling should allow for arm movement to the side and grasping. Ask the doctor about this option.

• Do not lift sweaters or buttonless shirts over the head with both arms. Slide the arm on the pacemaker side out of its sleeve, and use the opposite arm to pull the sweater over the head.

• A woman needs to slide bra straps down and slide the bra to her front to undo it.

• Do not sleep turned over on the pacemaker side of the body; body weight may impair healing.

• If no one can help with hair washing, it should be done using the arm on the unaffected side.

Pacemaker Checkups Are Essential

Your family member may at first feel insecure about wearing a mechanical device involved with the heart's pumping action. This leeriness is quite normal; it takes time for just about everyone to trust their pacemaker and get rid of fear that the device will give out.

It would be *extremely* unusual for a mechanical pacemaker to stop working completely. In occasional rare circumstances it can slow down. If it does, though, the wearer's natural rhythm will take over sufficiently to give one time to call the doctor or go to an emergency room. Very few pacemaker patients depend on their pacemakers completely.

You and the older person wearing the pacemaker must understand that if it is checked correctly and periodically, the device will indeed be very effective and will last many years. A pacemaker designed to fire into one chamber of the heart can last up to fifteen years, with an average of seven years. A dual-chambered device can last up to nine years, with an average of five years.

Occasionally, pacemakers are faulty. A wire may not work correctly, or some problem may arise in the workings of the circuitry in the pacemaker box. So that potential problems can be picked up and corrected early, all pacemaker patients are told to have their device monitored regularly, according to the doctor's instructions. They are also instructed to report any recurring symptoms, such as those they experienced before the pacemaker was implanted.

Most pacemaker patients are told to have the device checked every three to four months, from the comfort of home, through a telephone checking service, and to have it checked at the doctor's office once a year. Most important, pacemaker wearers and their families are taught how to recognize, between checks, the physical signs that a pacemaker is failing. Failure is not common, but everyone in the family must be prepared to recognize and handle such incidents sensibly, just in case.

Telephone Checking

Telephone monitoring is a real boon, especially for older people who have trouble getting themselves back and forth to the doctor's office. Although most people wearing pacemakers can rely on this method, some doctors prefer to check their patients at the office or clinic, especially those who have a pacemaker that performs complex functions.

To facilitate Medicare payment in full, the doctor's office will have or order appropriate checking equipment, and arrange for a monitoring center to check the older person's pacemaker. Most pacemaker patients receive their monitoring equipment through the mail, although some doctors provide the equipment at their offices, so that its use can be taught at first hand.

Most people have no difficulty setting up the equipment at home, following written instructions and supplementary directions from the doctor. If you're having trouble, though, do ask the doctor to arrange for instructions to be given either at the office or by a visiting nurse. The equipment consists of a special transmitter box into which the telephone receiver fits, and a magnet connected to the box, which is held over the pacemaker.

The older person, or you, will need to make regular appointments to call a receiving center for pacemaker checking. Do make sure that appointments are met; they take only a few minutes. If the technician doing the checking decides that the pacing system is not working as it should, someone at the center will contact the older person's doctor right away.

Self-Monitoring

Before you leave the hospital a nurse will show you how to take a pulse. A pulse equals a heartbeat, whether it comes from the heart's own pacemaker cells or from an artificial pacemaker device. Knowing how to take a pulse is vital so that the older person, you, and other caregivers can measure whether or not the pulse rate has dropped below, or is too high above, the rate for which the pacemaker is set.

If your parent, spouse, or friend experiences any return of symptoms felt before the pacemaker was inserted — such as fatigue and dizziness — the pulse must be checked. Although the required rate varies among patients, most pacemakers are set at rates above 60 beats per minute. If the pulse drops below this level, or above the

Tips for Pacemaker Safety

Questions about pacemaker safety can be confusing. Here are some basic tips to follow.

• Get written confirmation from the doctor of how many beats per minute the pacemaker is set for so that self-monitoring can be done at home.

• Get specific written instructions telling everyone in the family when to call the doctor and when to call an ambulance. You need a list including symptoms to look out for, the pulse rate that is considered too low, and the pulse that is considered too high.

• Ask your relative or friend to always carry a pacemaker identification (ID) card. This card is handed to patients before they leave the hospital and lists basic information about the type, model, and manufacturer of the pacemaker, as well as the name and telephone number of the doctor in charge of the pacemaker. The card can help medical personnel make decisions in case of serious illness, an accident, or a pacemaker malfunction.

• Although it rarely happens, the pacemaker box can slowly and painlessly erode through to the skin surface. If this erosion is caught early, the pacemaker can be repositioned in a minor surgical procedure. If the device is left to erode through the skin, however, a new pacemaker has to be implanted. Report any skin discoloration or any showing of the pacemaker's outline to the doctor. Also report any signs of infection, redness, puffiness, discomfort, or pain.

• Ask the doctor about any necessary precautions around high-voltage electrical equipment. Today's pacemakers are well shielded against interference from microwave ovens and most home and garden appliances, hair driers, electric shavers, vacuum cleaners, lawn mowers, and so on. Precautions do need to be taken around high-powered electrical equipment, found in industrial areas, and for some medical diagnoses and treatments.

• Always inform medical personnel who are not familiar with your relative's medical history about the pacemaker.

• The dentist should be told about the pacemaker before starting dental procedures so that an x-ray shield blanket can be worn over the chest during use of electric-powered equipment.

level the doctor has told you is safe, you must call the doctor immediately. Of course, if the older person blacks out completely, you must call an ambulance. Certainly too, if he or she experiences unusual fatigue and dizziness with or without a change in pulse rate, call the internist or general practitioner to discuss what your course of action should be.

Pulse taking becomes a valuable technique to use when illness comes, such as a cold or the flu. It is well known among pacemaker specialists that their patients often blame symptoms of illness on a malfunctioning pacemaker. A simple pulse check every day during illness can reassure the wearer that the pacemaker is working properly.

STROKE

A stroke is an event similar to a heart attack, but it is the brain and not the heart that becomes damaged. In a stroke a part of the brain is suddenly cut off from its blood supply because an artery supplying an area of the brain becomes clogged up, or the vessel tears and leaks blood.

If a tiny vessel goes wrong, then only a few brain cells lose their blood supply and the damage isn't noticed. But if a larger blood vessel — with many smaller vessels branching from it — has a stroke, then thousands of brain cells will start to lose their function. When many thousands of cells suddenly stop sending messages to each other and to areas of the body that they control, these parts of the mind and body can suddenly stop working.

Most strokes diminish the brain's control of the body's nerves and muscles, bringing on a feeling of lost sensation, weakness, or paralysis on just one side of the body. Also, they frequently leave people with emotional problems — swings in mood, with crying and laughing at seemingly inappropriate times.

Because a stroke can strike any part of the brain and in any size of blood vessel, the effects will be very different from person to person. More massive strokes usually affect a combination of functions at once, but milder strokes can knock out just one important function, such as use of an arm or a leg. One stroke may affect one's ability to swallow food and to see properly. Another, though, may influence speech and the ability to read and write, as well as memory. Some strokes also block one's ability to urinate and defecate.

Fewer Strokes Are Proving Fatal

About one third of stroke victims don't survive the initial stroke, making it the third leading cause of death in our country. Even though stroke is still up there next to heart disease and cancer, things are improving dramatically and the number of fatalities from stroke has been cut in half over the past two decades.

It seems that elderly people are having as many strokes as ever, but in easier-to-treat, milder, less debilitating forms. American Heart Association doctors attribute this changed picture to vast improvements in medical treatment and to the healthier habits that large numbers of people are practicing, among them follow-through on high blood-pressure checks and treatments.

Strokes mainly affect elderly people, because age brings on more of the advanced forms of heart and blood-vessel disease that cause them. A stroke is rare before age sixty, and when one does happen, it is often a complication of being born with a heart abnormality. They are commoner in men than in women and more frequent among black people than white people, probably because many more black people have high blood pressure.

Untreated high blood pressure is the most important cause of stroke. Having diabetes or a high red-blood-cell count are also risk factors. So too is a diseased heart, which becomes a source of clots that can travel to the brain. The person who has had a first stroke is also at high risk of having another.

What Goes Wrong?

As with heart attacks, most strokes are a result of atherosclerosis, or the buildup of plaque within the arteries. As we have mentioned, not all strokes are caused by blockage of the arteries, however. Some are hemorrhagic strokes, which occur when a defective artery within the brain bursts. Let's look at the four common causes of stroke and how they manifest themselves.

Cerebral thrombosis. The most common form, the thrombotic accounts for 70 to 80 percent of strokes. They usually occur at night or first thing in the morning, when a blood clot congeals on the walls of an artery that is already built up with fatty deposits or plaque. This kind of stroke is very often preceded by ministrokes or TIAs, which are strokes that last fewer than twenty-four hours.

Cerebral embolism. From 5 to 14 percent of strokes are precipitated by an embolism — a wandering clot of blood, or a globule of fat, or even an air bubble that originates outside of the brain. It travels to the brain and gets stuck in an artery. Most emboli causing strokes are blood clots. The commonest cause of such strokes is the heartbeat disorder called atrial fibrillation.

Hemorrhagic stroke. Bleeding into the brain from a ruptured artery accounts for about 17 percent of strokes. This form is the most dangerous, and people who have one are likely to die within twenty-four hours. When the hemorrhage occurs on the surface of the brain between the brain and the skull, it is a subarachnoid hemorrhage. When the hemorrhage occurs deep within the brain it is caused by an aneurysm, which is a blood-filled pouch that balloons out from a weak spot in an artery wall.

TIAs Are a Warning Sign

Most serious and damaging kinds of stroke usually come on suddenly and take their sufferers completely by surprise. But about 10 percent of such strokes are preceded by warning strokes called transient ischemic attacks (TIAs) that can occur days, weeks, or even months before a major catastrophic stroke. It is likely that small emboli arise from areas of damage in the arteries of the neck and travel through the brain, breaking up before any permanent damage is done.

A TIA occurs as a temporary stroke, usually for less than five minutes. The average is about one minute, although some can last several hours. When they occur several times they are very strong predictors of a major stroke. Like earthquake predictors, they are more useful for telling that the event will occur than when it will come. Often elderly people and their families ignore TIAs because their immediate consequences are brief.

But don't allow an older person to ignore TIAs. They merit prompt medical attention that can prevent a fatal or disabling stroke. The doctor can treat the underlying conditions causing TIAs with medications, sometimes with surgery. If you think the older person you are caring for has had a TIA, call the doctor immediately and insist on an evaluation of the trouble as soon as possible.

The symptoms of a TIA are very similar to those of a full-fledged stroke in progress. The difference is that the older person will have the symptoms and then say something like, "that's funny, I couldn't see for a while out of one eye," or "my arm felt completely numb last night for a few minutes," or "I was speaking on the phone and I had to hang up because my lip drooped and my speech got slurred." Sudden dizziness, confusion of thoughts, and a sudden fall are also signs of a TIA.

Signs of a Major Stroke

Most people who experience a stroke do not lose consciousness, nor do they usually feel pain, for the brain is not supplied with pain receptors. Later, if they recover, they usually can describe in vivid detail what it felt like to suddenly lose faculties and sensations. Hemorrhagic strokes can be painful, however, often causing a sufferer to grab his or her head suddenly and complain of an excruciating headache that feels very wrong.

Not uncommonly, an older person will wake up from sleep knowing that a stroke has occurred. About 18 to 20 percent of strokes happen during sleep. Otherwise, strokes can occur at any time, during any activity. If you realize the person you are caring for has had a stroke, call an ambulance. If the older person is wavering in and out of consciousness or has lost consciousness, turn him or her to the side to prevent the tongue from falling back, where it could block the airway.

According to the American Heart Association these are the warning signs of a stroke:

- Sudden weakness or numbness of the face, arm, and leg on one side of the body.
- Loss of speech, or trouble talking or understanding speech.
- Dimness or loss of vision, particularly in one eye.
- Unexplained dizziness, unsteadiness, or sudden falls.

The Wait-and-See Period

The first few days after a stroke are a time of anxious waiting, and only time will tell how much permanent damage has been done. In a major stroke — when one side of the body is totally paralyzed, or profound loss has struck several mental functions — the prognosis is not usually good for full recovery. Many stroke patients experiencing milder symptoms do recover fairly quickly, however, getting back to their full potential or close to it within a few weeks. For others, recovery means a slow and dragged-on relearning of lost functions and learning of new ways of coping.

Although you must be realistic, you also need to be optimistic. The person who has not quickly regained or started to regain functions within a few days needs an enormous amount of support during the hard work of rehabilitation. It's possible for extensively paralyzed stroke victims to revive a surprising proportion of lost capacities so that they can eventually return home from a hospital or rehabilitation center. Most stroke victims who are supported by good rehabilitation with professionals and with their families do usually get better in time, until they reach a plateau, usually within three to six months.

Recovery depends on the amount of brain damage, the patient's attitude and stamina, and the quality of support he or she gets from the professionals who run the rehabilitation. Your role as a family is also of utmost importance. Only you and other family members and friends can let the person you love know that it's worth plugging away at getting better, during the weeks after the initial stroke.

Treatment of the Acute Phase

Right after the older person comes into the hospital, he or she should be evaluated by a neurologist experienced in the vagaries of stroke management. The goal is to determine the location of the damage in the brain and the extent of the damage, as shown by evolving symptoms. A computer-aided tomography (CAT) scan should be done, photographing the brain. The scan is helpful because it shows if a brain tumor caused an apparent stroke, or whether there has been a hemorrhage. It also can show the area of the brain that has been damaged (the infarct).

Once the neurologist has determined the kind of stroke that has occurred, medical treatment can begin. The patient may be given medications — anticoagulants or blood thinners for a thrombotic stroke and drugs to lower blood pressure and encourage blood clotting for a hemorrhagic stroke. During the first three days following a stroke — the acute phase — the brain starts to swell. During this phase the patient is kept quiet on complete bed rest. If the danger is grave, the patient is put in intensive care.

During the acute phase, while the brain is swelling, further damage is threatened. This is the hardest time because it determines whether or not the patient will recover. Speech disturbances, mental confusion, and paralysis may improve for a day and then become worse. Some stroke victims rally during this time — to their joy and that of their families — and others become obviously worse, or slip into coma or death.

An experienced neurologist will be able to tell you whether you can probably expect improvement or whether you will just have to wait the acute time out. Frustrating as it is, no neurologist can give easy answers, unless the stroke clearly looks like a mild one.

What You *Must* Know About Rehabilitation

Rehabilitation Needs to Begin Right Away!

Once the immediate crisis of a stroke is resolved, for better or worse, the medical treatment ends and the rehabilitation begins. Most doctors who treat stroke medically do not have training in stroke rehabilitation, a specialty in itself, and so turn their stroke patients over to the care of physiatrists, physiotherapists, speech therapists, and others specially trained to help those who have experienced sudden damage to the nervous system.

In the past few years, many major medical centers and community hospitals have opened rehabilitation floors. Medicaid and Medicare will pay for in-hospital care of stroke patients — if it is restorative — for weeks, even months. Hospitals now see keeping stroke patients around as a profit-making advantage, rather than referring them out to rehabilitation institutes. Doctors working out of hospitals without specialized rehabilitation refer their stroke patients to other locations, or to home health agencies that are equipped to send specialized personnel into the homes of stroke victims who are able to go home following hospital discharge.

Any good doctor caring for a stroke patient will arrange for rehabilitation to start in the hospital as soon as the patient has "cooled out" from the stroke. Rehabilitation is crucial to someone getting better, rather than worse, from the consequences of a stroke. Early measures, such as turning the person in bed frequently and exercising paralyzed muscles, can be started in bed by the nursing staff. The nursing staff can also assist and encourage the patient to do as much as possible on his or her own, whether it is walking, eating, dressing, or using the toilet.

In a well-run hospital, rehabilitation staff are sent to see stroke patients as soon as their critical care is over. The staff then work as a team with the patient, the nurses, and the patient's family. Rather than looking at the stroke as a medical problem to be tracked down and treated, the rehabilitation team analyzes the damage done to the patient's physical and mental functions.

The goal of rehabilitation is to restore as many functions as can be, so that the patient can lead the most productive and independent life possible. Rehabilitation may mean teaching the patient how to walk again, regain bladder control, speak more clearly, regain balance, or write. It also involves teaching the family how to help in the rehabilitation and giving them a realistic understanding about how to plan for the future, when their relative gets beyond the rehabilitation stage.

If you find that your parent is left to lie in bed in the hospital with no signs that anyone is starting a program of rehabilitation, consider changing hospitals as soon as you can. Although most hospitals do an excellent job at providing stroke patients with appropriate care, there are exceptions. Your parent could end up neglected. Call the local chapter of the American Heart Association and they will put someone on the line who can tell you about the kind of care you should expect and where you can find it locally.

If you're having trouble arranging a transfer, contact the hospital's patient representative or patient services department for advice. If no one in the hospital is being helpful, contact the County Medical Society.

Who's Who on the Rehabilitation Team

Major medical centers and community hospitals (those equipped to rehabilitate stroke patients) will have on staff the experts listed here. During rehabilitation your parent is entitled to their services.

Physiatrist. A doctor who has studied rehabilitation medicine and taken exams in the specialty for certification, the physiatrist directs the medical aspects of rehabilitation care and prescribes treatments.

Psychiatrist or psychologist. Stroke patients often lose control of their emotions, crying or laughing inappropriately or expressing anger. This behavior can be a direct result of damage done to the brain, or of a depression in reaction to the disaster of the stroke. A psychiatrist or psychologist experienced with stroke patients will be able to diagnose the source of the behavior and recommend ways of treating it.

Physical therapist. Therapists work with a stroke patient's muscles and joints, usually of the hips, legs, and feet. The therapy consists of special exercises to prevent muscles from stiffening up or wasting, or to restore lost functions. The therapist also assists patients with walking, whether alone or with assistive devices, and can be very helpful in telling you about devices to order in advance for home use.

Occupational therapist. The occupational specialist teaches stroke patients how to relearn basic everyday tasks that are essential to independent living: how to dress, eat, prepare food, write, and draw. She can be a wealth of information about assistive devices — special eating utensils, writing gismos, dressing devices — and will know about all kinds of tricky ways of doing things so that they will get done somehow or other.

Speech therapist. Many patients need help to regain speech and communication skills or to make the best of the skills they have retained. The speech therapist can diagnose what is wrong with speech patterns and design a plan for treatment. She also explains to the family the whys and whats of the patient's speech impediments and how everyone can best communicate.

Social worker. An appointment with the social worker should be made as soon as possible, if it looks as if the recovery will be prolonged and difficult, or the stroke has caused extensive damage. The social worker can advise you about long-term planning and its cost. If necessary, she can help you find a place in a rehabilitation facility, or a nursing home, while you have time to look for a good one that is Medicare eligible.

Questions to Ask in the Hospital

Once you have settled down from the initial shock of your parent's stroke and made sure the sufferer knows you are there for support, our advice is that you try to read about the kind of stroke your parent has had. Many hospitals supply their own literature or publications by the American Heart Association and other groups. Stroke is a complex subject: you need to understand the dynamics of the one your parent has had so that you can participate in the rehabilitation and make plans for the future. If you can't get easy-to-read literature, then call the closest chapter of the American Heart Association for a packet of free information on stroke. Make sure it includes the excellent short book *Stroke: Why Do They Behave That Way?* It will clarify many of your parent's symptoms and how you can help improve his or her intellectual and behavioral functioning.

A stroke often hits a family without warning. Like most people you probably have only a cursory idea of what a stroke is and hardly any information about standards of care to expect from the hospital. The following questions will help you be an advocate for your parent. If they apply to your situation, use them to communicate with the doctor in charge and the nursing staff:

1. Will you tell us when our parent has passed the critical stage?
2. Do you have an idea about the extent of the damage that will be permanent? What advice can you give us about planning for our parent's care after hospitalization?
3. How do I meet with the social worker?
4. Will my parent need prolonged therapy? Any idea how long?
5. When will rehabilitation start? Who is in charge of rehabilitation? Will a physiotherapist see my parent? An occupational therapist? A speech therapist?
6. Can we meet and observe the rehabilitation specialists working with my parent?
7. Does the hospital have a stroke rehabilitation floor? If it does not, how do you recommend my parent get rehabilitation?
8. Can we be taught how to provide range-of-motion exercises in bed?
9. Why is my parent not being given range-of-motion exercises in bed? (If he or she is bedridden.) Why is she not being helped to move from bed?
10. Is my parent suffering emotional problems related to the stroke? Does she need to be seen by a psychiatrist?
11. Does my parent have any loss of bowel and bladder function? Do you expect this function to return? What is being done to restore bowel and bladder function? Has a program been started?
12. Why does my parent have a catheter now that the acute phase is over? (Left in for more than a few days, the catheter may interfere with normal reflexes and make recovery of bladder

control difficult or impossible to achieve. Catheters should be left in only if the patient has lost all control of bladder function. They should *never* be left in patients simply to keep the bed dry and nursing tasks simpler.)

13. Can we order a bedside commode, or have my parent put on a bedpan? If the staff expects "accidents," can we arrange for adult diapers to be worn? If the hospital will not supply adult diapers, can we bring in or purchase our own for the nurses to use?

Questions to Ask about Home Care

If your parent is being discharged from the hospital or from a rehabilitation facility, be sure you have answers to these next questions well before your parent goes home:

1. How can we best make arrangements to set up the house for safety and independent living?
2. What special equipment do we need to order?
3. Who will set up the equipment and teach the family how to use and care for it?
4. What medications is my parent taking? Can they be taken with the other medications he or she is already on? Can any medications be deleted from the drug regimen?
5. What do we need to know about physical care? Special exercises for joints and muscles? A program of bowel and bladder management? Deep-breathing exercises?
6. Will my parent need a special diet?
7. Is my parent eligible for Medicare-paid professional rehabilitation services through the Visiting Nurse Association or another home health-care agency?
8. Is my parent eligible for a home health aide paid for by Medicare funds? If not, do you advise we pay for an aide out of pocket?

11

Kidney and Bladder Problems Can Always Be Helped

KATHARINE JACKSON KNEW *from the acrid urine smell in the apartment why on the telephone her mother had seemed so unhappy and withdrawn for two months, and why a neighbor had written to say her mother hardly ever went out. Clearly, her mother was incontinent. Katharine found other telltale signs while her mother took a bath: towels were placed over the bottom sheet of the bed, the sofa was stained, and boxes of sanitary napkins were hidden at the back of the bedroom closet. "Mother, why didn't you tell me?" Katharine said tearfully while they made dinner. "I'm so ashamed," said Mrs. Jackson. "Besides, there's nothing anyone can do to help me and I didn't want to worry you."*

You have come to the chapter about urination difficulties, a subject still shrouded in darkness, ignorance, worry, and denial. The issue is often hard for families to deal with because embarrassment becomes a barrier to discussion and to working out ways of lessening problems, if not eliminate them entirely.

Urination problems, very common for older people, include difficulty in getting to the bathroom on time; having to "go" frequently; or for many like Mrs. Jackson, the burden of urinary incontinence that can range from the discomfort of slight urine leakages to the mortification of severe wetting. Even though these kinds of problems are prevalent, many older people, too embarrassed to inform their families or even doctors, seclude themselves because of worry and a sense of shame. Some give up their social contacts altogether, as well as outings to the supermarket, even visits to the doctor, rather than face the threat of accidents.

Untold and unnecessary suffering spoils life for too many older people, who could be helped if only they could put away their shame, seek the proper advice, and work with their doctor and their family. Research shows that only one in twelve people with incontinence seeks medical help — an appalling state of affairs — when incontinence is most often treatable.

If your mother or father, or anyone else you care about, is having trouble related to urination, understand that dignified solutions to every problem are available. Among these answers are: scheduling fluids and trips to the bathroom, eliminating medications that can irritate the bladder, giving medications at the right time, setting up the home to make the way to the bathroom easy, and seeking medical or surgical treatment if that is appropriate.

Millions of older people across the country are wearing adult diapers even though they've never sought medical attention for their bladder-control problems. You should encourage the person you are caring for to turn permanently to adult diapers only when all other alternatives have been diligently investigated and tried, under a medical specialist's supervision. Most people are not even aware that pleasanter and cheaper treatments for incontinence and alternative ways to manage it can be had.

The misconception that diapers are the only answer has been bolstered and encouraged in the past few years by the companies manufacturing them. Not only have adult diapers come out of the closet, they are also advertised extensively in magazines and newspapers and on television. Unfortunately, these advertisements prey on the public's ignorance about incontinence and the notion that nothing else can be done about it.

Please remember that every kind of problem related to urination, whether it is just irksome or serious enough to become a ruling force in one's life, has a cause and an appropriate treatment. We do not suggest that solutions are easy, for they often demand perseverance, efficiency, and organization. But they are there for those who want to know about them and apply them.

Breaking Through the Embarrassment Factor

As with Mrs. Jackson, the first sign that an older person is having difficulty controlling elimination is her beginning to stay home more, without divulging the reason. Many older people become obsessed with keeping their urinary problem secret, and they are difficult to help because they keep denying it's there. The great and devious lengths they can go to in hiding evidence can be masterful. Families can often mistake peculiar behavior, refusals to go out, and lack of participation in family activities as a sign of stubbornness, moodiness, and diehard independence.

If you have an inkling that your mother or father is suffering in silence with a urinary-tract problem, try different approaches to break through any wall of embarrassment. If you can involve your parent in a plan with which everyone in the family will help and persevere, the situation can be dignified so your mother or father can live a more normal life without fear of distressing situations. There are really no easy answers for us to give you, but to try and persevere.

First, realize that the older generation was brought up in a much more restrictive, puritanical time. For most, in their youth, talk about "bodily functions," especially elimination of urine or feces, was considered indecent. Acknowledge when you bring up the subject for the first time that you wholeheartedly recognize it is embarrassing, if not painful, to discuss. And make it clear that you are not passing judgment; you mention it because solutions to the problem can be found if the two of you seek them with a doctor's help.

Our society's attitude toward incontinence is another reason older people are often so difficult to help. Although this is a health problem profoundly disturbing life for millions of people, it may also be our last great taboo. In a time when the media delve into just about everything humanly possible, medical programs on television avoid the subject, as do women's magazines and newspaper lifestyle sections. And so far none of the major health societies has put on a national campaign to increase people's awareness of incontinence and how it can be helped. No wonder ignorance and denial of incontinence are rampant, and many older people are saddled with the mistaken notion that incontinence is normal with aging and that nothing can be done about it.

Even married couples can share a ban on the subject, always skirting it but ever aware of it. One partner, repelled by wet sheets during the night, may start to sleep in a separate room, but say nothing for fear of disgracing the other. Usually, though, when communication about incontinence is blocked, other communication breaks down too. Sadly, partners may stop being affectionate with each other, and the incontinent partner may be left at home alone for fear of "accidents." In this arrangement it is probably best to try communicating first with the person who has the problem, to help him or her seek treatment, and later to mention the subject to the partner, and to other family members if necessary. Talking behind the incontinent person's back, though, will only create paranoia and more shame.

One way to reduce an older person's embarrassment about the subject is to say, "You are one of 12 million Americans who have this health problem" and "In the over sixty-five age group, around 25 percent of men and 40 percent of women are troubled by incontinence in varying degrees of severity." Another approach is to explain that leakage is an honest-to-goodness symptom of a disorder that needs to be diagnosed and treated, and treated sooner rather than later because it may get worse. If the family simply finds it too difficult to confront an elderly relative reluctant to face reality, then make a call to enlist a doctor's help. Much easier said than done, for you have to make sure your doctor is sympathetic to this problem and knowledgeable about the diagnosis and treatment of urinary problems in the elderly.

Finding the Right Doctor

Another reason so few people seek help for urinary leakage has to do with doctors' attitudes. Doctors can be just as embarrassed by incontinence as anyone else, and quite a few would rather avoid the problem. A Harvard University Medical School study reported that when patients do mention incontinence, fewer than one in three physicians will initiate even the most rudimentary evaluation. Families trying to help an older relative cope with incontinence will often face a wall of embarrassment from their parent, only to come up against another obstacle in doctors who lack sympathy and knowledge of the subject.

The reasons for this abandonment are unpleasant. Many physicians have less than enough knowledge about geriatrics and consider incontinence an inevitable part of aging and an unfit subject for them to investigate. Overall, the subject has been neglected in medical schools, giving doctors in training little course work on managing incontinence, and leaving them to rely on stopgap measures such as catheters and diapers. Certainly in hospitals incontinence traditionally has been handled by the nursing staff, who are trained to teach patients practical methods for managing incontinence.

Even urologists, with years of specialized training in treating diseases of the kidneys and urinary tract, may not universally be interested in incontinence. Many find it uninteresting, and cumbersome to treat in their practice because so much time has to be spent talking and working with the patient to achieve a turnaround. Also, teaching patients how to help themselves is not a profitable business, Medicare and most insurance companies do not cover for teaching time, and many older people cannot afford frequent visits for the many hours of professional help they may need. Things are changing a bit as the population ages and doctors come to grips with the ever larger number of geriatric patients in their practice. A few medical schools are now offering courses on incontinence to students and doctors in practice.

All is not darkness and gloom: certainly some conscientious doctors make it their business to treat incontinence so that people can return to a life more nearly normal. It is your job to find one of these. If your usual doctor is obviously not qualified or interested in treating your mother or father, seek a doctor who is. Persevere and you will find one you like, who will achieve a cure or at least help manage the problem.

The ideal situation is for your doctor to refer you to a urologist, gynecologist, or family-practice doctor who provides specialized incontinence services, or to an incontinence clinic at a medical center close to home. Each year more board-certified urologists are taking an extra year of training in the field of incontinence control. Several teaching hospitals across the country offer such training programs, based on one that was started in 1980 at the University of California, Los Angeles, by Shlomo Raz, M.D. Otherwise your detective work is simply to call the nearest medical center or university hospital and ask if they have an incontinence clinic, or ask the secretary in the department of urology for names of doctors who treat incontinence.

If you have no success in getting to an expert, write to or telephone the organizations listed in the Appendix. All are excellent organizations, set up to help incontinent people understand treatment options and improve their lives.

Diagnostic Tests You Should Know About

The cornerstone of diagnosis is the patient's history. It is a good idea for anyone experiencing urination problems to go to the doctor's office with a record of his or her pattern of urination (see the urination record form on page 251). Just from clues in the record, the doctor may be able to spot the kind of problem.

At the initial visit, it is important that the incontinence specialist rule out the eight *reversible* causes of incontinence that will not require urodynamic testing or sophisticated treatment.* These causes can be remembered with the acronym DIAPPERS (with an extra P):

D Delirium due to acute medical illness such as pneumonia, heart attack, or heart failure.
I Infection of urinary tract.
A Atrophic urethritis and vaginitis that accompany menopause.
P Pharmaceutical causes:
　　Sedative hypnotics
　　Anticholinergics
　　Adrenergic agents
　　Calcium channel blocker
P Psychological causes, such as severe depression.
E Endocrine diseases that cause confusion and produce diuresis, hypercalcemia, or diabetic ketoacidosis.
R Restricted mobility.
S Stool impaction.

Before treatment is started a thorough urological workup is essential. The doctor should do a urinalysis in the office and a urine culture (results are back within forty-eight hours) to test for bacterial infection. Other tests can give the examiner valuable information about the underlying problem. These tests, which mimic the bladder's filling and emptying cycle, are part of a standard workup.

Urine-flow test. The patient is asked to urinate into a collection device that measures the amount of urine and the speed with which the bladder empties.

Cystometrogram. A narrow tube (catheter) is inserted into the bladder and the bladder is then filled with water or carbon dioxide.

---

* For this summary we are indebted to Neil Resnick, M.D., Harvard Medical School.

The person is asked to tell when the bladder feels full, when the urge to go is felt, and when he or she can't hold urine any more.

Cystogram. A catheter is inserted and the bladder is slowly filled with a dye to make the bladder visible; then an x-ray image is taken.

Daily Diary

The daily diary is a way for the older person and you as caregiver to participate in the diagnosis. After filling in the chart you will have a day-by-day record of daily problems in bladder control. The diary will help the doctor define the problem more clearly and provide a record of its progress.

Record for twenty-four hours a day:

Write U to record each time of urination
L to record each time of leakage
D to record each time fluids drunk

	DAY 1	DAY 2	DAY 3	DAY 4	DAY 5	DAY 6	DAY 7
6 A.M.							
7 A.M.							
8 A.M.							
9 A.M.							
10 A.M.							
11 A.M.							
12 N.							
1 P.M.							
2 P.M.							
3 P.M.							
4 P.M.							
5 P.M.							
6 P.M.							
7 P.M.							
8 P.M.							
9 P.M.							
10 P.M.							
11 P.M.							
12 M.							
1 A.M.							
2 A.M.							
3 A.M.							
4 A.M.							
5 A.M.							

Some Normal Kinds of Problems

Before we get started with practical advice about warding off incontinence and managing it if it does occur, you need an idea about how the urinary tract ages and the kinds of changes older people can expect. If your mother or father lives with you, the situations we describe will be familiar.

Why So Many Trips to the Bathroom?

Even by middle age we all make more frequent trips to the bathroom, and at night rudely wake up to the call of a full-feeling bladder if we have had a drink before going to bed. Ever so gradually, starting in middle age, the bladder begins to hold less urine. The capacity declines from two cupfuls at around age thirty to one cupful at around seventy, with perhaps even more reduction to come.

At the same time as the bladder loses ability to hold urine, the kidneys produce more of it as they age. Yes, more! An older person's urine is loaded with more water and less concentrated in proportion to the amounts of wastes it contains. The result: more trips to the bathroom, both day and night. This change happens because the kidneys lose up to a third of their millions of tiny filtering units — the nephrons and tubules — that concentrate urine while weighing how much water to send back into the blood stream. Also, the kidneys become less responsive to antidiuretic hormone or ADH, which regulates retention of water.

Very old people often become disturbed by the frequency of their urination. You need to explain that the change is normal. In their eighties some people probably set out for the bathroom twice as often as someone in early middle age. If you notice, however, that your mother or father changes the usual pattern of bathroom trips, be suspicious that a urinary-tract infection or other health problem is to blame. In this case, a visit to the doctor is needed as soon as possible to get the problem treated.

Older people all experience the annoyance of getting up in the night to urinate, sometimes two or three times, even after they have been careful to drink nothing after dinner, and even if they empty the bladder before going to bed. You may hear your mother or father trudge to the bathroom half an hour or so after falling asleep. Families who have to help their elderly members with toileting often become exasperated by having to get them out of bed again to urinate so soon after they have been tucked in.

This Jack-in-the-box behavior occurs because urine is made faster and more efficiently when we lie down. The artery supplying blood to the kidneys pumps faster in a prone or supine position and sends more blood through the system for filtration.

Falls are a big worry when a frail older person gets out of bed to urinate at night. Many elderly people experience their first broken bone while half asleep, heading for the bathroom.

You need to set things up to defend the older person against having a fall in the night. Besides putting night lights along the way, make every effort to arrange for the elderly person to sleep next to a bathroom. If this placement is not possible, purchase a bedside commode and place it close to the bed. Covered during the day with an attractive cloth, it can look like a piece of bedside furniture, or it can be hidden behind a decorative screen. Men can use a urinal placed by the bedside. Also, select nightgowns or pajamas that are easy to undo and take off; Velcro fasteners are by far the easiest to deal with in a hurry, and can be sewn into clothing to replace buttons and hooks.

Sleeping pills can cause an artificially deep sleep, masking the urge to urinate, and they can make one feel groggy and disoriented on the way to the bathroom. Sleeping pills and sedatives may well help the elder fall asleep, but they can be far more trouble than benefit. Our advice is to use sleeping pills occasionally at most — never routinely, and in the lowest effective doses.

Beware of Dehydration and Salt Overload

Because the aging urinary tract puts out a more watery urine, drinking enough water to keep the body in proper fluid balance matters more than ever. Older people are much more prone to dehydration, especially when ill with bouts of fluid-depleting diarrhea or vomiting. Many make the mistake of skimping on fluids in an attempt to go to the bathroom less. A big mistake, for the urinary tract needs its eight glasses a day to run smoothly and filter any wastes and substances, which can become toxic if left in the blood stream.

The aging kidneys filter wastes much more sluggishly than they did before, and salts, wastes, and medications can leave the body at a slower rate. The salt from a meal, for example, will take almost twice as long to leave the blood of an older person. We discuss this subject further in Chapter 13, "Managing Medications Safely." Medications need to be carefully juggled to be sure they are safely cleared by an older person's less-efficient kidneys.

Older people should be wary of too much salt. An overload of it in the blood stream causes water to be retained throughout the body, and holds back water that the kidneys need to filter other wastes from the body. Many older people have a heavy hand with the saltshaker and a strong desire for heavily salted food because their ability to taste salt may be out of order. This impaired ability to taste salt is now considered a normal aging change. The way to deal with bland-tasting food is to spice it up with lemon juice, herbs, and sauces containing small amounts of salt. More and more shakes of salt are the wrong way.

Urinary-Tract Infections Are More Common
The elderly are especially prone to bladder infections because of changes in the urinary tract that come with aging and their less-efficient immune systems. All older people need to take steps to prevent urinary-tract infections, and recognize the symptoms of an infection. Women usually get them more than men; the female urethra is much shorter than a male's, and germs have an easier time getting to a woman's bladder. (The urethra is the tube leading from the bladder to the outside of the body.) Infections can be a result of poor hygiene and too few baths or showers, but usually they start with bacteria growing in an inadequately emptied bladder.

At any age we all can prevent infections by practicing good hygiene, drinking plenty of fluids, and always trying to empty the bladder completely when we have the urge to urinate (normally every two to three hours). Sufficient fluids — about eight glasses a day — will trigger normal bladder emptying, if someone's nerve reflexes are intact, and also keep the urine diluted, acidic, and less hospitable to bacteria. A safe and pleasant way for an older person to ward off urinary-tract infections is to drink a glass of cranberry juice every day. It is one of the few fruit juices that does not change from its acid state to an alkaline one as it passes through the kidneys. Buy bottled or canned juice, not cranberry-juice cocktail, which is loaded with sugar and artificial ingredients. Not many supermarkets carry pure juice, and so you may have to buy it at a health-food store. Chill and sweeten it with an artificial sweetener, or mix it with apple juice if the taste seems too sour.

Usually symptoms of a urinary-tract infection are all too obvious. A full-grown colony of bacteria, invading the lining of the urethra and maybe the urine in the bladder, can cause such symptoms as frequent, painful urination, a feeling of warmth or burning during urination, itching, and perhaps foul-smelling urine. Another symptom may be urge incontinence, which involves having to go to the bathroom frequently, with difficulty in getting there in time.

Some old people can have a low-grade infection and be incontinent for weeks with no other symptoms. If an infection becomes severe, fever and chills may develop. If any symptoms occur, call the doctor and make an appointment so that a urine test can be done and antibiotics started. Do see that your mother or father takes the full course of antibiotics to be sure the infection is kicked out of the body. Don't allow him or her to stop just because the uncomfortable symptoms of an infection are gone.

Types of Incontinence and What Can Be Done About Them

Incontinence, the uncontrollable release of urine, is not a disease in itself. It is a symptom, either of an underlying disease or of a weakness in some aspect of the muscles supporting the urinary tract. The different kinds of incontinence have specific causes and treatments, although some people have a combination of types, complicating their treatment. Women are subject to incontinence more than men, but it is common in men, especially if they have a prostate condition. We next discuss the five kinds and the treatments available for them. By putting the subject in perspective, we hope to demystify it for you — it is a straightforward health problem.

> Stress incontinence
> Overflow incontinence
> Urge or gush incontinence
> Prostate-surgery incontinence
> Drug-induced incontinence

Stress Incontinence — Usually a Women's Problem
Stress incontinence, which has nothing to do with psychological stress, causes small bursts of urine to leak from the bladder when the abdominal muscles are stressed, as in lifting heavy objects, getting up

from a chair, exercising vigorously, or coughing, sneezing, or laughing. "Please don't make me laugh" is a familiar plea from those who have stress incontinence.

They usually make a habit of going to the bathroom frequently, for they leak urine more easily with a full bladder. Often they gush a small burst while getting up out of bed in the morning, as their abdominal muscles push against the bladder, usually full after several hours of sleep.

This type of incontinence occurs when the bladder has lost its support from the muscles of the pelvic floor. The weakened muscles cause the pelvic organs — the reproductive organs and the bladder — to slip from their original place into a lower position. In this downward position the bladder neck loosens and, if squeezed by the abdominal muscles, or jarred open as occurs when the person with stress incontinence moves vigorously, opens easily. People with stress incontinence also lose urine when sphincter muscles surrounding the urethra weaken. Normally the sphincter muscles can be controlled by thinking a command for them to contract and hold in urine, or relax to let urine out.

Stress incontinence is by far the most frequent kind of incontinence in women, especially those who have delivered several children, and it is predominantly a women's problem: six out of seven people with this type are female. Because men don't have a uterus and childbearing to support, the muscles holding their pelvic organs in position are rarely stressed and stretched. They can run into trouble with stress incontinence, though, after radical surgery for prostate or colon cancer.

Many women experience weakened pelvic muscles as production of estrogen hormone wanes after menopause. Alone or combined with other factors, this change can contribute to the problem. Estrogen in sufficient quantity keeps the muscles of the pelvic floor and the tissues of the urethra strong and in tone.

Both men and women can have stress incontinence caused by excessive weight, constipation, constant coughing (from smoking and chronic lung problems), nerve trouble with the lower back, or disruption resulting from abdominal surgery.

Surgery is the preferred treatment if the older woman can withstand it, but should be held off until exercises to strengthen the pelvic muscles, weight loss, medication, or other nonsurgical techniques are tried. (We'll spend more time on surgery later.)

Overflow Incontinence

People with overflow incontinence dribble small quantities of urine on and off all day, and when they do go to the bathroom their urine stream is weak. Small quantities of urine can leak with activities like coughing, lifting, and laughing, but this leakage, unlike that caused by stress incontinence, occurs even when the body is relaxed and at rest. Those with overflow incontinence never get the satisfaction of feeling they have completely emptied the bladder. The reason is clear: their bladder is never completely empty.

This type of incontinence occurs when the urethral tube leading from the bladder is narrowed by prolapsed organs, scar tissue, or an obstruction of some other kind, or because of a neurological problem. Elderly men with enlarged prostates that have been neglected are the ones who most often have the problem, although it is not uncommon among women. Because the bladder never gets an opportunity to empty, it gradually stretches larger and larger. Finally, all this stretching makes the muscular sphincter, at the bladder's outlet, too weak to hold back urine, and it has difficulty receiving conscious messages from the brain to stop and start the flow of urine. The result is uncontrollable dribbling of urine, the classic symptom of overflow incontinence.

Besides being terribly embarrassing, this is the most potentially dangerous type of incontinence. The urine trapped and pooled in the bladder frequently becomes infected, and left untreated can lead to a serious bladder or kidney infection, even one that could travel throughout the blood stream. In fact, often an older person's overflow incontinence will be diagnosed because a urinary-tract infection brings him or her to a doctor's attention. In severe cases of overflow incontinence the urine can back up out of the bladder into the kidneys to create an extremely dangerous medical crisis.

In the long list of causes behind this type of incontinence, some are temporary and easily treated, others more complicated but still treatable in some way. Conditions narrowing the urethra include prolapsed organs, prostate enlargement in men, urinary-tract infections, sexually transmitted diseases, tumors, and chronic use of medicines that constrict the urethra. Over-the-counter and prescription medications for cold and hay-fever symptoms, and many other medications as well, can cause urethral tightening. Another cause is self-induced: some elderly people hold their urine because getting to the bathroom is difficult, and their bladder becomes overstretched.

Treatment of overflow incontinence depends on the cause. If the urethra is obstructed by prolapsed pelvic structures, scar tissue, an enlarged prostate, or a tumor, then surgery may be the answer. In some cases medications can be used to relax the sphincter so that it opens and closes easily. Then, replacing medications that cause overflow with others that do the same job without that side effect is always a good idea. Urinary-tract infections can usually be treated with antibiotics. The person whose sphincter has some control left can benefit from bladder retraining, which may bring improvement and cure. Another technique that is proving helpful in managing overflow incontinence is self-catheterization, draining the bladder by inserting a small tube in the urethra at every attempt to urinate. More about these treatment options later.

Urge or Gush Incontinence
The most frequent incontinence among the elderly is said to be the urge or gush type. People with this disorder have an overly "sensitive bladder," and discover that each drink — water, coffee, cola, or alcohol — causes urination disproportionate to the amount they actually drink.

Besides having to go to the bathroom frequently, people with urge incontinence have difficulty getting there on time. Often they have only a few seconds from the first warning that the bladder is ready to "go" to the time it empties. The bladder does not have to be even close to full for the urge to be felt; sometimes just a few drops will stimulate bladder contractions and emptying.

Normally we can suppress the sensation of a full-feeling bladder and temporarily put the need to urinate out of our minds. With urge incontinence, however, the message to hold off on urination never makes it to the bladder because of damage or disruption to the nerve pathways running from brain to bladder. A number of conditions can cause such disruption, among them lasting diseases to which the elderly are prone, such as stroke, multiple sclerosis, Alzheimer's or other dementing illnesses, or Parkinson's disease. More short-lived causes include urinary-tract infections and the effects of multiple drugs. Sometimes the bladder becomes overly sensitive and quick to contract if prolapsed pelvic organs or an obstructed prostate puts pressure on it.

Surgery is not usually an option for this kind of incontinence because generally its origin is not structural but connected to the nervous system. The usual treatment consists of medications to relax the bladder, either alone or in conjunction with bladder-training techniques.

Prostate-Surgery Incontinence

Why Is Prostate Surgery So Common? The prostate is a walnut-size structure, present only in males, situated deep in the lower abdomen beneath the bladder and surrounding the outlet from the bladder like a doughnut. The gland secretes fluid that carries sperm during ejaculation. The cells of the gland become larger (called hypertrophy) with age and normal hormonal changes, and by age sixty all but a few men have an enlarged prostate.

. Often, enlargement occurs without causing troublesome symptoms, requiring no treatment. But with increasing age, many men gradually notice that urine flows, not in a constant stream, but in stops and starts. Most men can tolerate an interrupted flow of urine, but urination can become troublesome, with dribbling during the day, a very weak stream, difficulty in starting, and increased frequency, especially during the nighttime sleeping hours. Then it is advisable to have part of the prostate removed by prostatectomy — that is, prostate surgery.

Going for a cancer cure is another good reason for prostate surgery. Cancer of the prostate is age-related, for about 80 percent of men who have it are over age sixty-five. In fact, 30 percent of men over fifty and 40 percent of those over sixty have some form of prostate cancer. According to the American Medical Association, almost every man over eighty has some form of the disease.

The behavior of prostate cancer is variable. Although it certainly always deserves attention, cancer of the prostate usually grows slowly and is highly curable, compared to many other cancers. The best advice is that every man over age fifty should have a digital rectal examination as part of the annual physical. Cancer of the prostate is usually easy for an experienced examiner to detect. Additionally, doctors are able to detect early cancer of the prostate by two techniques: transrectal ultrasound, a painless x-ray technique; and a new blood test called PSA (Prostate Specific Antigen).

Can Prostate Surgery Cause Incontinence? Prostate surgery done to resolve troublesome urination does not normally cause permanent urinary incontinence. Almost every man who has surgery for prostate enlargement needs six weeks of healing time before everything returns to normal, and that includes normal urination and normal sexual activity. During recuperation, some temporary dribbling of urine may appear. Socklike drip-collecting devices can be worn so that urine does not wet clothing and cause embarrassment.

Unfortunately, however, approximately one of 200 men who have prostate surgery that is not done because of cancer do become incontinent.

If your father does become permanently incontinent after prostate surgery for a nonmalignant condition, you should know that further surgery may be needed to cure the incontinence. Do not take the surgeon's "there's nothing we can do" as the last word on the subject. Your father may be a candidate for an artificial-sphincter operation. Urologists can surgically implant this medical device in the body so that a man can regain control of his urination. The operation and device are not suitable for men who are in poor health or mentally confused, but the majority of generally healthy men who have the device implanted by an expert surgeon find it provides relief from incontinence.

Prostate-cancer surgery is always more radical than routine surgery for an enlarged prostate, and a few men who have this more invasive kind of surgery never regain natural bladder control. Most men, though, regain control within a few weeks, although a few do take about six to nine months, including a program of exercises and medication. Those who have permanent incontinence after prostate-cancer surgery should consider the artificial sphincter. If it is inappropriate, they can examine the much-improved urine-collecting devices now available.

To find out if your father is a candidate for the artificial sphincter, arrange for him to be examined by a urologist who has successfully implanted several. American Medical Systems, the company manufacturing the device, sells it only to urologists trained in the surgery required and the followup routine of care. If you write to or telephone the company at Incontinence Information Center, P.O. Box 9, Minneapolis, MN 55440, they will provide you with material on incontinence and the artificial-sphincter device, and a list of board-certified urologists in your area. The American Urological Association's state sections will also send names of board-certified urologists.

Drug-Induced Incontinence

If you look through a drug manual (such as the Physician's Desk Reference) you will see that incontinence is listed as a possible side effect ascribed to hundreds, if not thousands, of the approximately 25,000 Federal Drug Administration (FDA)-registered drugs on the market. Incontinence among the elderly is often caused by drugs they are taking, a fact often overlooked by the doctors who prescribe those drugs. Elderly people are especially sensitive to the effects of drugs, and when it comes to aging and medication, lack of information about the subject is the rule rather than the exception.

Of course, doctors often need to prescribe several drugs for their older patients, for otherwise their lives would be in danger or life would be miserable because of discomfort and pain. It is no secret, though, that the elderly are living amid a drug crisis: many of them are given too many drugs simultaneously by doctors who have too little understanding of how they work, individually and in combination, in the body. Part of the problem too is that older people often see different doctors for different ailments, without consulting a primary doctor who will take charge and coordinate the medical program.

The more drugs one takes, the greater the potential for side effects, including loss of bladder control. The average person over sixty-five uses two or three drugs a day, but plenty of older people take many more. Too many elderly people clearly lose control of the bladder, while taking ten or even more medications every day. Chances are that so many medications will cause more collective harm than individual good. Sometimes it takes just one more medication, such as a tranquilizer, added to the usual regimen, to tip an elder into incontinence.

When incontinence is or threatens to be a problem, medications need to be very carefully reviewed by the physician who is trying to determine the cause. When you and your parent go to the doctor's office, bring along a list of all medications taken routinely and intermittently. Include over-the-counter medications such as laxatives, sleeping pills, and vitamins, as well as prescribed drugs. Even better, if you can swing it, put all your parent's medications in a bag for the doctor to see. Upon reevaluation, the doctor may be able to cut out some drugs altogether, prescribe different drugs, or set lower dosages that will work without causing incontinence. Drugs commonly causing incontinence include some tranquilizers, antihistamines —

even those sold over the counter to treat colds and coughs — heart medications, and diuretics.

Treatments

Yes! Incontinence can be treated, and often cured. The experts now say that incontinence can be one-third cured, one-third improved, and one-third managed. "Managed" means that people remain just as incontinent, but certainly are more comfortable and functioning better than they could before seeking medical attention. Understand, however, that if someone is very ill or severely demented, it is not realistic to think that incontinence can be cured or turned around. Some cases are incurable and best managed with collection devices and absorbent pads.

In this section we look at some of the common forms of treatment. Without getting into too much detail, we give you enough information that you can start to be an informed consumer, able to select a doctor who is up on state-of-the-art treatments for incontinence — a specialist you can trust who will help your mother or father. Do not become one of the eleven out of twelve people who does not seek help. Do go after help, and the best you can get. These are the treatments to consider:

- Exercises to strengthen and train pelvic-floor muscles.
- Surgery
- Bladder training and toilet scheduling
- Intermittent self-catheterization
- Medications
- Indwelling catheterization
- External collecting devices
- Absorbent products and special clothing

Exercises
Kegel Exercises Do Work. Women with mild to severe stress and urge incontinence have the advantage of being able to try correcting their problem by practicing an exercise that strengthens the muscles of the lower pelvis. Called Kegel exercises, after the doctor who developed them, they really do work for mild cases of stress incontinence. The muscles involved act as a sling to keep the bladder and bladder neck supported, and they also form the outer sphincter, the

stopgap muscle at the exit of the bladder where it meets the urethra. Because these muscles are under our voluntary control, we can exercise them to build their strength and bulk, just as a body-builder builds up outer muscles.

Kegel exercises can indeed restore stronger, thicker pelvic-floor muscles so that no more leakage occurs. But anyone who tries the exercises has to take them very seriously and buckle down to the commitment of doing them. Kegeling takes about three months to have an effect. We know numerous patients of all ages past sixty-five who have benefited from the exercises, but these are predominantly motivated women determined to help themselves. If your mother is very frail or mentally confused, you probably are not in a position to get her to do Kegeling exercises, but if you think you can encourage her to do them diligently, so much the better. She may well be able to restore her bladder control and experience the joy of accomplishing a physical feat.

If your mother does not want to talk with you about such an intimate form of exercise, or if she thinks you are out of your mind for suggesting a seemingly absurd pursuit, enlist your doctor's help in getting her to realize the great benefit to her of following the routine. Any doctor who sees many older people should have written instructions on Kegel exercises for all women patients, and of course any worthwhile doctor will discuss the benefits of Kegeling with patients, and not just the ones who are already incontinent. Ideally the exercises should be done by all women over thirty-five as a routine health-maintenance measure, giving it the same status as tooth-brushing and flossing.

At first it can be difficult to isolate and flex the correct muscles, but the more one does the exercises the easier they become. The best way to find the muscles and get the feel of the exercise is on the toilet: Try to stop the flow of urine in midstream by contracting the pelvic-floor muscles, the same ones that stop a bowel movement. Repeat several times until you are sure of the action and sensation of consciously contracting the muscles. Do not tense the muscles of the abdomen, legs, or buttocks. Once one is clear about how to do the exercise it needs to be done daily, for three sets of twenty-five repetitions, holding each contraction of the muscles for a count of five seconds, and then relaxing for five seconds.

The beauty of the exercise is that it can be done silently and discreetly, during just about any relaxing pursuit: watching television, lying in bed, or sitting in a chair. Quite a few older women have a great deal of difficulty finding the right muscles to squeeze, until they do the exercise while urinating in the toilet. They should get in the habit of stopping and starting the flow of urine a few times every time they go.

Some women think that Kegeling while urinating will cause urinary-tract infections because of a backup of urine. Not true; the exercises are hygienic and safe, and all women should stop and start the flow of urine as a matter of course, and do the exercises if they are able throughout the day.

Men Can Exercise, Too. Although Dr. Kegel originally designed the exercises for women, men too can benefit from them. Many urologists now recommend that men do the exercises after prostate surgery, especially if they experience mild dribbling of urine in the weeks after surgery. Just as women do, men can do a routine of exercises and learn to stop and start their stream of urine. With perseverance, they can strengthen the pelvic muscle supporting the bladder.

Surgery

Surgery is an option if exercises, medications, and bladder training are not working, or for someone who obviously has a blockage in the urinary tract. Even frail elderly people can tolerate a number of newer minimally invasive, corrective procedures. When all else has failed to restore continence, the artificial sphincter can be discussed.

Usually, deep abdominal surgery is not required; rather, the surgeon works through the vagina, or uses the endoscope (a narrow tubelike instrument with a light at the end), to see and operate inside the bladder. In this way the surgeon can relieve an obstruction, lift up pelvic-floor tissues to return a sagging bladder neck and urethra to normal position, or repair a constantly opening bladder outlet so that it closes efficiently. The hospital stay usually is only two or three days for a procedure that does not involve an abdominal incision.

Surgery is the most popular treatment for women who cannot correct stress incontinence with exercises. Approximately 90 percent of the time the problem is a sagging bladder neck, which the surgeon can lift to its normal position by an operation performed through the vagina. Occasionally, a suspension or lift operation is inappropriate because the bladder neck is unable to close. The surgeon then creates a sling to compress the bladder so that it can close. The Raz sling operation accomplishes this compression, also without the need for abdominal surgery. The hospital stay can be from two to four days with these operations; after six weeks of healing time, sexual relations usually can be resumed.

An abdominal operation may be recommended if a woman has incontinence as well as other gynecological problems that are best corrected abdominally. The standard abdominal operation for stress incontinence, the Marshall Marcheti Kranz procedure, has been all but replaced in recent years by the through-the-vagina procedures.

The outcome of surgery is of course most successful if the surgeon has plenty of specialized training in urologic surgery. Such a surgeon is more likely to work at a medical center that has a department of urology equipped to run urodynamic tests. A surgeon with special fellowship training in control of incontinence will certainly have the necessary expertise, although all urologists are by definition specialists who treat problems of the urinary system medically or surgically.

Most women who have had the surgery regret that they had not undergone a corrective operation sooner. We can say generally that nationwide too few women are having the surgery who could clearly benefit from it. General anesthesia and surgery of course have their risks, and elderly people, depending on their state of health, may or may not be good candidates for surgery. Certainly surgery should be considered, no matter how old one is, but the benefits must be discussed and weighed against the risks. One of the risks is that the surgery can be done too tightly so that incontinence remains. A skilled surgeon, however, will know how to avoid this complication.

Bladder Training and Toilet Scheduling
The most frequent form of management and treatment for incontinence is "retraining" the bladder. This method is especially helpful for those who have urge or gush incontinence. People who have lost control can condition the bladder to hold more and more urine so that they urinate on a schedule. In a sense the bladder is exercised by being told to regain its volume and muscle strength.

The ultimate aim is to train the bladder to take two to three hours to fill before emptying completely. Some people can achieve this goal, and others are able to reduce the number of times they need to urinate, and also gain the comfort of knowing approximately when they will urinate.

Doctors who treat incontinence often have a nurse or urology technician working with them to teach patients bladder training. A kind, tolerant nurse skilled in teaching bladder training can make the difference between success and failure, as long as she has a willing and earnest student. The method does work, but not without considerable effort.

The incontinent person is asked to follow a strict schedule specifying the amount and type of fluid she is to drink, and when she is to go to the bathroom. The schedule is established after the patient has provided the nurse with a log recording her pattern of urination, and the times at which she is incontinent. It is important to write in the quantity of fluid drunk as well as the type of fluid, such as water, coffee, or milk. People with sensitive bladders may have sensitivities to specific drinks, which the pattern in the log can indicate.

Please refer to the easy-to-fill-out Daily Diary on page 251. The bladder-training schedule is based on this record. The incontinent individual is encouraged to urinate at specified intervals, whether or not the desire to do so is there. The schedule is adjusted as time goes on and as the bladder starts to regain control.

Intermittent Self-Catheterization

In recent years, self-catheterizing has gained in popularity because it allows people to empty the bladder "artificially" on a schedule without the constant threat of accidents. The treatment is usually prescribed for those who have overflow incontinence, because they have the problem of never being able to empty the bladder completely, as well as the risk of leftover urine becoming infected. The technique is sometimes recommended for those who have urge incontinence that cannot be managed with medication and bladder training. Sometimes too it is used as a temporary adjunct to bladder training, to prevent the bladder from overstretching.

Self-catheterization involves inserting a narrow tube into the urinary opening and up into the bladder to drain the urine. People are usually taught to do the procedure at home while sitting on the toilet, at scheduled intervals. It may sound unpleasant and somewhat frightening, but people who have been doing self-catheterization get used to it quickly and like the control it gives them. Unless they followed the treatment routinely they would have to wear a permanent indwelling catheter and a collection bag, or diapers; given the choice, most prefer self-catheterization.

The procedure is painless and safe; infection is far less likely than with a permanent indwelling catheter, and in fact, if used correctly, the risk of infection is very low. The person using the catheter exposes it to his or her own germs, which are "self" germs and generally not harmful. More bacteria will appear in a urine sample than someone normally has, but the amounts are tolerable.

The same catheter can be used for up to several weeks, as long as it is washed with soap and water after each use. The hands *must* be thoroughly washed before and after inserting the catheter. Good hygiene is also required after bowel movements so that fecal material does not contaminate the area where the catheter is inserted.

Catheters come in small kits that can be carried in a handbag or a pocket. Older people who have arthritis in their hands or other problems with manual dexterity can learn to self-catheterize with a customized catheter.

Medications

Medications are frequently used along with other methods to control bladder problems. For mild cases of stress incontinence, specialized drugs help the bladder outlet stay closed; the active ingredient is the same as in many cold remedies. For urge incontinence, medications relax the bladder and make it less sensitive and less quick to expel urine. For overflow incontinence, several drugs occasionally increase the strength of bladder contractions; others just relax the sphincter muscle at the bladder outlet, allowing the urine to drain more freely. Women with problems related to low estrogen, urethral inflammation are sometimes given estrogen creams to insert in or around the vagina, or oral doses of estrogen.

All these medications have side effects. For example, those designed to relax muscles sometimes can cause dry mouth, constipation, and blurred vision. The use of estrogen in women is controversial, and many doctors will not prescribe it for women who have a family history of some types of cancer. Some medications work well initially but may eventually fail to work as the body becomes used to them. It is very important to keep in touch with the doctor prescribing medication and to change it, or lower dosages, if problems come up.

Indwelling Catheterization

Indwelling catheterization — keeping the catheter in the body — is considered the last choice of treatment for incontinence. Until recently catheterizing was the main treatment, so that nursing homes once were full of incontinent old people with catheter tubes running from inside their bodies to bags on their beds and wheelchairs. With the kinds of techniques we have just described, many of these people could have been helped in other ways. Probably the worst aspect of permanent catheterization is its very high risk of infection. Those who are catheterized for more than a few weeks also may lose the tone of the urinary sphincter and their natural ability to urinate. This loss is tragic for people who are catheterized because of a temporary condition that was mistaken for something untreatable and permanent.

Permanent catheters do have their place, however. They are used to drain urine if the bladder cannot empty itself because of an obstruction or nerve damage, or if one is unconscious or so terribly confused that no other alternative makes sense. They are also used if the skin is dangerously and painfully broken down by moisture and prolonged bed rest. But in general be extremely leery of any doctor who wants to catheterize a patient for more than a few days or weeks. Always ask if other treatments can be tried instead.

External Collecting Devices

A number of devices on the market collect urine as it comes out of the body, through a tube leading to a collection bag. The catheter tube does *not* enter the body but is attached to a man's penis or a woman's crotch, so that the risk of infection is low. The bag can be attached to a leg and hidden underneath pants or a long skirt, providing the wearer with mobility. People of all ages are wearing these devices while at work or joining in social activities.

These devices should be used only when other methods have been tried, or while one is waiting for surgery, or waiting for other methods to work. No one should rely on an external collecting device for their life, unless absolutely necessary. The longer the device is used the more difficult it is to bring back bladder control. And no one wants to carry around a collection bag unless they have to.

Men can easily wear a catheter tube attached to a condom and if needed a belt to hold it in place. Women's devices have been available for only a few years. They are held against the body with adhesive or suction. One new device, the Hollister Female Urinary Incontinence System, is gaining in use and popularity. The system uses a pliable silicone cup, the pericup, which funnels urine away from the body into a collection bag worn against the body. A small piece of the pericup is inserted in the vagina for anchorage and the rest of the cup is held against the body by suction.

Absorbent Products and Special Clothing

No one should be encouraged to "just wear adult diapers" around the clock if other methods are clearly more suitable. But absorbent briefs and pads certainly have a place for people who need them, and as a security backup for those worried about wetting themselves and their clothing, while they use other methods to control incontinence.

Do work with a nurse specialist or a doctor to decide on the most effective and affordable product. Adult diapers and incontinence-related products are now a big business. Scores of companies manufacture different products, many of them now sold in supermarkets and through catalogues. Finding out which products are available and how to order them can be a dizzying experience without well-informed help. Wearing absorbent incontinence products also necessitates meticulous skin and odor control, both best taught by someone with expert knowledge.

Diapers and pads vary tremendously in quality and capacity for absorbing urine and controlling odor. Pads have been invented that absorb many times their own weight and hold fluids in suspension. Stay away from sanitary napkins, which are not designed to hold urine and control its odor. Diapers, often called briefs, are an all-in-one disposable or washable garment, and pads are worn with specially designed pants with a waterproof crotch. Less bulky and cumbersome under clothing, pads are useful for people who dribble but do not gush urine. Other products give extra protection, such as slips with a waterproof back panel, and pads for furniture and bedding.

How to Foil Skin Irritation

Anyone wearing adult diapers for more than a day or two should have instructions on how to take care of his or her skin. Urine can quickly irritate the skin, and the diaper creates an ideal environment for bacteria and fungi. Good-quality diapers are designed to wick or draw urine away from the skin, but even so proper skin care is of utmost importance.

Some Practical Advice

Here are some practical tips to make life easier at home for yourself and the person you are caring for. You want to set things up at home so that the older person can carry on a routine of activities without discomfort and embarrassing accidents.

• Provide about eight glasses of fluid during the day.

• Cut out drinking three hours prior to bedtime.

• Offer the older person a chance to pass urine at regular intervals, usually around every two hours. That's how long it takes for the bladder to fill with 120 to 240 cubic centimeters (cc), or about 1/2 to 1 cup. Also, the bladder is best emptied before uninhibited contractions begin at about 300 cc.

• Discourage frequent trips to the bathroom, unless absolutely necessary. Hold urine for a predictable length of time, for otherwise the muscles will shrink and the bladder will become conditioned to frequent urination.

• If accidents are common, keep a chart of drinking and urination patterns and ask the older person to sit on the toilet half an hour before urination usually occurs.

• Choose clothing that is easy to remove in the bathroom — wide, lift-up skirts, lapover skirts, and elastic or tie pants for women and men. Replace buttons at the waist with Velcro strips.

• Discourage rushed bathroom sessions. Provide time and privacy for urination so that the bladder empties completely.

• Try to give diuretics on a schedule that will keep their peak action from occurring during the night. If one dose is prescribed every day, give the drug in the morning with breakfast. If two doses a day are prescribed, ask the doctor if they can be combined, or if the second dose can be given with dinner, *not* before bedtime.

• Seat the older person closest to the bathroom, and if possible free one up for the older person's exclusive use. At night, provide a toilet close to the bed. Analyze how long it takes her to get to the toilet. Accidents can easily happen if someone has poor mobility and more than 40 feet to travel to the toilet.

• If sitting down on the toilet is difficult, buy a raised toilet seat and install a grab bar or bars on the wall next to the toilet. One bar should run parallel to the floor at a height of 33 inches.

• Unnecessary pressure is placed against the bladder if an older person strains to get in and out of bed or a chair. Make sure the bed is easy to get out of by seeing if the person's feet touch the floor while sitting on the edge. Most elderly people can get out of a 17-inch-high chair without unnecessary stress and strain.

- Eliminate drinks that seem to irritate the bladder and cause it to empty quickly. Common culprits are caffeinated beverages, including coffee, tea, diet and regular colas, grapefruit juice, and alcoholic drinks.

- Eliminate foods that seem to irritate the bladder, such as grapefruit, asparagus, sugar, some spicy foods, and chocolate.

- Constipation can cause incontinence. Be sure the diet is sufficient to maintain bowel regularity — high in fiber and high in bulk, with eight glasses of fluid throughout the day.

- Stop any smoking in the house. Inhaled cigarette smoke irritates the bladder and can make it more sensitive. And smoking causes bladder cancer.

- If absorbent briefs and pads are worn, provide the bathroom with an unobtrusive pail that has deodorant in the lid.

- Remove wet clothing or bedding as soon as possible after accidents happen. As urine sits outside the body it changes chemically, releasing strong-smelling ammonia. If it is difficult to rinse items right away, store them out of the way in a special pan with deodorant in the lid.

- If furniture becomes wet, use specially designed cleaning agents to prevent lingering odor.

Here are some general tips for skin care:

- Change the diaper soon after it has become wet. If dribbling is a problem, change to a clean diaper several times a day.

- The skin needs to be washed with mild, nonperfumed soap and warm water every time a diaper is changed.

- After rinsing, the skin must be thoroughly dried with a soft cotton cloth or towel.

- Before putting on a clean diaper, apply a thin film of moisture-barrier cream. Too much cream, though, will contribute to skin breakdown.

- Don't use powder. It can chafe the skin, congeal with urine into irritating lumps, or trap moisture in skin folds.

- Call the doctor if the skin feels burned, or looks irritated, overly pink, or bright red. The symptoms may signify a fungal infection, treatable with an antifungal cream, or a bacterial infection, treatable with prescribed medication. An easily treated vaginal infection could also be present, producing irritating secretions.

A patch of skin can become sore even if the measures listed above are carefully followed. The person suffering the problem may find out the reason by answering these questions: Is the diaper too tight? Does it need to be changed more frequently? Is the diaper surface too rough? Is the diaper's plastic outer layer in contact with the skin?

12

Facing the Challenge of Cancer

NOT MANY YEARS AGO, cancer was one of the worst words anyone could hear. Even today, we seem to fear cancer more than any other disease, equating it with pain, terrible suffering, and imagining that treatment will be as bad as or worse than the disease itself.

Rarely do people connect *cancer* with *cure* — even though about 40 percent of adults who have cancer *are* cured of it and about 10 percent of cancers that were considered incurable just ten years ago can now be remedied.

Most people, when they hear that they must now deal with this dread disease for themselves or for someone they love are distressed, terrified, and numb with shock. The realization that cells in the body are not growing properly and, in fact, are dividing rapidly to crowd out and destroy normal cells that the body needs is terribly upsetting. No one can help but dread having to make decisions and manage the disease, no matter what the prognosis.

It may be comforting to realize, however, that within the past ten or fifteen years such great strides have been made in the cancer field that we may have less to fear from cancer than we think. New discoveries are coming rapidly and may dramatically alter the way in which patients can either cope with or recover from this disease.

Better Treatments

To begin with, a great deal more is now known about various cancers and how they can best be treated. Although everyone used to think that cancer was just one disease and the only effective way to deal with it was to cut it out, doctors know today that they're up against something much more complex and specific. Cancer is not simply one disease; it is an umbrella label for more than a hundred types of the disease — some more virulent than others, some more responsive to treatment than others.

Today's cancer doctors (oncologists) know very precise details about the many types of cancer that originate in any one site or in many systems in the body. They know how to pinpoint the specific types of cancer and their behavior. With this knowledge they can more precisely tailor treatment, taking into account the patient's unique hormonal patterns, immune strengths, previous illnesses, and disabilities. They know, for example, that one kind of breast cancer may be thwarted by hormone therapy but another requires specific chemotherapy. They also know that one kind of prostate cancer responds best to surgery, but another is best treated by hormone therapy alone.

Above all, many people don't realize that most cancer treatments are much more effective than they used to be, and what's more, they're easier to take. Chemotherapy began to be widely used only in the 1960s, and at that time was a last-ditch effort resorted to when other treatments hadn't worked. Severe side effects, such as nausea and vomiting and lowered blood counts couldn't be controlled, making chemotherapy almost always difficult, and even dangerous. In the early days of chemotherapy, doctors and nurses used to stand by after giving the chemotherapy and cringe in anticipating the side effects. Most older people remember gruesome stories about what horrible side effects did to their friends or neighbors who got radiation treatments or chemotherapy — and they remember thinking that the cure was definitely worse than the disease.

Today, treatment does not necessarily make patients sick at all. Small, easily tolerated doses of chemotherapy are often given in the very early stages of cancer as insurance against any possible spread. But even with the treatment given for more advanced cancer, many patients can tolerate an entire course of chemotherapy or radiation for six months or a year without ever experiencing major reactions or side effects. Some people can drive themselves home after having their chemotherapy and then continue with their usual activities. In some cases, oncologists can prescribe chemotherapy in pill form that patients can take at home, along with their regular medication.

Hundreds of drugs are now available to oncologists to treat specific cancers. Research has devised better ways of delivering these drugs to the cancer cells, which they destroy with much less damage to healthy surrounding tissues in other systems of the body. Whereas in the past only massive doses of one drug at a time were given for treatment, today oncologists often give three or four drugs together in lower dosages that individually and in combination are less toxic to the patient. After years of clinical trials, they also now know which drugs work best in eradicating or reducing specific cancers.

Many forms of chemotherapy are relatively easy on the body but damaging to cancer cells; others are not so selective. Some cancers respond only to strong chemotherapy agents that are accompanied by nasty side effects. On the positive side, doctors and nurses have learned many ways to help patients manage the side effects of such drugs.

Preventing side effects is now the name of the game. For instance, patients are given new, very effective medication for nausea *before* receiving treatment, and they are often asked to drink many glasses of water before coming in for chemotherapy. During chemotherapy, they are often put on intravenous fluids (saline solution) to help flush out the toxins after they have done their work in the body. New medications, known as blood-stimulating factors, can be given to lessen the destructive effects of chemotherapy and radiation therapy on the bone marrow, where blood cells originate. These medications reduce the need for blood transfusions and the risk of infections and bleeding during cancer therapy.

Patients are also encouraged to have dental work done before treatment in case the chemotherapy damages the extremely delicate tissue of the mouth. Chemotherapy can exacerbate preexisting dental problems. If side effects do occur, doctors and nurses can help patients recover from them.

Better Pain Control

People often fear not just the treatment, but also the pain of cancer. Cancer, though, is not always painful. Pain is rarely a problem in the early stages, and even in advanced stages it's not always present. If pain does occur, oncologists have many ways of reducing it, and these days, they are quite willing to do so.

It used to be that doctors discouraged or denied narcotics to cancer patients, for fear they would build tolerance to them before they really needed them. They also feared that their patients would become addicted to drugs. That thinking has proved wrong. Now physicians and nurses believe that patients should get as much medication as they need to dull pain, because the patient's comfort is more important than the remote possibility of physical or psychological addiction.

Any good doctor who cares for a patient with cancer knows how to manage pain so that the patient never has to suffer intractable pain at any stage in the disease. The doctor who doesn't know how should refer your parent to a pain specialist who works with cancer specialists. According to the National Cancer Institute and the American Cancer Society, the days of patients rocking in agony while awaiting their next dose of painkillers should be gone forever.

Make Sure Your Older Family Members Get Checkups and Report Symptoms

Old age is not a time to slack up on vigilance about cancer. In fact, cancer is primarily a disease of the elderly. According to the National Cancer Institute, people over sixty-five are 100 times more likely to get cancer than their younger counterparts because of years of exposure to toxins and other environmental insults to the body that lead to the development of cancer cells. Also, aging has its effect, especially in individuals who have a genetic susceptibility to the disease.

Despite the prevalence of cancer in their generations, however, older people are not nearly as good as they ought to be at reporting symptoms that would lead to early detection and effective treatment. Often the cause is that older people confuse symptoms of cancer with aging itself or with the chronic diseases they so often have.

Some older people also take symptoms lightly and don't report them out of dread that the signs might indeed mean cancer. These are some of the symptoms that are ignored all too often:

- A sore that won't heal
- Obvious changes in a mole or a wart
- Blood in the urine or persistent difficulty in urinating or having bowel movements
- Diarrhea alone, with no sign of intestinal flu
- Unusual and persistent constipation or a change in the usual frequency of bowel movements

- Persistent indigestion or stomach discomfort
- A sore throat and difficulty in swallowing
- Unusual bleeding or discharge anywhere in the body
- A nagging cough, hoarseness, difficulty in breathing, and coughing up blood in the sputum
- Pain that is persistent and without apparent cause
- A thickening or lump in the breast, vulva, neck, head, or other part of the body

Another problem that interferes with early detection is that older people don't routinely examine themselves for signs of cancer. Because of the mores with which they were raised, some older women find it particularly difficult to touch and examine their breasts for lumps or to search the vulva and genital area for sores and irregularities. (Vulva cancer is uncommon, but if detected early, it's curable.) Similarly, older men rarely follow their doctor's directions to do a monthly exam of their testicles that would lead to early detection of testicular cancer. Make sure to encourage your parents to check themselves for any cancer symptoms and to go for annual checkups. If they're seeing specialists for chronic problems, such as diabetes, arthritis, or heart disease, don't let them become complacent about having thorough, full-body, all-system checks every year with a general practitioner who will keep records of their health changes and test results.

Remind your parents to be on the lookout for symptoms and to insist on discussing them with their doctor, expecting that treatment for cancer will be considered. If they do have cancer, chances of cure are maximized if it's discovered early.

How Serious Is the Cancer?

If your parent or older friend does have cancer, the doctor, using tests and pathology studies, will determine the size and type of tumor, where it is, and whether it has spread. The doctor will also identify the stage to which the cancer has progressed; that means talking about how much cancer is in the body and how far it has spread to other areas.

Staging numbers are used by physicians to indicate how far the disease has advanced. Stage I is the most curable, stage IV the least. Doctors also use other designations that include "T" and "N" and "M" categories. You may see these designations written on your parent's charts. The T stands for tumor, and the number, I through IV, indicates the size of the primary tumor and how extensively it has invaded the surrounding tissues. The higher the number, the larger the tumor, or the depth or amount of involvement in the local area, or both. The N stands for lymph nodes, and, along with the numbers I through IV, indicates how extensively the tumor has spread to the closest lymph nodes and the size and number of the nodes involved. (Because the lymph system is a network carrying fluids throughout the body, if the cancer has spread to the lymph nodes, treatment is much more likely to be systemic.) The M, which stands for metastasis (the medical word for "spread"), with a zero (o) or a plus (+) sign indicates whether or not the cancer has spread to distant parts of the body.

Doctors and national and international committees are constantly working at standardizing and refining language describing the kinds of tumors and their behaviors so that all doctors can interpret the labels accurately. Identifying the stage of cancer makes it easier for doctors to communicate with each other and thus decide on the proper course of treatment. The labels also make it easier for doctors to inform families about treatment options and how they need to plan for care.

Be sure to ask your doctor to translate the medical description of staging so that you and your parent will know what they mean. When you call for information or second opinions, you can use these medical labels yourself to make sure you communicate exactly what is going on.

Is Treatment Worth It for an Aged Person?

Your parents or older friends may believe that if they were to be treated for cancer, they'd be subjected to unproved experiments at a stage in life when they would be best left alone. When it comes to treating older people who have cancer, many people, including some poorly informed doctors, think, "What's the point? They don't have long to live anyhow; why put them through an ordeal during the last years of their life?"

Even if cancer is discovered too late to be cured, treatment is worth the aggravation if it can prolong life and alleviate symptoms. No one should be sent home to die unless perfectly sure that this is what he or she wants. Remember that there are many options —

even if it's not a knockout cure — no matter what the age. Your parent may be old and frail and afraid of feeling miserable because of cancer therapy, but if treatment is tailored to his or her state of health, it can ultimately reduce discomfort from disease, or, even better, put it into remission. In remission, the symptoms would disappear, even though the disease is not totally eradicated.

Even when remission or a cure does not seem likely, attention still needs to be given to the length of survival for an older person. In today's constantly changing and more positive climate of cancer care, it is important for older people, like younger people, to pay attention to the length of time they have left to live. It seems most unfair and cruel for anyone to deny or discourage an older person from accepting treatment that can reduce a cancer's spread into vital organs and nerves, or treatment that can bring worthwhile months or years to a person's life.

Many cancer doctors believe that elderly people should disregard their age when aggressively seeking treatment. They say that older people should look at cancer therapy as an "investment in life." Sometimes a few months of discomfort from treatment can mean years of high-quality living — a benefit that is well worth the trouble if that's the result.

Besides thinking cancer treatments are not worth going through because they're afraid of them, people also avoid cancer therapy because they assume that it's an all-or-nothing choice. But drastic treatment is not always necessary or advisable, especially for an already frail older person. Treatment usually can be tailored to fit the older person's physical tolerance.

Generally, radiation is tolerated much better than other methods. In radiation therapy, high-energy rays damage cancer cells so that they're unable to multiply. Like surgery, radiation is a local treatment that affects only the cells in the treated area. For chemotherapy, anticancer drugs are given intravenously, by injection or sometimes by mouth. These drugs, though targeted for specific cancer cells, are distributed to them through the blood stream.

Sometimes the doctor and an older patient will decide not to use the full arsenal of treatment. They'll forgo the standard chemotherapy and surgery, and will use radiation alone. At other times, they'll decide to use only chemotherapy in lieu of surgery, or to simply remove a lump and not follow up with radiation or chemotherapy.

A doctor examining a frail older person may determine with the patient and the family that gentle treatment is called for. Everyone may agree that it will be worthwhile to add time to the older person's life. For instance, with a frail eighty-five-year-old woman who has breast cancer, a lumpectomy with mild chemotherapy by pills at home may be all that's needed to ensure that she lives out her life span without being debilitated by the disease. A standard, more aggressive treatment, including surgery and a full course of chemotherapy, may be appropriate for the extremely hale and hearty seventy-eight-year-old woman who swims twenty laps a day and wants to fight for a complete cure.

Another misconception that works against treatment is that cancer grows so slowly in the elderly that treating it is pointless. Generally, that argument is wrong. Most often, cancer presents itself in the elderly just as it does in younger people. Nevertheless, some tumors do grow furiously; some progress less rapidly in the elderly body. For instance, some forms of prostate cancer are so slow-growing that his physician may choose to do nothing to treat the cancer if a man is in his late eighties or nineties. Some forms of breast cancer do appear to be less aggressive in very old women. But these are rare exceptions.

Above all, cancer needs to be discovered early and biopsied so that its type and stage of growth can be determined. Treatment is based on these factors, which are independent of age. For the most part, cancer *should* be treated the same for the young and old, if the patient wants to live longer and is in good enough health to withstand the surgery, chemotherapy, or radiation.

The Patient's Right to Know

In most cases, it's very important for patients to know their diagnosis so that they can make plans accordingly and understand and manage any physical changes they're experiencing. Some doctors and families are inclined to "protect" older people from the truth. In the hallway outside the older person's room they whisper to the staff not to tell the patient about the cancer. The family may mean to protect their relative from shock or despair, but this approach usually is a mistake. The lie can also be quite cruel because it denies any knowledge the patient may already have and demeans his or her ability to take part in issues that involve the core of dignity and self-determination.

On the other hand, some people truly may want to be spared the medical details and gloomy predictions. If your mother or father is one of these people, you should intervene with the medical staff to discourage medical and nursing staff from trooping through the room talking about test results and the purpose behind every investigation. If the doctor in charge orders a CAT scan, it is his or her responsibility to explain why; other doctors who come by should not say, "We're arranging a CAT scan because we want to look for spreading cancer."

If your parent has a strong cultural bias against the doctor-tell-all way of thinking, or is very ill, is mentally confused, has Alzheimer's disease, or is terribly debilitated from other conditions, you may choose to get involved with the physician in charge to discuss how much your parent should be told about his or her condition. This is a very individual issue. Some people want to know every aspect of their diagnosis and plan for treatment; others do not.

Your mother might be mortified if her doctor took to the limit modern thinking about the patient's right to know — telling her all the medical details that the staff knows — including, to her horror, the prognosis of just how long she has to live. Although most people want to know the general outline — that they have cancer of the lymph system, for example — it would defeat their spirit to hear a young resident state that they have only three months to live. In fact, doctors can't always be sure about how long a patient has to live; they *guess*, from experience and studies they know about. Most often it is not advisable to share these guesses with the patient — unless, of course, the patient asks for the information in detail.

Even when the news is bad, a sensitive physician can find ways of telling patients the truth that still let them have a say in their own destiny without turning off hope.

Of course, some physicians communicate life-and-death issues to their patients with less than the required sensitivity. Some, in fact, are extremely uncomfortable discussing death — how it may happen and the stages involved. They may then mask their own discomfort by bluntly presenting statistical odds and excessive medical information that is only frightening. Sometimes the patient's perception of the facts communicated is so terrifying and confusing that it creates depression, anxiety, and a quick decline in the patient's health. This new stress comes at a time when the patient needs to muster maximum emotional and physical strength.

To settle issues of communicating medical information, you need to tell the head nurse and the physician in charge how you want things handled, perhaps leaving the job to this physician and to you as a family. The head nurse will write your request into the nursing notes, relaying it to the nurses at each shift change. Specialists called in on the case will usually check in at the nursing desk and review the chart before meeting the patient.

Questions for the Doctor

If your frightened parent calls you up and tells you that cancer has been diagnosed, or if you are in the doctor's office when the verdict is given, you will have a lot of questions. You should find out some details so that you, together with your parents, can make decisions about the best doctors to work with, the hospital to use, and the appropriate course of treatment.

When you talk to the doctor, take notes on all that is said so that later you will have everything straight. The shock and burden of the news may leave you and your parent confused and troubled in focusing on all the sudden answers. If you want to be really careful about getting everything recorded properly, take a tape recorder along for the interview.

Among other questions you may have, be sure to get answers to those listed here. Get responses for your own use and for discussions with other doctors and health professionals whom you may consult in the near future.

1. What is the medical name of this cancer?
2. How do the name and the disease it represents translate into everyday language?
3. How did the doctor conclude that this cancer is indeed the one your parent has? (What tests were run? Was a biopsy done? Blood tests? Physical exam? X-rays? CAT scan? Angiogram? Ultrasound?)
4. Is the cancer localized in one place, or has it spread to the surrounding lymph nodes, or to other parts of the body (metastasized)?
5. If it has spread, where did it originate?
6. At what stage is the cancer? (Stage 1, 2, 3, or 4. See the next section for further information on stages.)

7. Is the cancer curable?
8. What is the standard treatment for this cancer in younger adults?
9. For my parent, what would be the wisest, safest, most effective, and most tolerable treatment?
10. What is the goal of treatment? (Will they do all they can to cure the disease with the standard, aggressive treatment? Will they use a less aggressive one in an attempt to cure it? Or will they simply do all they can to reduce the cancer so that my parent suffers less discomfort than without treatment?)
11. What are the side effects of this doctor's recommended treatment?
12. How well might my parent tolerate these expected side effects? How will they affect his or her normal functioning, daily pleasure, and ability to live independently?
13. How will this treatment affect management of my parent's other medical problems? (For example, arthritis, diabetes, heart disease, Parkinson's.)
14. How will this treatment be paid for? Will it be covered by Medicare or Medicaid? Do you accept Medicare or Medicaid? If not, how much will you charge? If so, do you charge beyond the Medicare or Medicaid payment, and if so, how much?

How to Help Your Parent Ensure the Best Treatment

How do you know that the diagnosis and advice your parent is given is accurate? And how do you know that your parent's doctor knows what he or she is doing? Is the treatment plan that's been recommended the best and the safest?

You can recognize a doctor's lack of expertise if he or she advises your older parent *not* to seek any treatment at all. Doctors who believe elderly people shouldn't bother with cancer treatments beyond going home and being comfortable are out of touch. They are either misinformed about possible treatments for older people or they're too quick to dismiss seventy-, eighty-, or ninety-year olds who don't want to be written off because of their age.

An excellent source of information is the National Cancer Institute's telephone hotline: (800) 4-CANCER. At no charge, you can obtain information about your parent's cancer, including methods of diagnosis, staging, and treatment. The NCI can also provide you with information on clinical trials that may be appropriate for your parent and the names and phone numbers of nearby physicians who take part in those trials.

Whether or not you have doubts about your parent's treatment, it's important to get a second opinion. The NCI Network can tell you over the telephone places they have designated as Second Opinion Centers. You and your parent can go to a center and meet with a team of specialists who will review your parent's diagnosis, medical history, pathology reports, biopsy slides, and other details and provide a sound second opinion about the best course of treatment. Don't be afraid or embarrassed to ask the doctor who made the original diagnosis for records, x-rays, and test reports as well as pathology slides. You may have to do some footwork for a day or two gathering everything to take to the second-opinion center, but understand that access to reports and other materials is your legal right and is well worth the effort. If you run into any problems, be sure to contact the patient representative at the hospital.

The American College of Surgeons also can provide a list of hospitals which treat cancer and which have met program standards of the American College of Surgeons. The local chapter of the American Cancer Society will provide the names of doctors and their cancer specialties.

If you are in a health-maintenance organization (HMO) that requires you to use the doctors they have selected, tap into the NCI Network to determine whether treatment that the HMO doctors recommend is indeed considered the latest and the best. If it is not, put your HMO doctor in touch with the NCI and consider paying for a second opinion from an oncologist working out of a major hospital or cancer center. This oncologist can then work in tandem with your HMO doctor.

If free to do so, your parent may want to choose an experienced oncologist either to treat the cancer or to take charge of treatment by other specialists — surgeon, radiologist, pathologist, hematologist, or chemotherapist. Oncologists should always be consulted before treatment begins because they have the knowledge and the tools to either cure or provide palliative treatment rendering the disease less destructive to vital organs and nerves.

How to Use the NCI Network (Do Use It!)

The best way to ensure excellent treatment for your parent is to contact the telephone service of the National Cancer Institute: (800) 4-CANCER.

The NCI's Cancer Information Service is an electronic telephone network that weaves together the latest and best information on cancer treatment. Started in 1976, the service is our government's attempt to bring all important information and discoveries on cancer to doctors, nurses, and patients in every corner of the country, rather than keeping it in pockets of exclusivity at the National Institutes of Health in Washington or scattered in research labs or doctors' offices.

Around the country hospitals are NCI-designated cancer centers. Although many hospitals refer to themselves as "cancer centers," they may not meet the same high standards required for designation as an NCI Cancer Center. The telephone service will tell any caller throughout the country where to find the nearest cancer center, and the best place for treatment that is less than a day's drive away. If your parent has a common cancer with an established treatment protocol, you will probably be referred to your community hospital. But if it is a rare form of cancer, you will probably be advised to go to a research-oriented, cancer center where the staff knows all forms of cancer. The NCI goal is to ensure that no one has to drive overnight to get effective treatment.

Seventy-eight-year-old Elizabeth Pickens used the NCI information service, and her experience shows what a difference it can make in someone's life. Mrs. Pickens lived in a small Kansas town and had been seeing the same doctor for thirty years. Finding that she had cancer of the colon, this doctor recommended surgery by his colleague at the local hospital, and said that the surgery would probably include a colostomy, which would mean Mrs. Pickens would have to wear a bag for emptying her bowels, over an opening on her side, for the rest of her life.

Before surgery was scheduled, however, Mrs. Pickens and her daughter wondered if this was the best or the only route to take, and whether such surgery alone would be the most effective. They also wanted to find out if a colostomy was absolutely necessary.

They called (800) 4-CANCER, gave the name of the cancer, and said they had been told it had spread to her lymph system. The NCI staff member on the line learned from her computer that the latest clinical trials showed that Mrs. Pickens's cancer was best cured by surgery that did not involve a colostomy, and that following surgery she should have a combination of two anticancer drugs. She also found that her community hospital was not an NCI-designated center but that two hours away, in Wichita, was a designated cancer center where doctors routinely gave this combination of treatments.

After consulting with an oncologist and surgeon whom they sought through the Wichita hospital's referral service, Mrs. Pickens and her daughter decided to follow their recommendations. They were to ask Mrs. Pickens's home doctor if he would be willing to give her chemotherapy treatments prescribed by the NCI oncologist and to have surgery in Wichita that would not require a colostomy.

Not only did the home doctor agree to give Mrs. Pickens the chemotherapy, but he also visited her soon after her surgery at the NCI-designated cancer center.

Doctors and community hospitals also use the NCI network regularly and find it particularly useful for asking questions about what is being done for cancers they haven't previously encountered or that they're not up to date on. Physicians sometimes refer to the Physician Data Query line as the Pretty Darn Quick line. They're told information about the latest clinical trials and preferred treatments for most types of cancer. Many doctors work closely with the NCI and are thus able to treat their patients knowing about the most recent thinking in this rapidly changing field.

Thinking of your parent, you'll find that the NCI can help you further clarify what the diagnosis means, and give you information about the disease and side effects of treatment. If you've been so eager to receive the news that you haven't listened to the details, a staff member at the NCI network will explain it all again. They will tell you the treatments that are established and considered worthwhile for the cancer your parent has. They also help you determine what your parent might expect in the future, especially if the doctor is uncomfortable talking about difficulties or other bad news. They may also be able to refer you to people who can help with questions about insurance coverage and let you know how your parent can apply for clinical trials. They will also refer you to people who can discuss the financial management of your parent's case, which could become quite complex.

Tips for Dealing with Side Effects after Chemotherapy

As we have said, side effects of cancer treatment are better managed today than ever before. Doctors and nurses are very knowledgeable now about what to recommend to relieve the negative effects of chemotherapy, radiation, surgery, and other cancer treatments.

Oncologists often recommend that their patients emphasize adequate caloric intake and good nutrition, with a nourishing high-protein diet, before having chemotherapy and other treatments. They can then maintain reserves of storable nutrients and body fat and bolster the immune system in helping the body recover from insults received from the disease, chemotherapy, radiation, and surgery. They also provide fluids to patients before and during chemotherapy to diminish damage to the liver, bladder, and kidneys, and to flush toxins from the system. And they give antinausea drugs to relieve sickness produced by chemotherapy or radiation.

Although cancer treatments are better managed and are less toxic than they used to be, the stronger treatments will produce predictable side effects that are uncomfortable and problematic. These are among the commonest problems that people come home with after treatment:

- Fatigue
- Nausea and loss of appetite
- Constipation or diarrhea
- Sores in the mouth
- Fever, chills, and sweats
- Hair loss
- Radiation enteritis, an inflammation of the intestines that sometimes results from radiation applied there
- Swelling

If any of these side effects is severe, the person you are looking after may have to return to the hospital for treatment. To avoid this trouble, refuse to take the person home if he seems too ill to leave the treatment center. Many older people are given cancer therapy as inpatients rather than outpatients so that the doctors can watch their condition following chemotherapy. This technique is helpful because the elderly are more susceptible to side effects and unusual, less-predictable responses to cancer treatments.

It can be quite difficult to take care of these problems at home without a medical professional in attendance. Make sure the doctor or nurse tells you what to expect when your parent comes home from treatment and how to deal with the problems that arise. It can be frightening to care for an older person after treatment if she is frail, or if you're worried that pre-existing problems will flare up or worsen from the stress of it all.

Here are some tips that may help you with the problems we have mentioned:

Fatigue

This is a common problem and should be expected after chemotherapy or radiation because the body is exhausted from getting rid of destroyed cancer cells and toxins used in the treatment. Some treatments can also harm blood cells, leaving patients with anemia, which shows up as weakness and tiredness.

Ask the doctor how long to expect fatigue to last, and report back if the fatigue goes on longer. Overcoming excessive or extended fatigue from anemia may require that the older person have blood transfusions or iron therapy. The patient should get lots of restorative rest and sleep and have help with daily tasks while fatigued. This is important: No one recovers from fatigue by becoming more fatigued from having too much to do.

Nausea and Loss of Appetite

To prevent nausea and vomiting at home, ask the doctor if it would be a good idea for the person you are taking care of to be put on an antinausea drug for a few days. Once begun, a cycle of nausea and vomiting is hard to control.

If the older person does come home nauseated and vomiting and cannot hold liquids, and this siege lasts more than a few hours, call the doctor. Dehydration in an elderly person can become extremely dangerous in a hurry.

Allow the older person to relax, with few or no responsibilities. Distraction by music, television, or self-hypnosis often helps.

If the sight or smell of food brings on nausea or lack of appetite, do the cooking while your parent, spouse, or friend is in another room or taking a walk.

If there has been vomiting, offer salty foods such as crackers and salty soups. Vomiting causes depletion of salts and other necessary minerals as well as food.

Have your patient eat dry foods such as toast and crackers, especially after waking up in the morning. These foods seem to settle the stomach.

Offer as many liquids as your patient can handle. These can be clear soups, gelatin, or carbonated beverages (ginger ale is a good one).

Avoid citrus drinks and tea, coffee, or other caffeinated beverages, all of which can be highly irritating to the stomach. When fruit juices are given, they should be clear and diluted with water. Apple juice is always a good choice.

Have your patient frequently eat small portions that are low in fat, rather than three meals a day.

Have the patient try to wait at least two hours after eating before lying down flat. If he or she wishes to rest, however, set up an easy chair. Keeping the head at least four inches higher than the feet may actually decrease nausea and indigestion.

Offer liquids through a straw if it's helpful. For some reason, this trick reduces nausea for many people.

Constipation
This can be a problem after some chemotherapy drugs are given. Be sure your parent is given foods that will prevent it, if possible. Foods should be high in roughage or fiber — fruits, green leafy vegetables, and whole-grain cereals and breads. Large quantities of water — two to three liters a day should be drunk.

Encourage your spouse, parent, or friend to use the toilet or a bedside commode *as soon* as he or she is able to get out of bed.

If necessary, a laxative or suppository can be given — but do so *only* under the doctor's direction. The NCI telephone network has good information on a variety of choices.

Whereas constipation is annoying and uncomfortable, fecal impaction can be dangerous if not life-threatening. An impaction, which is a complication of constipation, occurs when the patient accumulates dry, hardened stool that cannot be passed, whether in the rectum or farther back in the colon.

Signs of an impaction are lack of a bowel movement for several days, or explosive diarrhea, or leakage of diarrhea with coughing, or other changes in the bowel movement. An impaction pressing on the nerves in the back will cause back pain. If it presses on the kidney area, urinary symptoms can follow, including incontinence, frequency and urgency of urination, as well as retention of urine. The older patient may also have nausea, vomiting, or abdominal pain and be in a terribly disoriented mental state.

It's imperative for the person who has a fecal impaction to be seen immediately by a visiting nurse or by a doctor in an emergency room. The impaction can be removed by a nurse or a doctor who knows precisely what to do.

Mouth Sores, Inflammation, or Thrush

After rigorous chemotherapy, mouth sores, inflammation, or thrush (a fungal infection that looks like patches of cottage cheese on the tongue or throat) may appear. If these problems arise, they usually do so from five to fourteen days after treatment.

As a caregiver, you should look into your patient's mouth if he or she is unable to do so. Signs of problems are redness and swelling; white patches along the lining of the mouth, tongue, or throat; dry mouth, unpleasant taste in the mouth, burning sensations, sensitivity to hot and cold food, and occasionally, bleeding sores. If the doctor has not told you to expect these problems, call the doctor or nurse immediately. A prescription for an antibiotic may be needed to prevent infection, an anti-inflammatory to reduce swelling, or even a medication to stop bleeding.

Generally, however, these tips will help take care of the mouth.

• DO keep the patient's lips moist with petroleum jelly or a moisturizer.

• DO tell your patient wearing dentures to remove them if gums become sore. They should stay out most of the time until the mouth heals. (Of course, he or she will want teeth in for eating or for seeing visitors.)

• DO offer soft foods, such as mashed potatoes, yogurt, egg custards, milkshakes, creamy cereals, pasta and cheese, scrambled eggs, foods soaked in milk, and blenderized stews and casseroles.

• DO encourage plenty of fluids — eight to ten glasses a day.

• DO suck on hard, sugarless candies to stimulate saliva.

• DO use baking soda in solution for brushing the teeth instead of abrasive, over-the-counter toothpaste. Mix one teaspoon of baking soda to one quart of water to create this solution.

• DO rinse the mouth every two to four hours to remove debris with a solution of 1 teaspoon of salt diluted in one quart of water. Do not use a commercial mouthwash.

• DO use a humidifier in the house, if it is heated with dry heat.

- DO NOT offer alcoholic beverages.
- DISCOURAGE cigarettes, which can be very harmful to the mouth.
- DO NOT offer citrus fruits, tomatoes, or foods that are spicy, coarse, or hard.
- DO NOT use a toothbrush if the mouth is raw, because doing so will be very painful. Instead, use a clean, damp washcloth or bandage pad with bicarbonate of soda in solution or saline solution.
- DO NOT use lemon or glycerin swabs from the drugstore to refresh the mouth, because they increase dryness.
- DO talk to the doctor and ask for a medicine to numb the gums and tongue, if your patient's mouth is so painful that eating is difficult.
- DO apply pressure with a piece of gauze dipped in ice water to any spot in the mouth where bleeding occurs. If the bleeding doesn't stop, call the doctor for medications that can be helpful.

Fever, Chills, and Sweats

Fever, chills, and sweats are dangerous to older people because they can easily be thrown into hyperthermia (raised body temperature), heart arrhythmias, or heart failure by this increased metabolic activity. Such symptoms could also be the signs of a serious infection in need of *immediate* medical attention. The doctor should tell you what to do for an unexpected fever. But if fever does arise, keep the elder cool but free from drafts while the doctor is called. During periods of chills, wrap warm blankets around the patient and keep the room warm.

Hair Loss

One of the most upsetting side effects of cancer treatment is loss of hair. Not all patients experience the loss, however, even when given the same drugs. Usually any loss that does occur comes within two weeks after therapy starts. It gets worse over one to two months, but the loss is temporary. People who do lose their head hair usually find it comes out in clumps when they're brushing or shampooing. Bunches of hair may be on their pillow in the morning when they wake up.

After chemotherapy is completed, patients' hair *will* regrow. Some people report that their hair grows in thicker and softer than it ever was before.

Before treatment starts, it's a good idea to buy the best wig or toupée that the budget allows. Consult with a beautician who has worked with people who have lost hair during chemotherapy. (You can call your local chapter of the American Cancer Society for names.) These people can also help your older parent or friend with hair styles as hair grows in.

Doctors are experimenting with ways of preventing hair loss during the chemotherapy session. They put a cap on the patient's head ten minutes before the drug is given. The cap contains coolants that narrow blood vessels in the scalp, lessening the amount of the drug that reaches the hair follicles. The cap works best for people who are receiving low doses of drugs. It can't be used for patients who have cancers that might spread to the scalp, such as leukemia or lymphoma.

Radiation Enteritis
Sometimes the large and small bowel are extremely sensitive to radiation when aggressive cancer treatment is given to the abdomen, pelvis, or rectum. Some people have trouble with their bowel function for several weeks after chemotherapy or radiation. They may have cramping, nausea, loss of appetite, or watery diarrhea. Food isn't easily absorbed into their intestinal tract. Of course, when bowel symptoms are this severe the doctor must be involved with home care and continuing medical treatment of the problem. The doctor will prescribe antidiarrhea medications, drugs to prevent bowel cramping, and special salts.

Usually a lactose-free diet is recommended (see Chapter 7) that is also low in fat and residue (low-fiber). Have the person you are helping AVOID these foods if he or she has radiation enteritis:

> Milk and milk products (exceptions that are often tolerated better include buttermilk, yogurt, and processed cheese. Milkshake supplements such as Ensure are lactose-free and may be used)
> Whole-bran bread and cereal
> Nuts, seeds, coconuts
> Fried, greasy, or fatty foods
> Fresh and dried fruit and some fruit juices, such as prune juice
> Raw vegetables
> Rich pastries
> Popcorn, potato chips, and pretzels

Strong spices and herbs
Chocolate, coffee, tea, and soft drinks with caffeine
Alcohol and tobacco

These foods should be encouraged:

Fish, poultry, and meat that is cooked, broiled, or roasted
Bananas, applesauce, peeled apples, and apple and grape juices
White bread and toast
Macaroni and noodles
Baked, boiled, or mashed potatoes
Cooked vegetables that are mild, such as asparagus tips, green
    waxed beans, carrots, spinach, and squash
Mild processed cheese, eggs, smooth peanut butter, buttermilk,
    and yogurt
Food at room temperature

Drink 3,000 cubic centimeters of fluid every day. Allow carbon-ated beverages to lose their carbonation before drinking. Start a low-residue diet on the first day of radiation-therapy treatment.

A few helpful hints: Add nutmeg to food to help decrease mobil-ity and spasms of the bowel. Serve food at room temperature rather than hot or chilled. Offer plenty of fluids. Start encouraging a low-residue diet on the first day of treatment.

Swelling

The swelling known as lymphedema can be caused by the disease or can follow surgery or radiation to the lymphatic draining systems of the body. These systems are in the armpits, the pelvis, and the area where the hips and the thighs meet at the front of the body.

Usually lymphedema resolves a few days after treatment, but not always. The swelling is not usually noticed until fluid fills up in the tissue 30 percent above normal. The skin then looks turgid and taut, like a fluid-filled balloon. Signs to watch out for and report to the doctor include feelings of tightness in hands, arms, legs, and feet; rings or shoes that don't fit; weakness; pain; aching; redness; swell-ing; or signs of skin infection.

Patients at risk for edema are those with advanced testicular can-cer; advanced gynecologic cancer; prostate cancer when the whole pelvis is radiated or subjected to surgery; malignant melanomas of the arms or legs, if they've undergone node removal or radiation therapy; and breast cancer, if lymph nodes have been removed and radiation has been given.

If your parent has lymphedema, either short-term or chronic, the doctor must know. The self-help tips listed here can control and manage this condition. Besides providing comfort, they will help prevent the older person's especially delicate skin from breaking down or forming pressure sores.

- Keep swollen arms or legs above the level of the heart whenever possible.
- Avoid tight elastic around the waist, ankles, or arms.
- Wear loose-fitting shoes around the house and follow the foot care recommended for diabetic feet (Chapter 9).
- Avoid extremes of hot and cold on the area that has edema.
- Avoid weight or pressure on the arm or leg.
- Don't let the older person sit in one position for thirty minutes or longer without moving.

Make Sure That Pain Is Managed Well

Cancer is not always painful, but it often is when in its advanced stages. According to the National Cancer Institute, 60 percent or fewer of patients with advanced cancer do have pain. When the pain is there, however, it can *always* be alleviated.

As the spouse, adult child, or friend of an older person you love, it may fall into your lap to make sure that this person doesn't suffer unduly from the pain.

The first criterion for proper pain management is to find if the patient is reporting the pain he or she is experiencing. Some older people don't want to talk about their pain because they don't want to be complainers. They're stoic and they think it's their responsibility to tough it out and not be a burden to anyone. Others also fall into the trap of worrying that they'll bother or alienate the doctor if they call up to report that they're in pain.

Another important consideration is to see that the physician and other caregivers don't share the misconception that older people avoid the extremes of pain that younger people suffer. Some evidence in the literature suggests that pain response is somewhat dulled for some older people, but perception of pain is a highly individual sense. To believe the myth that pain decreases with age is to set the stage for abuse and cruelty.

If you have questions about your parent's pain management, again call the NCI Cancer Information Service (800-4-CANCER) or the local chapter of the American Cancer Society and ask them how to find pain specialists nearby.

Pain has many causes and depends upon how the cancer affects the functioning of the older person's body. Pain can be caused by colonies of cells that spread to the bone and exert pressure against the sensitive membranes that surround the bone tissue. It can be caused by a tumor in the abdomen that presses against a nerve, or by extraordinary swelling that forms as fluid shifts from a blocked duct in the lymphatic system.

The pain that patients with advanced cancer experience can be chronic, with no specific beginning or end. This kind of pain is often a dull, gnawing, relentless ache that can depress the person and change personality. With chronic pain, a bright, cheerful woman who thrills to the sound of bird song and other simple pleasures can turn into a withdrawn, stay-at-home recluse who would rather sleep than engage with the world. She may lose weight, become irritable, go on crying jags, or even feel suicidal. If the family is not alert to these symptoms the person suffering this kind of pain may go without greatly needed treatment.

Acute pain is impossible to ignore, and usually people do seek help for it. This kind of pain is stabbing, burning, penetrating, and excruciating; no one can stand it long enough to function at all normally. Pain like that affects sleeping, eating, talking, and all other aspects of life, and demands immediate attention.

It's quite helpful for any older person who's experiencing pain to keep a pain diary, recording the degree of pain experienced on a six-point scale. The American Cancer Society suggests this rating scale:

0 = no pain
1 = discomfort
2 = mild pain
3 = distress
4 = severe pain
5 = excruciating pain

This diary should be kept daily, whether or not pain is there, and taken to the doctors at every visit and used in telephone conversations with the doctor or nurse. The diary should reflect

when the pain started
what triggered it
what the person was doing at the time
what relieved the pain, if anything
how long the pain relief lasted
how the pain is rated on a scale of 0 to 5

This information will give the physician a picture of the older person's pain. The doctor will then be able to determine how to alleviate the pain with medications or other techniques.

It's fairly standard practice for physicians to work up a pain-management ladder, beginning with, perhaps, Tylenol (acetaminophen) or aspirin, which are surprisingly effective against chronic pain if given without interruption. At the next level are the nonsteroidal, anti-inflammatory drugs such as Motrin. Then come the weak narcotic drugs such as codeine, propoxyphene (Darvon), and oxycodone (Percodan, Percocet). Strong narcotics such as morphine, hydromorphone (Dilaudid), or levorphanol are pulled out only when they're absolutely necessary to keep people free of pain during the advanced stages of disease.

Older people are sometimes reluctant to take morphine or any other narcotics because of fear they will become addicted to drugs. But they should be assured that they will not become addicts. Although the patient may build tolerance for the drug, this problem can be managed by switching medication at an appropriate time.

The side effects of narcotics, often a problem in the past, are more manageable today. Drowsiness and nausea, in particular, can now be treated with drugs that weren't available a decade ago. Antagonists, the drugs that block side effects of a drug as it is being given, are a big boon to pain management. Doctors used to have to be extremely careful not to give enough morphine to depress the breathing center in the brain. Now antagonists are available to block that negative aspect of some morphine drugs.

One of the best things about pain management today is the great development in pharmacology that allows doctors such a wide choice of options in treating pain. In each drug family, many more choices are on the market, especially among drugs designed to treat acute pain. These can be given alone or in combination to reduce side effects and increase comfort and safety for the patient.

Another significant change is in the delivery of drugs to the body.

In the old days not long since, narcotics and other potent painkillers could be injected only at spaced intervals, a real problem for two reasons. First, it was impossible to keep enough of the drug in the patient's blood to prevent peaks and valleys of pain control. The patient would usually start to feel the drug wearing away and endure pain while waiting for the next injection. The other problem was that patients who needed powerful injectable painkillers for chronic or acute pain had no choice but to become pincushions with no places on the body that weren't sore from previous injections.

Today, injections are still given in the hospital and patients and their families are taught to administer injections at home. But when injections are no longer suitable, better ways are at hand to deliver the painkiller. These methods allow patients the relief of being able to stay at home, whereas before, they often had to go to the hospital to get treatment for intractable pain. Now, long-acting morphine, for one, comes in a pill that lasts twelve hours. This revolutionary invention means that a patient like Dan Stucky can take two pills of morphine every day at home while he watches the National Basketball Association playoffs in an easy chair with his grandchildren and other neighborhood visitors. Not long ago, he would have been confined in the hospital.

Another major improvement is the portable infusion pump that allows long-term use at home. The latest version of this pump, called a Patient Controlled Analgesic (PCA), is worn like a beeper on the patient's waist, much as doctors and nurses wear a beeper wherever they go. The difference is that this pump has a tube that inserts into a vein and gives a continuous drip of painkiller into the blood stream. The patient does have to insert medication into the pump every day and make sure that it's properly cleaned. Not all older people are candidates for the device. It takes manual dexterity that might be difficult for arthritis patients, and requires good vision and mental acuity.

For people who cannot tolerate pills or use an infusion pump, an option at home or in the hospital is continuous intravenous infusion from an IV pole at the patient's bedside. This relatively new arrangement allows doctors to give continuous pain relief. For an IV to be used at home, the family must be very carefully taught by a qualified visiting nurse from a home health agency recommended by the doctor. They need to know how to change the intravenous solutions and recognize when things go wrong with the IV or the patient. If your parent is sent home on an IV drip, you MUST make sure you have adequate training in how to manage it. If you or your parent don't feel you can manage an IV, insist on having a nurse come to the house to set it up and take care of it every day. At-home IVs are usually arranged through hospice programs when the patient is considered incurable. Medicare and other insurance coverages apply to hospice services (see Chapter 15).

Noninvasive pain-management techniques, such as meditation, guided imagery, biofeedback, relaxation, and other techniques can also be helpful complements to pain medication. All such techniques require training and practice to become effective. Unlike pleasant distractions such as a good videotape, television, or great music, they're not a quick fix. Remember, however, that for most people any of these techniques is not a substitute for pain medication. They are simply helpful adjuncts that give patients a real sense of control over their experience. Some people report that they add a much-needed spiritual feeling to their days.

If you help someone with pain medications at home, here are some useful tips.

• Give medications on time and in the precise dosages recommended by the doctor.

• If your patient is on a drug regime, call the doctor if pain comes on before you give the next dose.

• Be sure you report any nausea, dizziness, drowsiness, constipation, or other side effects so that the doctor can change either the medication or the dosage or provide the older person with another drug that will counter those negative effects.

Support Groups Can Help

Support groups can help both you and the person you love cope with the emotional fallout of dealing with cancer. The American Cancer Society sponsors groups in most places where they have a local chapter, and they can refer you or the person with cancer to other groups not affiliated with them. In a group, you as caregiver can share your fears, feelings, and frustrations, learn about nearby resources, and find out how to give home care that you may need to know about.

Sometimes the person who has cancer can also get a great deal of support by meeting with other cancer patients. He or she can also make new friends among people who are having similar stresses and experiences. After recovering from treatment they may enjoy getting involved in helping other cancer patients cope with the disease.

In the meantime, be sure to call or write the American Cancer Society for a free copy of *Caring for the Patient with Cancer at Home: A Guide for Patients and Families,* an invaluable resource. For other information on cancer and cancer organizations, see the Appendix.

13

Managing Medications Safely

HANDLING MEDICATIONS PROPERLY will challenge your knowledge, alertness, and common sense; it can also make an enormous difference in the health and safety of the older person you care for. Although they save lives and do miraculous things, medicines are just as dangerous as diseases and must be watched just as closely.

Drugs are a serious business at any age, but older people, who often need them for chronic conditions, also run a great risk of experiencing side effects or adverse reactions. Because the drugs move more slowly through the older body, elders are also much more susceptible to toxicity (poisoning) and drug overdoses than younger people.

It's rare to find an older person who doesn't have at least one tale to tell of a medication that created an illness at least as bad as the original disease. All too often, they have fallen into a medication—illness spiral, begun when an adverse reaction to a drug is incorrectly interpreted as a new illness. That misdiagnosis in turn leads to another prescription, which may create a new side effect that is then interpreted as another disease . . . and so on. Sometimes people are taking so many pills that it's almost impossible to sort out the condition that started a pharmaceutical chain reaction.

You'll want to do all you can to prevent the disasters that happened to the following individuals.

• Eighty-one-year-old Gladys Parker was usually a happy, independent woman who had arthritis in her hip. She became so weak and dizzy that her son was sure she was going downhill fast with some hidden disease. When he called the doctor, however, he was told not to worry; his mother was having "balance problems and feeling tired, like so many people do at her age." The doctor told the son to ask his mother to be sure to come for her annual physical, which was due in a few weeks. But before the appointment Gladys fell on the bathroom floor and broke her hip. In the emergency room her son was told that her blood test showed her to be anemic. The doctors determined that the round-the-clock doses of an aspirin substitute that she took for her arthritis pain had caused a slow bleeding condition in her stomach. The bleeding had caused anemia, with its symptoms of weakness and dizziness.

• John Zaleski, a kind, gentle, brilliant man, a former engineering professor, wandered through his house and garden talking to himself and screaming at the neighbors. At night he woke several times in a cold sweat, terrified by dreadful nightmares in which he saw bridges and other structures he had designed collapsing. His usual doctor being out of town, the secretary instructed his family to take him to the nearest emergency room. There he was so abusive to himself and others that the doctors ordered him to be put in restraints and on sedation. When the family showed the doctors a list of medications and said the behavior started after their father's last visit to the doctor, they concluded that John Zaleski's behavior could most probably be blamed on a heart medication he had started that week. Within three days he returned to normal, though exhausted and humiliated by the ordeal. It turned out he had been taking double the prescribed daily dose of the drug.

• Eighty-seven-year-old Mary Thurmond suddenly had to provide hands-on care for her husband after he experienced a stroke. Although she had been frail for several years, she insisted on taking care of him, except for a few hours a day when a woman she hired on a friend's recommendation came to dress and bathe him and take him downstairs to their building's lobby. Besides organizing and giving him thirteen medications, she had to remember to take the seven that various doctors had prescribed for her. She became thin, extremely dizzy most of the time — no doubt from all her own medications — and depressed under the arduous strain of caring for her husband. Her doctor put her on an antidepressant. The next week she was found in her apartment lying in bed, in and out of consciousness. She was a victim of polypharmacia — too many drugs at once — her kidneys had failed. On the way to the hospital she died of a heart attack, which was listed as the cause of death.

These are not just exceptional horror stories; they are coming up more and more often.

Reasons for the Problem

Drug misuse among older people is so widespread that it is referred to as "the other drug problem." Explanations are numerous and interwoven. The problem is the doctor, the patient, and the caregiver, making it unique to this day and age. Many more medical conditions (and let's not forget emotional ones) are treated with medications than ever before. The elderly person not on medications is a rare bird.

To help an elder avoid the pitfalls of drug taking, you need to understand what can go wrong.

Drugs Are Complex Concoctions

Medications are composed of potent chemicals that do not always act as intended. Not even the best doctors can precisely predict how the drugs they prescribe for elderly patients will work. For doctors, the choices are especially perplexing and snagridden when the older person has several chronic conditions at once.

Another difficulty in prescribing drugs for the elderly is that standard dosages of drugs are usually tested in middle-aged people, not those in their seventies, eighties, or nineties. If you thumb through the drug manuals that doctors commonly use, you will see that dosages are recommended for adults and children, but no special category is set for the elderly. When doctors prescribe for them, particularly new drugs, in a sense they are experimenting.

Only in recent days have drug companies begun to test new drugs for safe use by the elderly and to publicize their results. So far mandatory requirements have been applied so that drugs will be tested in older as well as younger people.

Making things worse are the drugs flooding the marketplace. Doctors can't keep up with interactions among all these drugs. Typically, they know the expected workings, side effects, and combinatory interactions of the drugs in their specialties. Knowledge of drugs in areas beyond their own is usually based on hearsay and reading in drug manuals.

Drugs Are Processed Differently in the Aging Body
The elderly, like the very young, usually need to have drugs prescribed for them with extreme caution. Bodily changes with aging alter the way in which drugs are processed in the body.

In its journey from entrance to exit, a drug goes through four steps as it is absorbed, distributed, metabolized (broken down), and eventually excreted. A drug's harmless progress through the body depends on all these steps working according to the expectations of the scientists who designed it. Expectations are usually adjusted for drug takers in the prime of life. Let's see how drugs are processed in the aging body.

Altered Absorption. A drug taken through the mouth and into the stomach can be absorbed at varying rates, for an older person's stomach is usually slower at churning up and digesting its contents. Sluggish absorption of drugs is not usually significant, but it can be if a drug works only with exquisitely fine tuning of the dosage. Stomach irritation is a much greater worry. Drugs known to be caustic to the stomach lining certainly will more easily irritate it, if they stay in the stomach longer.

Altered Distribution. On their way through the circulation, drugs have varying affinities for different tissues. Some drugs are especially attracted to water, some to fat, some to muscle, and some to bloodstream proteins called albumin. As the body gets older the proportions of the tissue types shift. Usually, fatty tissue increases, muscle mass decreases, and less water is carried in the circulation. The blood stream also carries less albumin — a binding site for some drugs — especially if the older person is ill or undernourished. All these changes in body composition make internal drug processing more complicated.

Unless this altered body map is worked into the drug dosing plan, the possibility is strong that too much of a drug will be retained at the wrong place in the body. An example is Valium, (diazepam) which is highly fat soluble, or attracted to fatty tissue. An eighty-five-year-old given Valium according to standard dosage may retain it in her fat tissue beyond the time it was supposed to have left the body. After several doses she could easily experience signs of Valium toxicity because the drug has built up in her body.

Altered Metabolism. Drugs and potentially poisonous substances are metabolized — chemically changed — by enzymes in the liver and broken down into compounds that can be safely used. An older person's liver often receives less blood flow and loses significant amounts of enzymes. This slowdown means drugs given at normal adult dosages remain more potent and more capable of causing toxicity.

Altered Excretion. With age the kidneys slow considerably and lose their ability to quickly and easily flush medication from the body. Some studies show that by the eighties, kidney function has diminished as much as 50 percent. When drugs leave the body at a slower rate, they can build up to a blood level higher than might be preferred.

Polypharmacia — Too Many Drugs at Once

"It seemed something had to be done for mother. She was on thirteen medications that were making her dizzy, forgetful, and nauseated some days. She wasn't the same person she'd been a year or so before.

"We called her gynecologist, her internist, her cardiologist, her arthritis specialist, and her eye doctor, and each said that if she went off the medications they had prescribed, her symptoms would return. None of these specialists seemed to want to take the time to talk to the others about mother's medications. We felt hopeless; it was all so clear to us that all those drugs were a disease in themselves.

"Sure, she needed to take heart and high blood-pressure medications, but did she need to be on seven drugs for these conditions alone? along with a diuretic? What about the cortisone she was taking for her rheumatoid arthritis, along with the aspirin she took every day? Was cortisone necessary? Her arthritis didn't seem that bad. We wanted to take her off the antianxiety medicine; somehow this seemed one that would not be dangerous for us to withdraw. But she wouldn't even consider the idea, and told us she needed it for the jumpiness she felt from the medications.

"The last straw came with the skin rash, which formed all over her back and arms. Her internist prescribed an expensive cream, which tipped her monthly bills for drugs up to $300. When the rash didn't go away we were told mother should see a dermatologist.

"Fortunately, we live in a big city. Los Angeles has several uni-

versity hospitals with geriatrics departments. We called the hospital closest to us and asked if they had a walk-in clinic. When we made an appointment the secretary told us to put all mother's medications in a bag and bring them in.

"If only we had taken this step sooner, mother would have been saved untold suffering. A geriatrician hospitalized her for three days for detoxification and observation. Now she's on five prescription medications, and aspirin as needed for her arthritis pain when it flares up. She is feeling a whole lot better. So do we; we have our mother back."

That's James Coltran, sixty-one, talking about his eighty-three-year-old mother.

This woman was lucky that she had a caring family able to intervene and set her drug taking on the right track before things got completely out of hand. No conclusive studies are reported on the elderly people who die of polypharmacia — too many drugs at once — but certainly the number must be high. Droves of elderly people are being hospitalized because of drug-related symptoms. One study showed that about 12 to 17 percent of hospital admissions are prescription-drug related.

Of course elderly people have plenty of health problems and usually do need to take several medications at once; if they don't, their health can worsen. But multiple health problems lead to multiple medications. The likelihood of adverse reactions increase in direct proportion to the number of drugs one takes at any age.

And yet, no one needs to take a slew of medications — twelve, fifteen, or twenty of them — one on top of the other, every day. The doctor who keeps prescribing more and more drugs for a patient, without weeding some out, is putting the patient on a fast track to danger. A thoughtful physician will prescribe a new drug only after carefully examining the patient to see if the illness the drug is intended for is really present. And if the illness does merit drug treatment, this physician will keep a careful eye on all the other drugs this patient is taking and how these may interact with each other and the new drug.

But though it is a doctor problem, polypharmacia is just as much a patient problem. The elderly person as drug consumer should let the doctor know about other doctors being seen, and exactly what drugs these doctors have already prescribed. This is the patient's responsibility much more than it is the doctor's.

Your parent as consumer and you as his or her advocate should be sure that, first, you agree with the doctor's opinion that a new drug is necessary. In an acute situation, family members usually have little time to consider what drugs are being used. But a chronic disease gives time to carefully look at the need for a drug and how it will affect the older person's ability to function. If it affects mental coherence, emotional or physical stability, or vision and hearing, a drug may be worse than the disease.

Noncompliance

A patient's failure to take medications according to specific directions is called noncompliance. The refusal is an obvious danger in itself, just as harmful as a doctor's not caring about aging changes, how they affect prescribing, or how many drugs a patient is already on. Compliance starts in the doctor's office. The doctor should give clear directions, but the patient should send up a mental red flag as each prescription is written, and not leave unless directions are written down and thoroughly understood. If the older person is incapable of following directions, then it's a caregiver's responsibility to get proper directions and see that they are carried out.

Anyone who ministers to elderly people knows that more than a few can be lax about taking the medications they really do need to take. Studies show that more than half the people over sixty-five don't take their prescriptions according to their doctor's instructions. Often patients don't know the names of the drugs they are taking, how to use them, or even why they're taking them. Many patients skip dosages, neglect to refill prescriptions, and take their medicines at the wrong time in the wrong dosage with the wrong foods and drinks. Many elderly people also swap medications with friends and decide to take drugs from friends, without even telling their doctors.

Usually you can find a good reason, or several reasons explaining why someone doesn't take medications according to specifications. Only when these reasons have been identified can the lack be corrected. One of the main reasons elderly people fail to take important medications is that their other medications cause confusion and disorientation. Another is cost: many people, rich or poor, give up on high-priced drugs. Another reason is befuddlement over having to juggle several medications at once, perhaps several times a day. Without an organized schedule and system for taking drugs, the whole business becomes a setup for mistakes and frustration.

Safety

Now that you know where the trouble spots are, you need practical advice about how to make the best of medications so that they are a help rather than a hindrance — a benefit to the older person's quality of life, rather than a deranger of mental and physical abilities. In the rest of this chapter we map out for you how drug taking should be approached. We suggest solutions to the problems we have just discussed, and a way out from under problems that may already be afflicting your parent or anyone you care for.

Working with the Doctor

One Doctor Must Be in Charge. Your parents, for example, will be far less likely to run into trouble with medications with a good primary doctor. Even if different specialists are consulted infrequently or regularly, this doctor can act as gatekeeper for the plan of care and as protector of your parents' best interests.

This primary doctor must thoroughly understand geriatric medicine in order to safely prescribe medications and monitor the medications given by other specialists. Your parents should respect and like this doctor and fully believe he or she cares about them as patients as well as people. Communication is vital to proper drug taking. Going to a doctor who rushes through appointments can make them feel uncomfortable asking questions and talking about their worries. A caring doctor encourages patients to get on the telephone when they experience side effects, or when they grapple with some detail they don't fully understand.

If your parents are not seeing any one doctor who is obviously in charge of their care, we suggest you help them find one. In shopping around for a general practitioner, an internist, or a geriatrician, make it clear that you're looking for someone to take on the job of commander-in-chief of their health, including all their medicines. When you go in for an appointment, bring all the drugs your parent takes. The doctor can then do a "brown-bag review." Remember to include over-the-counter drugs as well as those prescribed by doctors.

Because medications are usually part of medical management for just about any problem, evaluating a doctor's approach in prescribing medications will give you a pretty good idea of overall ability. If the doctor seems "free" with medications and unwilling to accept challenges to his or her way of prescribing for and taking care of your parents, then he or she is not the best doctor for them.

The Geriatrician's Golden Rules for Prescribing. Beyond a doctor's manner and willingness to communicate, how can you judge if he or she is prescribing judiciously? Prescribing is a tricky business that depends on many variables, especially the patient's health and number of complaints. But we suggest these points of reference in looking at how your parent's illnesses are being handled, some golden rules that doctors should follow when prescribing medications for the elderly. Although complex medical problems don't allow of simple solutions, nevertheless basic principles of doctoring for the elderly do always apply. You can find these principles in any basic geriatric medical or nursing text.

Rule 1. Stopping a drug is generally more beneficial than starting one.

Rule 2. Use as few drugs as possible.

Rule 3. Manage medical problems without drugs, as much as possible.

Rule 4. Don't give a drug if its side effects are worse than the disease.

Rule 5. Keep dosages low and go slowly if increasing them.

Rule 6. Monitor the effects and toxicity of any drugs frequently.

Rule 7. Stop useless drugs.

Rule 8. Keep a profile of all the drugs the patient is taking, including those from other doctors and nonprescription drugs.

Rule 9. Help the patient keep drug costs down.

Rule 10. Monitor the patient's compliance and make sure medications are taken according to directions.

The Patient's Part. When the doctor hands over a prescription to a patient, it is the patient's responsibility to ask some basic questions. No one should go rushing off to the drugstore to get the order filled without knowing the fundamental reasons why the drug has been prescribed and the consequences of taking it. If you are managing your parent's, or another older person's, overall plan of care, be sure these questions have been asked about any drug being considered. If your parent hasn't asked them, call or make an appointment with the doctor and ask them yourself.

- What will the medicine do for the problem?
- Is the drug necessary?
- Can nonpharmacological approaches to the problem be found?
- How does the drug work?
- Will it interact with other medications?
- What are the side effects? Common, expected ones, as well as severe ones?
- Can this drug easily cause toxicity?
- Should the drug be taken with meals? after meals? on an empty stomach?
- When is the best time of day to take the drug?
- Should any foods be avoided?
- Should any activities be avoided?
- How long does the drug need to be taken?

Anyone who has a health problem or several at once should keep a medications record. (We show a sample later in this chapter.) Take this record to every doctor's appointment. It can be filled in each time a new drug is prescribed and altered as the drug plan changes. Most important: show the record to all doctors at all appointments so that they know from one time to the next what your parent is taking and in what quantities, among other considerations. Think of it as a written agreement between doctor and patient, a contract based on the doctor's prescribing appropriately and the patient's complying by following directions.

Reading the Prescription

One vital aspect of being a drug consumer is to be able to read the prescription before the pharmacist translates it and labels the container. Doctors and pharmacists usually are very careful, but as a consumer getting your parents' prescriptions filled, or helping them with the job, you should become part of the team and take responsibility for double-checking.

Mistakes can happen along the way. The doctor can slip up and write out the wrong dosage or the wrong concentration, even the wrong name of the drug. The pharmacist can make errors in translating the doctor's orders. After years of writing notes on patients and hundreds of prescriptions every week, quite a few doctors have a rapid-fire shorthand that is difficult to read. Anyone handed a prescription to fill should look at it before leaving the doctor's sight and be sure the words and letters are legible beyond doubt. Besides being a safety practice, doing this proofreading will save time at the pharmacy. We have all seen pharmacists scratching their head over the meaning of a prescription, and calling the doctor who wrote it for an over-the-telephone decoding.

Reading the prescription is simply a matter of (1) deciphering the handwriting, and (2) learning the symbols doctors have used for centuries to communicate with pharmacists. Most symbols are abbreviated Latin words, left over from the bygone days when medicine was taught in Latin. If you are faced with a prescription that you can't understand, don't be intimidated — just refer to this list, and if it's still not clear, ask the doctor.

a.c.	before meals	**O.U.**	each eye
A.D.	right ear	**p.c.**	after meals
A.L.	left ear	**p.o.**	by mouth
b.i.d.	twice a day	**p.r.**	by rectum
c.	with	**p.r.n.**	as needed
cap.	capsule	**q.h.**	every hour
cc	cubic centimeter	**q.2h.**	every two hours
ext.	external use, extract	**q.3h.**	every three hours
gt., gtt.	drop, drops	**q.i.d.**	four times a day
h.	hour	**s.l.**	under the tongue
h.s.	at bedtime	**sol.**	solution
int.	between meals	**susp.**	suspension
ml	milliliter (30 ml = 1 ounce)	**tab.**	tablet
	(5 ml = 1 teaspoon)	**t.i.d.**	three times a day
O.D.	right eye	**top.**	apply topically
O.S.	left eye	**ut dict.**	as directed

Reading the Label. As a saving gesture to us English speakers, pharmacists type up labels for drug packages in plain, easy-to-read English, as in the label illustrated on page 311.

As a service to customers many pharmacists add information the doctor may have left off the prescription, about how a drug should be taken. Some pharmacists post colorful stickers on the vial or package, such as:

Medications should be taken with plenty of water.
Take with food.
Do not drive — may cause drowsiness.

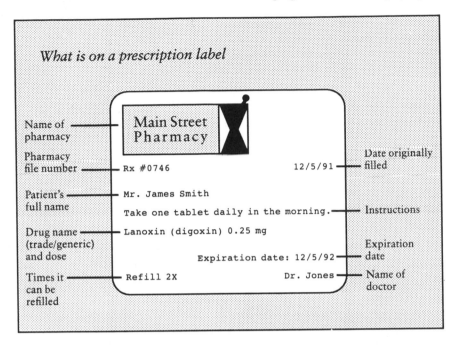

What is on a prescription label

Name of pharmacy — **Main Street Pharmacy**

Pharmacy file number — Rx #0746   12/5/91 — Date originally filled

Patient's full name — Mr. James Smith

Take one tablet daily in the morning. — Instructions

Drug name (trade/generic) and dose — Lanoxin (digoxin) 0.25 mg

Expiration date: 12/5/92 — Expiration date

Times it can be refilled — Refill 2X   Dr. Jones — Name of doctor

Do not drink milk or eat dairy products with this medication. Take medication on an empty stomach.

Or, as with many diuretics, "It may be advisable to drink a full glass of orange juice or eat a banana daily with this medication."

The Local Pharmacist
When they step behind the counter, pharmacists aren't just dropping pills into containers and mixing solutions. Their job carries a lot of responsibility and they are trained professionals who have put in at least three years of specialized education in pharmacology. They learn about toxicity, metabolism, and the absorption of drugs — in short, everything about how drugs behave in the body. They also learn how to help patients manage their drugs and doctors to prescribe the best treatment.

A good pharmacist will prove helpful to your parents in all aspects of drug taking. Finding a local pharmacy, where your parents like the pharmacists, is just as important as picking a good doctor. It's a good idea to select just one in the neighborhood, and to stick with it for drug purchases, including those bought off the shelf. In a responsible, well-run pharmacy, records are kept on every patient. The pharmacist will include a patient's allergies, chronic illnesses, and frequently used over-the-counter drugs, and will check all new prescriptions against the record. Many pharmacies have set up a computerized record system and have bought sophisticated programs that read out how different drugs will interact in combination with each other. To cut costs you may want to combine using medications purchased in a local pharmacy with some purchased at lower cost through a mail-order service (see below).

The pharmacist has a legal obligation to catch mistakes on prescriptions and to call the doctor if filling the prescription means danger to the patient. Pharmacists also are legally obligated to tell the patient the drug is dangerous, and not fill the prescription if the doctor won't change it. Although they don't have the authority to change a prescription, they do have the knowledge to advise patients and make recommendations that have to do with safety and all aspects of drug taking.

Any "good" pharmacy will offer a range of helpful services, which include:

- Keeping drug profiles on patients
- Checking drug interactions on a computer or in manuals
- Drug counseling about when medications should be taken, side effects to look out for, how to manage side effects, foods to avoid, and activities to avoid
- Cost-cutting advice
- Advising about storage
- Giving out written information published by manufacturers of drugs
- Providing easy-to-open containers for people with arthritis
- Providing a liquid form of medication for those who have difficulty swallowing tablets or capsules
- Typing directions in larger print for the visually impaired
- Itemizing information for insurance and tax records
- Offering delivery for the homebound
- Offering charge accounts

Mail-Order Pharmacy Services
Although the ideal is for an older person to use one pharmacist, it is not the cheapest way to go. Many company health plans include through-the-mail catalogue service for discount drugs. So too does

the American Association of Retired Persons (AARP) Pharmacy Service, which is the largest private mail service by far, processing more than 8 million prescriptions every year.

These catalogue services offer drugs at low prices. Ordering drugs from a catalogue can mean considerable savings, perhaps as much as 80 percent on some drugs particularly if in generic versions. They are ideal for the person who needs to take drugs every day for maintenance in chronic illnesses. Drugs can be purchased in bulk and stored for long-term use.

Mail-service pharmacies take prescriptions sent by consumers and process them just as does any neighborhood pharmacy. The prescription is checked by phone with the doctor, if necessary, and computer records are kept on patients just as in a retail-store pharmacy. Toll-free telephone lines allow customers to call in orders for and ask questions about their drugs. The AARP Pharmacy Service sends out easy-to-understand leaflets on drugs sent to customers, and it will fill any prescription that can be sent through the mail.

If your parents do use a mail-order service, they will still need to find a pharmacy in their neighborhood. Catalogue services usually take about a week to deliver and so are not able to meet short-term demands for drugs. The person who needs a medication that very day, such as an antibiotic, a painkiller, or an anti-itch cream, will not be able to wait for a catalogue order to come through. Some drugs can only be purchased from drugstores, and some have special storage requirements and so will not travel well. So-called state-controlled substances, such as narcotics and amphetamines, are not allowed to be sold through the mail.

If your parents believe ordering from a catalogue will work well for their condition, then they need to find out if their health plan has such a service. The AARP service is available to all its members. To find out about membership, which costs only $5 a year, contact the AARP (see Appendix for details). Their pharmacy service operates out of thirteen satellite pharmacies across the country. It has an excellent reputation.

Getting Medications Organized

Medications have to be taken on time, in the correct dosages, and according to special instructions. If your parent needs to take several preparations, doing so can become not just complicated but boggling. To keep medications straight, you need to set up a system that makes the task easy and sure. If remembering to take them is a problem, the system must also include reminders — mind joggers — telling when it is time to take each medication.

The Basic Chart System. Keeping checkoff charts is by far the best method for anyone who can easily write and read. The best approach is to copy and keep two charts.

The Medication Record (page 315) is a quick summary of all the drugs being taken, including

- Name of the medication
- Reason for taking it
- Name of doctor who prescribed it
- Date on which it was started
- What it looks like
- When to take it
- How to take it

This chart can provide space for the name of each drug, what it's for, its shape and color, directions for taking it (how many times a day it should be taken, with meals or on an empty stomach, and any special warnings), and the time of day when it should be taken. You can copy this chart and hang it near the place where the medicines are kept so that your parents can refer to it. It's a good idea to keep a copy to take along to doctors' appointments.

The "Medications I Take" chart (page 316) is handier and designed to be portable in a handbag or pocket for outings from home. It's simply a handy chart for keeping track of when medicines are taken and for marking the times when they are supposed to be taken. The chart can be copied on a small card for weekly use, or on a larger sheet to be hung up at home near the store of medications. This chart functions more as a reminder than a record, and for this reason it can be thrown away once filled out completely.

The Color-Coded Chart System. If your parent is visually impaired or mildly confused, try working with a color-coded system. Write out a poster-sized chart with large block letters, giving the name of each medication and when it's supposed to be taken. Next to each drug's name, place a colored sticker that matches one you put on the drug's container. To follow up drug taking, make a large chart with oversized writing like the one we show.

Medication Record

MEDICATION NAME REASON FOR USE	DESCRIBE MEDI- CINE HERE	WHEN TO TAKE MEDICINE				SPECIAL DIRECTIONS

REMEMBER
BRING THIS CHART TO ALL DOCTOR APPOINTMENTS.
INCLUDE ALL THE MEDICATIONS YOU ARE TAKING.
DO NOT CHANGE THE WAY YOU TAKE THE MEDICATIONS WITHOUT
CALLING THE DOCTOR.
DO NOT SHARE MEDICATIONS.
IF YOU HAVE ANY QUESTIONS, CALL THE DOCTOR.

The Daily or Weekly Pillbox. You can buy a compartmented pill dispenser from a drugstore or surgical-supply store. These containers are helpful for people who have trouble counting out pills for the day and remembering at what time each gets taken. The several designs on the market include some with built-in beeper alarms that go off at times you can set. Most people select a weekly pillbox with seven compartments, each divided into four that can be marked for different times of the day. A daily pillbox can simply be marked to hold a day's medicines. The advantage of this method is that you or another caregiver can count out the pills for the day or the week, or the older person can do so at a routine pill-sorting time.

Two cautions apply in using any container method. First, some drugs lose their strength when taken out of an airtight container, and others may have to be kept refrigerated. Before setting up a con-

Medicines I Take

Name of drug and what it's for	Color and shape	Directions and cautions	Times

tainer system, ask the pharmacist if drugs will be adversely affected. Second, this approach involves leaving medications out of their capped containers, where they are more easily accessible to small children.

Generic Drugs

The best way for your parents to cut down on the cost of their drugs is to turn to generic versions, whenever they are available. Most drugs that have been around for more than fifteen years are on the market in generic form. You or your parents will find generic versions of drugs in the local drugstore, or through a mail-order pharmacy service.

Your parents should always ask their doctors if a drug is available in generic form. In some states, even this step is not necessary,

Memory Joggers

The forgetful or confused person needs more than a well-organized system showing which pill to take when. If your parent is unable to remember, consider these approaches.

- You will be responsible for saying when it is pill-taking time.
- You can call your parent at the appropriate times.
- Put medications in front of several alarm clocks set to appropriate pill-taking times.
- Staple plastic bags with a day's worth of pills to a large-print calendar. Ask your parent to cross off the date after all pills have been taken for the day.
- Place pills where your parent is likely to be at pill-taking times. Put morning pills at the breakfast table, after-lunch pills next to the armchair, and evening pills in a container near where your parent sits before going to bed.
- Keep nitroglycerin and other emergency pills in a container above the head of the bed.

for laws allow pharmacists to automatically fill a prescription with the cheaper generic version of a drug, unless the doctor has specifically written down that only the brand-name version is to be used.

Don't fall into the trap of thinking that generic drugs are second best to their brand-name equivalents, just because generics are so much cheaper. Most generic drugs are just as safe and effective as their brand-name equivalents.

What is a generic drug? Any drug has two names: its generic name, which is a simplified version of its chemical formula, and its brand name, which is given it by the manufacturer who innovates and first markets it under an exclusive patent. Once the patent expires, after fifteen years, other companies are free to manufacture the drug under the generic name or under another brand name. The antibiotic tetracycline is advertised and sold as tetracycline, but also under brand names such as Achromycin and Sumycin.

In shopping for generic versions of drugs it is helpful to know the generic names as well as the brand names. The table on page 318 will familiarize you with the generic names of fifty-two brand-name drugs that, according to AARP Pharmacy Service statistics, are most commonly prescribed for those who are age fifty and over.

Brand (trade) name	Generic (chemical) name
Aldomet	Methyldopa
Aldoril	Methyldopa and hydrochlorothiazide
Apresoline	Hydralazine
Ativan	Lorazepam
Calan	Verapamil
Capoten	Captopril
Cardizem	Diltiazem
Catapres	Clonidine
Clinoril	Sulindac
Corgard	Nadolol
Coumadin	Warfarin
Deltasone	Prednisone
DiaBeta	Glyburide
Dilantin	Phenytoin
Dyazide	Triamterene and hydrochlorothiazide
Feldene	Piroxicam
Halcion	Triazolam
Inderal	Propranolol
Isordil	Isosorbide dinitrate
Lanoxin	Digoxin
Lasix	Furosemide
Levothroid	L-thyroxine (Levothyroxine)
Lopid	Gemfibrozil
Lopressor	Metoprolol
Lorelco	Probucol
Maxzide	Triamterene and hydrochlorothiazide
Mevacor	Lovastatin
Micronase	Glyburide
Micro-K	Potassium chloride
Motrin	Ibuprofen
Naprosyn	Naproxen
Nitro-Bid	Nitroglycerin
Norpace	Disopyramide
Nolvadex	Tamoxifen
Persantine	Dipyridamole
Premarin	Estrogens, conjugated
Procardia	Nifedipine
Quinidex	Quinidine sulfate
Sinemet	Levodopa and carbidopa

Brand (trade) name	Generic (chemical) name
Synthroid	L-thyroxine (Levothyroxine)
Tagamet	Cimetidine
Timoptic	Timolol
Tenormin	Atenolol
Theo-Dur	Theophylline
Trental	Pentoxifylline
Valium	Diazepam
Vasotec	Enalapril
Ventolin	Albuterol
Voltaren	Diclofenac
Xanax	Alprazolam
Zantac	Ranitidine
Zyloprim	Allopurinol

Source: *AARP Pharmacy Service Prescription Drug Handbook*, 1992.

14

Caring for
the Convalescent at Home

WHAT WOULD YOU DO if you had to take care of your parent or
an elderly friend during a brief illness of a week or so, such as the
flu, or during convalescence from an injury or surgery? Would you
know how to set up the sickroom, make the bed, and provide personal care so that you could step in and handle basic caregiving tasks
for a short period?

If not, don't worry unduly. Most people don't know how. The
essentials are not hard to learn. We'll give you the basic steps in making
your family member or friend feel as comfortable as possible and
psychologically at ease, so that all energy can be channeled toward
feeling better. Then you'll get a crash course in preventing the complications that can occur when people are confined to bed for a few
days for more than a good night's sleep — complications purely related to lying in bed, not to the original illness that put them there in
the first place.

Get Directions from the Doctor

Directions on how to manage medical routines related to the original illness need to come from the doctor and nurses involved in the
older person's case. If it's been determined that the illness can be
treated at home, see that the doctor has informed you about the kind
of recovery that is expected and how to recognize problems that may
arise. Report any symptoms that are not an expected part of the illness. Anything new and unusual for the condition should be reported, such as pain, diarrhea, constipation that does not respond

to natural treatments, dizziness, confused behavior, depression, loss of appetite, or fecal or urinary incontinence. Find out too how to get through to the doctor in an emergency, and how to make routine reports if wanted. Learning how the individual doctor's system works will save a lot of hassles.

If you're bringing the patient home from the hospital for convalescence, understand fully what you are getting into. Well before the discharge, talk to the doctor and nurses in charge of the hospital care. Get precise directions on how to take care of your patient, with a clear picture of what the patient can and cannot do. Find out when and how to give medications, how to take care of a surgical wound, and learn special dietary and exercise possibilities. If special treatments have been prescribed, find out how to give them.

Preparing for the homecoming of someone who is severely debilitated — by a stroke, a broken hip or other bone, a complicated operation, or a severe illness — means you'll be in an entirely different level of involvement from the one we prepare you for in this chapter.

If you find yourself a caregiver for someone who needs rehabilitation of lost functions, or skilled nursing tasks, you must talk to the hospital discharge planner. This person's job is to consult with the doctor and nurses about what you can and cannot take on, and how to organize a home health-care team to carry out difficult tasks. You will find out how much payment for services you can expect to get from the older person's Medicare, Medicaid, and private insurance policies.

Nothing like Tender, Loving Care

Emotions and feelings are essential to healing. They are indispensable for controlling pain and discomfort, even the new, unwanted symptoms that can confound recovery from an illness or an injury. In a sense, positive feelings are the nutrients of the mind, just as necessary as the nutrients we must all have to stay well and to build up nutrition and strength as we recover.

You will need to take any steps you can to fill the older person you are caring for as full of good feelings and comfort as possible. Besides encouraging your family member to follow medical directions, you need to set things up for plenty of uninterrupted sleep, rest and relaxation, relief from pain, and nourishing meals to bolster the immune system. Your job is to help your family member feel as comfortable as possible so that his or her energies can be free for healing and getting back to the level of functioning the doctor considers a realistic expectation.

You and other caregivers will be doing a lot more work during the early stage of convalescence than will be required later. You may have to help your patient with bathing, toileting, and moving around the room. While doing these tasks, don't lose sight of your patient's need to feel in control. Your goal is to help the older person get back on his or her feet and to recover lost functions. Ask: What clothes would you like to wear? What time for a walk? What would you like to eat?

Although the tasks you perform and the comforts you provide are all-important, recovery is ultimately up to the person who is sick or injured. You need to encourage the older person to take an active role in recovery; being passive will only stall or deter progress and contribute to profound frustration. Plenty of tender, loving care from you and other family members will be an immeasurable boost to the older person's morale, but so too will encouragement to take control of getting better.

The convalescing older person may be quite anxious and afraid to resume activities such as getting out of bed to a chair, or to the bathroom, dressing, and taking meals again at the table with the rest of the family. Using any newly introduced assistive devices may seem prohibitively difficult. Your moral support will show best if you try not to rush the older person into new activities. Everything that is going to happen should be explained in detail, and you should repeat instructions as they are carried out. It may be helpful for you to talk about activities the day before you plan to introduce them.

Remember that the words "I can't" are usually another way of saying "I'm afraid." Instead of getting into a battle of words that might end up with you accusing the older person of stubbornness and defeatism, try to be reassuring and say you and other helpers will be close by to help with the new activity slowly, step by step. You may find yourself frequently saying "take your time."

Besides keeping the bedridden person comfortable in clean, fresh, wrinkle-free sheets and preventing all the problems that can arise from time spent in bed — pneumonia, circulatory disorders, constipation, and bedsores — you can find plenty of ways to hearten your patient and expedite recovery. The atmosphere you create should be one of calm and solace, and the tempo of days and evenings slow-paced, but not dragging into boredom and inertia. Here are some suggestions.

The Bedroom

• If you can choose, decide which room in the house to set up as a sickroom. Try to use a room that is cheerful, with a window which has good light and which allows the older person to see the changing world outside. Windows should have light-blocking curtains or blinds so that you can darken the room for naps and cut out glare when the sun is intense. Decide whether it is best to use a room away from the center of activity, or one close to it, so that the older person will not miss out on participating in family life. A room near the center of activity may make caregiving easier for you and other helpers, because serving meals and bringing things back and forth will be less cumbersome. Also, the convalescing person will be easier to hear.

• Consider renting a hospital bed, over-bed table, or wheelchair.

• Keep the room orderly by setting aside a corner for special supplies and equipment. The room should be as homelike as possible. Most convalescing people don't want to constantly look at sickroom supplies and containers of medications.

• Put a large calendar and a clock near the bedside, for it is easy for an ill person to lose track of time and days.

• Bring in flowers and plants to liven up the room and freshen the air.

• Put a pitcher of water and a glass at the bedside.

Meals

• Find out from the doctor if the older person needs a special diet. One may need to be designed for the physiologic demands of the illness and interference by any drugs with the body's production and utilization of vitamins and minerals. During illness the body's need for a balanced diet increases dramatically. So too does the need for nutrients such as vitamin C, of which the body needs more to counter emotional and physical stress.

• Illnesses and surgery can deplete the body's protein stores, leading to tissue loss and weakening the immune system. Ask for suggestions that will add protein to the diet. These may include offering high-protein liquid supplements; adding skim-milk powder to cooked dishes, cereals, and desserts; and adding diced or ground meat to soups, casseroles, and vegetable dishes.

• When the diet provides too few calories, the body draws on its stores of fat for fuel. Then it begins to break down protein, leading to tissue loss and weakened immune functions. Ask the doctor if you need to offer high-calorie dietary supplements and high-calorie, even high-fat foods.

• If you do need to offer a liquid dietary supplement, it may be more palatable chilled.

• Try to keep a routine mealtime schedule that is close to yours and that of the rest of the family. If the older person can't join the family at the table, family members should rotate taking meals in the older person's room. This strategy may motivate the older person to eat what he or she is served.

• If appetite is low, try serving small meals frequently at times you identify when appetite peaks. Breakfast may be the ideal time to provide a bigger meal, because the older person has all day to convert it into calories. Anticipate the effects of medications and treatments in your meal planning.

• Always try to follow the older person's food preferences and vary the color and texture of food.

• Presentation is an effective appetite stimulant, especially if the illness has dulled smell and taste. Arrange food and drinks on the tray as pleasantly as possible. Use varied, colorful napkins and place mats, and bring out the "best" china every now and then.

• It's best to start out planning small servings with an option for seconds. Large, heaped servings can deter even someone whose appetite is coming back.

• If the older person tires easily, save their strength for eating. If necessary, caregivers should butter the bread, cut food into pieces, and pour liquids.

• If the older person is visually impaired, be sure to put the food where they can see it. If necessary, you can describe where food is on the plate by comparing its location to hours on a clock face.

• Look into special assistive eating utensils if the older person has difficulty using standard ones. These include plate guards that keep food from spilling off the plate, suction cups on plate bottoms to prevent them from sliding off a tray or table, special easy-to-grasp spoons and forks, long-handled utensils for those who have limited range of motion in elbows and shoulders, and weighted mugs and cups for those who have trouble with holding.

• Drinking straws that are flexible at the top are helpful for those who easily spill drinks from cups. Snap-on lids for cups will hold a straw easily.

Fighting Boredom and Irritability

• Bring in visitors if the older person is well enough to socialize.
• Provide music. It can be a great mood elevator. Upbeat music can lift mood, and soft, calm music can be relaxing.
• Television or the radio, and book or short-story tapes can be entertaining.
• Ask grandchildren and other family members and friends to come in and play games with the older person.
• Ask grandchildren and other family members and friends to come in and read to the older person as a daily routine.
• Put a telephone next to the older person's bed. Make sure the ringer can be turned off, for times when he or she prefers quiet or sleep.
• Give the older person a backrub or foot massage. The touch you and other caregivers provide will increase circulation to the skin and help the older person feel good all over.

Know the Hazards of Bed Rest

Nurses and doctors used to say "Get back into bed!" to their patients recovering from illnesses and surgery. Now they say that staying in bed is a prescription for illness, *not* recovery.

A walk through the floors of any good hospital will show you scenes of obviously sick people shuffling slowly through the halls on the arms of attendants and relatives, and other obviously sick people sitting in the armchair next to the bed. Although such patients often look forward plaintively to getting back into bed, their staying out of bed and on the move as much as possible is part of a grand design. "Up to the chair" and "ambulate in the halls" are now a hallmark of proper nursing care, applied to patients soon after surgery and during illnesses of just about any kind.

Turning away from bed as the best place for convalescing people became a matter of policy after a landmark article in *The American*

Journal of Nursing in April 1967. This famous article, "The Hazards of Immobility," is still required reading for nursing and medical students and just about anyone taking care of sick or immobile people.

The authors of the article considered how confining someone to bed can force nearly all systems of the body to become sluggish and eventually shut down. The authors gathered information from many physiological studies to make their point. They showed that calcium leaches out of bones, insulin production drops, blood pressure goes up, fluid shifts out of its usual body compartments, and hormones stop working properly. They also pointed out that the kidneys malfunction, muscles waste away, reflexes dull, and signals between the nervous system and the cardiovascular system give out.

All these changes, they demonstrated, can become evident in just a few days. Anyone who tries to get out of bed after being there too long feels weak, dizzy, and prone to fainting. Anyone who doesn't move at all in bed risks joint stiffness, bedsores, and muscles that can't take orders from the brain.

We will spare you intricate details on this fascinating subject. Instead, let's get down to the problems you'll be working to prevent if your parent or other older family member is laid low for a while. Simple home-nursing techniques that you can apply will really make a difference in preventing the following problems.

Pneumonia
The lungs work best when we stand upright and in motion. In this position they function as efficient two-way bellows, bringing in oxygen and expelling carbon dioxide, and also ridding themselves of numerous built-up secretions. In the lying-down position, though, the lungs compress and the muscles of respiration must work in an entirely different plane. Studies show that after three weeks of bed rest the lungs take in 26 percent less oxygen.

Your most immediate attention should go to the lung secretions that can quickly build up with too much lying down. Anyone confined to bed is at risk for pneumonia, and if need be you should make yourself a real nag about helping the person you are caring for to do coughing and deep-breathing exercises every two to four hours, and to move around in or out of bed. Take a look at our discussion of pneumonia and the coughing and breathing techniques we describe in Chapter 8, "Managing Lung Disorders and Preventing Pneumonia." You can help your patient do the exercises by propping him or her up against pillows and offering support to the back with your hands.

Movement promotes lung health, either in or out of bed. Encourage the older person to turn over in bed frequently and to shift position and get out of bed several times a day — to a chair and to the bathroom. If your patient is in bed for more than a few days then you need to ask the doctor to recommend exercises to do in bed. Ask too if it might not be a good idea for a nurse to come in and show your patient how to use breathing devices that give the incentive to breathe deeply and fill the lungs.

Circulatory Problems

The most dramatic physical changes affect the cardiovascular system. Bed rest causes a pooling of blood in the extremities, thickening of the blood's components, and increased workload for the heart. These changes can have an especially profound effect on an older person who already has heart or circulation problems.

But the biggest danger is a condition called thrombophlebitis, which is inflammation of a vein and formation of blood clots or emboli. These clots can become dislodged and travel quickly to the heart or the lungs, where they can cause a life-threatening emergency. Thrombophlebitis most often occurs in the lower legs.

The way to prevent circulatory difficulties and keep clots from forming is to get your patient out of bed! Besides encouraging walks around the room and trips every four hours to a chair and the bathroom, you can make sure he or she wears loose clothing in bed, avoiding tight elastic waistbands, sleeves, socks, and stockings. When the older person sits up in a chair for more than several minutes, elevate the legs on a stool from time to time. When in bed encourage him or her to change position frequently and to wiggle the toes and move the feet.

If your patient is unable to move around the room at least every four hours or so, and if it looks as if the illness will carry on for more than three days, ask the doctor if you should not purchase special antiembolism elasticized bed stockings to stimulate leg circulation and get blood flowing upward toward the heart. Clean stockings should be put on each morning after sleep, before the older person gets out of bed to a standing position.

Constipation

Vigorous circulation, and muscular activity, relaxing and contracting around the bowel, stimulate it to churn and move food through the system. Anyone on bed rest is bound to be plagued by constipation, unless steps are taken to prevent it. (See Chapter 7, "Managing Digestive Disorders.")

Step one is to find out if your patient is on any constipating medications (either prescription or over-the-counter) that could be making the condition worse. Numerous medications alter the proper workings of the bowel. Constipating medications should be taken only if absolutely necessary. This limitation includes laxatives or cathartics, which can diminish normal bowel reflexes if used too often. Many doctors prescribe stool softeners for bedridden patients, to be taken daily; however, careful attention to diet and fluid intake will accomplish the same benefit, without adding another medication to the older person's regimen.

The next step is to provide a diet high in roughage and fiber — if it is allowed by the doctor and can be tolerated. These foods include fruits and vegetables with the skins left on, prunes, and whole-grain cereals and breads. Provide plenty of liquids, too. Exercise is needed as well. Encourage movement in bed and walking around the room, as much as your patient's state of health allows.

If diet, fluids, and exercise don't seem to work, call the doctor and ask if you should offer the older person an over-the-counter bulk-forming laxative, such as Metamucil or Senokot, if he or she isn't already taking one. If a bulk laxative doesn't help, ask the doctor if you should administer a laxative or an enema. Using such preparations, your patient may be able to have a bowel movement and feel relief. But be careful to avoid excessive use of laxatives and enemas, and always rely on other measures as primary treatment for constipation.

See the list in Chapter 7 of medications that cause constipation.

Bedsores

Sores Can Quickly Become Serious Ulcers. Any older person constantly lying or sitting still on the same pressure points in bed, a chair, or a wheelchair is at very high risk for skin ulcers. The older person's skin is usually fragile, thin, and inadequately cushioned with fat. Skin breakdowns can start in just a few hours over any bony part that supports the rest of the body.

Bedsores form because unrelieved pressure blocks the skin's blood supply, allowing the skin to deteriorate. The buttocks area is especially susceptible in the lying-down or sitting positions, but the elbows, heels, toes, and hips, even the fingers are also susceptible. Besides pressure from the weight of the body, other factors can contribute trouble. Shearing motions against the sheets and friction of any kind will cause skin to break down. Any kind of fluid — sweat, urine, or feces — can also provide a medium for irritation and bacterial growth.

The first signs of a pressure sore are redness and inflammation, NOT necessarily accompanied by discomfort or pain. If a sore at this stage is not immediately tended to it will quickly turn into an area of blistered, broken skin that will heal with difficulty. Skin ulcers can quickly become very serious, progressing into deeper and deeper layers of the skin and then to muscles, tendons, and bone, each becoming infected and damaged.

Once a sore has progressed beyond the early stages of skin breakdown, it can take months for new tissue to grow back into the wound, even with the best treatment methods and daily care. Any wound that extends deep below the skin may become so badly infected that the patient has to go to the hospital for treatment, which may require surgery.

Prevention Is the Key. The very best treatment for bedsores is to make a commitment to prevent them. Here's what to do. First, you need to reposition the person in your care every two hours during the day, and during the night if he or she is not going to be shifting position and turning. You have to use common sense to determine whether or not you or someone else will have to wake up to do repositioning.

If the convalescing person wants to lie in bed most of the time, simply ask him to shift position — from back to side and stomach to side — and to alter the angles of arms and legs. Put pillows and cushions between the legs and under the ankles to soften pressure and give comfort. If the patient is wheelchair-bound or confined to a chair, ask him to shift every two hours. Cushion the back and buttocks with a pillow or wheelchair cushion, and pad the footrest if the elder cannot move the legs frequently.

Consider getting an egg-crate mattress or a mattress cover made of synthetic sheepskin to cushion the bed. These items can be rented from a surgical supply store. Such bed cushioning, though, is no substitute for repositioning to prevent bedsores. The products have a marginal effect on preventing sores, and are most useful simply in providing comfort for those who don't like lying many hours on a hard mattress.

Bedcovers really have weight, which starts to be felt when one has to lie flat for days. You can improvise a bedcovers lifting frame by cutting the bottom out of a box and putting it under the covers with the bedridden person's feet inside.

The older person needs to be moved in bed very carefully and positioned so that skin is not subject to rubbing and shearing forces. Always move your patient slowly and deliberately off the sheets, without dragging him or her up or down against the bed. The sheets need to be kept clean and wrinkle-free; even crumbs and creases can create irritation and friction. If the older person is too difficult for you alone to move, *get help*. If necessary, ask a nurse or a home health aide to come in and show you how to use a drawer sheet. When you move your patient to a sitting-up position, prevent a slide back down the bed by comfortably bolstering with pillows.

Another point of resolution is seeking professional help as soon as an area reddens with the beginnings of a bedsore. Sometimes sores can form — particularly in someone with very frail skin — despite conscientious nursing care. If you do spot a bedsore, call the doctor's nurse to arrange for a visiting nurse to start restorative therapy. While waiting for professional advice, of course readjust your patient's position off the broken-down skin and see that it is clean and dry. Restorative therapy, for an ulcer that has broken through the skin's surface layers only, consists of special cleaning techniques, dressings, creams, granules and powders, and perhaps massages and a high-protein diet.

The Caregiving Basics

Now that you know how someone can keep getting sicker just from being in bed, consider how to set things up so that you can provide basic care, aiming to prevent complications of bed rest and unnecessary discomfort for your patient. You should know the ins and outs of how to make a comfortable bed, and if necessary, how to do it with an ill person in it; how to move the person out of bed and around the room; how to arrange toileting, bathing, and general cleanliness, in or out of bed.

If the older person you are caring for is unable to move around the room without your help, you or another family member will need to see that activities are done safely, without the danger of falls. Helping a frail, unsteady, and doddery person move can be a surprisingly difficult job. Your family member will feel every bit as heavy as his or her weight, especially if he or she is in a very weak condition. For this reason, please do practice the movement procedures we describe with another caregiver or a friend. Above all, be very careful not to go beyond your ability to perform lifting, supporting, and moving jobs. Enlist others to assist you, if you can't handle some procedures alone without clearly putting you and the patient in jeopardy of injury and falls to the floor. A great help can be to try to arrange for a visiting nurse to come in to teach you how to do such procedures.

Bed Making

How About a Hospital Bed? If the bedbound person is soon going to be up and about the house, you have every reason to use the usual bed. But if it looks as if your family member will be spending quite a bit of time in bed over the long run, consider renting a hospital bed with electric controls and side rails. The bed allows its occupant to raise feet, head, and height at the push of a button, changing the position of the body with little effort. A hospital bed also makes providing care in bed — meals, bed baths, positioning — easier on you and any other caregivers. Making a bed from the height of your waist is also easier on your back.

Although a hospital bed may be easier for caregivers, not everyone enjoys being in one. The mattresses are usually harder than those designed for home use, and some people don't like the feel of the plastic mattress upholstery, especially in summer or during fevers.

Falls from bed are a common accident among the frail elderly, especially when confused or lightheaded from an illness, or on medications that cause drowsiness or dizziness. If the older person is using the usual bed to convalesce, and is in danger of falling, think about lowering the bed by removing the frame or even putting the box spring and mattress on the floor. You can rent side rails for a home bed, but a hospital bed will have built-in rails that you can lift or lower according to safety needs. Recognize, however, that a mentally confused older person may climb over the side rails and have a worse injury than falling from the mattress would. Also, most hospital beds have wheels that make them easy to move; always be sure they are locked when the bed is supposed to be stationary.

Making an Unoccupied Bed. If your relative or friend can get out of bed, it is of course much easier to make the bed when empty. A good time is after breakfast and the morning routines of washing and toileting. Getting back into a freshly changed bed after cleaning up is a morale booster for anyone who is not feeling well.

Natural fibers — cotton for sheets and cotton or soft wool for blankets — are best for a sickbed. They allow air to circulate and sweat to evaporate more freely than synthetic fibers do. You want no hothouse environment under the covers, which can overheat your patient and also contribute to skin breakdowns. When you wash the sheets, rinse all soap residue out; you may have to run the washing-machine rinse cycle twice. Don't use fabric softener, for even the un-scented kind contains potentially irritating substances; static removers too are to be avoided.

Protecting the Mattress. If your relative or friend is apt to be incontinent you need to protect the mattress with a plastic cloth. The sheet can be an old shower curtain or tablecloth. It should stay tightly fitted over the mattress with no crinkling. Likewise, keep all other mattress cloths and sheets taut and smooth at all times.

Don't let the older person lie directly on any rubberized or plastic surface; doing so will cause skin breakdown. For padding, always sandwich an extra bedsheet, a mattress pad, or a rubberized cotton sheet between any plastic and the bottom sheet that your patient will lie on. A drawsheet, which is a sheet folded in half and stretched across the middle of the bed, is also a good idea, because it can be changed easily without disrupting the entire bed. If you use a drawsheet for an incontinent patient, place a rubberized cotton sheet or a disposable plasticized bed-protector pad directly under it. You can buy rubberized sheets and disposable incontinent bed-protective pads at drugstores and surgical supply stores. You will need several rubberized sheets and bedsheets so that you can change them frequently as they are soiled.

Your best bet is to use a fitted sheet for the bottom layer, so as not to fiddle with an oblong sheet that has to be secured perfectly every time you make the bed. The top sheet needs to be tucked into the bottom of the bed so that it doesn't slip away, but loose on the sides so that it is not too snug and restrictive. Your patient needs to be able to lie in bed flat with the feet pointing toward the ceiling and able to move freely.

Making an Occupied Bed. Making a bed with someone in it is an everyday chore in hospitals. It's easy to get the hang of it at home with a partner if you go slowly using these steps:

1. Two people, one on either side of the bed, are needed if the patient has no side rails to roll against and grasp. One person makes the bed, the other holds on to the patient.
2. Collect all bed linens: pillowcases, bottom sheet, top sheet. If necessary use a draw sheet, protective padding, and plastic or rubber mattress covers.
3. Loosen the tucked-in linens on each side of the bed.
4. Ask your patient to roll toward your bed-making partner or to the side rails as far as possible. Explain exactly what you are doing, step by step.
5. Pull out from under the mattress all the used sheets and neatly roll them under your patient as far as comfort allows.
6. Next, ask your patient to roll back toward you and over the hump of sheets. Now reach over to the other side and pull the roll of sheets off the bed, or have your partner do it.
7. Ask your patient to roll over again, back toward your bed-making partner or to the side rails.
8. On your side, make your half of the bed with the fresh sheets. Pull the unmade lengths of the sheets over toward your patient and tuck them under him or her as you did with the soiled ones.
9. Next, ask your patient to again roll toward you over the hump of clean sheets.
10. Again prevent the patient from falling out of bed. Either use side rails to lie against or ask your partner to make the other side of the bed.
11. Now make your patient comfortable at the center of the bed with loose top covers.

If your patient can lift up only at the hips and cannot comfortably roll over, then you can adapt the technique by making the occupied bed from the foot to the head. You will roll the sheets crosswise, toward the center of the bed from its foot, and have your patient lift up over them so that you can continue making the bed from the head end.

Moving a Frail Patient

In the hospital, nurses and nursing assistants always try to find partners to help move patients who can't help themselves. In this way they hope to save the vulnerable muscles in their own back and safely transfer the patient. Although you can learn how to transfer your parent, spouse, or any older person on your own, it's best to get someone else in the house or a neighbor to help, especially if your patient is very weak.

Here are steps designed to enable you to move someone without help. Before following the procedure, again we recommend that you must practice — until you get the hang of it — with someone else who can act weak and dizzy. Call in a nurse to instruct you, if you are unsure of your ability to move someone.

Check your own body mechanics before starting. Keep your center of gravity low by bending at the knees. Keep a wide base of support by spreading your legs about twelve inches apart.

To help your patient move from a lying to a sitting position, follow this sequence:

1. Turn your patient onto one side, facing you, and ask him to bend his legs.
2. Swing patient's legs over the side of the bed.
3. Place your hand under his shoulders and gently pull him upright. Be careful not to injure the shoulder joints by pulling too forcefully. Older people's shoulder joints are not as durable as those of young middle-aged people.

To make the move from bed to chair:

1. Determine if one side of your patient's body is stronger. Many elderly have one side that is better able to support its weight, especially after having a stroke or suffering from arthritis. You can test for strength by asking your patient to squeeze your hands or to extend both legs up as you push them down.
2. Transfer your patient on his strongest side first. If the right side is strongest, place the chair on his right so that he can

support himself from a position of strength. You can be helping with the weaker side.

3. Wake up his feet by asking him to wiggle toes and flex the ankles. Make sure the feet are not crossed over each other; they have to support him once on the floor.

4. Move in close to your patient. Your patient is sitting facing you on the edge of the bed. The chair is nearby with nothing in the way. Assume the good mechanics described above. Brace your knees against his or hers. Ask the older person to hold your shoulders (easier on your back). If he or she is extremely weak, ask him to lock hands around your neck (harder on your back, but safer for the transfer).

5. Put your hands around his or her waist.

6. Straighten yourself up while bringing him or her up to a standing position.

7. Stand together a minute or so. Your patient may be dizzy and need to equalize both senses and blood circulation. What's more, he or she may be tense, fearing a fall.

8. Never lose contact with the patient's knees. If you do, they may buckle under yours into a fall.

9. Pivot the patient with back close to chair and "good" arm on the chair.

10. Ease patient into the chair.

To help your patient walk from bed:

1. Always hold on to your patient. Place your arm around his or her back and offer prime support to the weaker side. Your other arm can hold the closest forearm.

2. Offer a cane to the strong side, if necessary.

3. Go slowly.

Toileting

The Bedpan or Urinal. If your patient simply can't get out of bed to a bedside commode or bathroom, then you will have to offer a bedpan or (to a man) a urinal. Body elimination — for almost everyone — is a highly private and personal act. You may find helping your patient — especially a parent — embarrassing, and handling the bedpan and urinal unpleasant. You may never quite get used to the chore.

How to Break a Fall

If your patient does start to fall:
- Don't necessarily try to bring him or her back up to prevent the fall; the sudden pressure may injure your back and bring you to the floor. Instead try to break the fall and slowly guide the older person safely to the floor, bending your knees, not your back.
- Get help if necessary to move the patient back to bed, or to the chair.

When doing the job, try to dignify it. If you think of it as an act of kindness and love, perhaps this attitude will help you. Provide privacy whenever possible. Here's how to make the best of toileting someone in bed:

1. If odors will occur, open windows and create a crossdraft (although not if the room will become cold).
2. Warm the bedpan by running warm water inside and along the rim. Be sure to dry the outside.
3. A little cornstarch or talcum powder will make sliding onto the bedpan easier.
4. If your patient can easily move, ask him or her to lift up onto the bedpan, or to turn slightly to one side. Next, gently push the pan underneath.
5. Use bed rails for your patient to hold on while using the bedpan, or provide hard pillows on each side of him or her. If necessary, provide support with your hand to his or her back.
6. If your patient can use a bedpan only lying down, follow these steps: have him or her roll over onto the side, next place the top of the bedpan (the rounded seat area) against the top of the buttocks, below the tailbone; have your patient roll easily onto the bedpan and position over the middle of it. If you have positioned it correctly, a four- to five-inch gap should remain in the narrowed front area of the bedpan.
7. Position your patient comfortably over the center of the bedpan so that it won't tip. Very important!

8. Offer toilet paper and provide privacy if the patient can be left alone.
9. When your patient is finished, ask him or her to lift off the bedpan.
10. Cover it with a cloth and remove to the side.
11. Provide your patient with soap and water in a basin, a washcloth, and a towel.
12. If your patient is unable to do so, clean the soiled area between the legs. Wash gently with soap and water, if necessary. Never allow urine or feces to stay on the skin; they are highly irritating and will contribute to skin breakdowns. Make certain too that all soap residue has been removed from the skin.
13. Empty the bedpan and wash it out with soap and water. If necessary soak it in disinfectant and clean later with a special toilet brush.

The Bedside Commode. A commode is a portable toilet that can be placed near the bed so that the older person doesn't have to go as far as the bathroom. You can buy or rent one from a surgical supply store. If the older person can get out of bed to use a commode, it is a much better alternative than a bedpan. The job of emptying and cleaning the bucket does need to be done with every use, though. To prevent odors and make cleaning the bucket easier, keep water in it after replacing it. Cover the commode with an attractive cloth, or behind a screen if your patient, family, and visitors don't like seeing it standing in the bedroom.

Bathing and General Cleanliness
Helping your patient stay clean and refreshed will do wonders to keep an optimistic outlook going. A bath in or out of bed and even a freshening-up session provides more than just cleansing for the body. A bath can be a relaxing, enjoyable experience and even relieve fatigue. It also gives you a chance to touch the older person and interact beyond just talking. A gentle touch from you — applications of soap and water, a warm cloth to the face, a soothing backrub, applying skin lotion — can be very therapeutic and pleasant.

General Tips for Bathing. Whether it's a bath in the tub, a shower, a bed bath, or a sponge bath at the sink, some basic principles apply to the care of an older person's delicate skin. Remember they have fewer hair follicles and oil-secreting cells and much thinner skin than younger people (see Chapter 5). Older skin is easily injured and susceptible to infection, and can also dry out, unable to easily lock in moisture.

To prevent injury and infection to the skin:

1. Use warm water. Never use hot water on the skin; it washes away natural body oils and contributes to dryness.
2. Rinse the skin carefully and thoroughly to remove all soap and water.
3. Don't use soap daily, except to clean the genitals, the armpits, and the hands. Water can be used daily, soap once or twice a week.
4. Use soap that is superfatted or glycerin-based. Avoid perfumed soap and antibacterial soap.
5. Completely dry all areas, especially under the breasts, in the skin folds, and between the toes. Bacteria thrive in moist, dark places.
6. Apply a nonperfumed emollient moisturizer to the skin after the bath to lock in moisture left within the skin's layers.

The Bed Bath. In the worst stage of an illness, or early in convalescence, you may see fit to give the person you are taking care of a bath in bed. But give a bed bath only if your family member cannot tolerate getting out of bed to the bathroom or the sink. Remember that the modern nurse's watchword is "up and about" whenever possible. To promote recovery you want your patient to be as active as can be, and not overly dependent on you.

Giving a bed bath requires you to be organized and unrushed. Choose a time when you can allow half an hour for the job from start to finish. After the bath you will need to change the linens, extra time that must be planned into the half hour.

The essentials. Gather the supplies listed here next to the bedside on a table. You don't want to have to go here and there looking for items you have forgotten while your patient is undressed.

Washbasin or bucket filled with warm water
Three towels
Two washcloths
Fresh linens for a bed change

A bath blanket (use a lightweight cotton blanket)
Soap
Lotion
Toothbrush
Toothpaste and mouthwash, if necessary
Hairbrush and comb

Include a razor and shaving cream for a man. An electric razor will be easier for you to handle if your patient can't safely shave himself.

The bed bath step by step. The correct way to give a bed bath is to wash from "clean" parts to "dirty," doing the genital area last. If your patient has the energy and the agility to wash his or her own genital area in privacy, though, it may be easier to offer a basin of water and a washcloth at the start of the bath. In this way she can exert herself, and then relax while you do the rest using a fresh basin of water and a second washcloth.

1. Make sure the room is warm and free of drafts.
2. Offer the bedpan or urinal before starting.
3. Take the spread, blanket, and top sheet off the bed.
4. Remove all clothing and cover with bath blanket.
5. Uncover each area as you wash it. Keep the other areas covered with the bath blanket.
6. Wash and dry the face and neck. Using no soap, start with the eyes, using a different corner of the washcloth for each eye.
7. Wash and dry the chest and both arms. Place a towel under the arms as you wash them to keep the bed from getting wet.
8. Place a dry towel across the chest. Fold the bath blanket down and wash and dry the abdomen.
9. Remove the towel from the chest and pull up the bath blanket.
10. Fold the blanket back from one leg at a time and place a towel under the legs to keep the bed from getting wet.
11. Wash and dry each leg.
12. Get a clean basin of water for cleaning between the legs. Place a towel under the buttocks and cover the torso with the bath blanket.

13. Clean the genital area first and the rectal area last. Be careful not to cross-contaminate the genital area.
14. Cover your patient with the bath towel, and if necessary more bedding.
15. Provide mouth care.
16. Provide a shave, if necessary.

Moisturize the skin in the same sequence, using the bath blanket along the way to prevent your patient from becoming chilled.

The Bathroom Sponge Bath. A sponge bath at the sink is a good alternative to a tub bath if your patient is too weak to manage the tub even with your support.

Seat your patient near the sink on a chair, or on the toilet, covered with a large towel for warmth. Slowly and methodically help the older person wash from head to toe, or do the job yourself. Safety permitting, stand just outside the door, while he or she washes between the legs. Remember to fill the sink with clean water and to offer a second washcloth for the job.

The Tub Bath: Questions of Safety. More accidents happen in the bathroom than anywhere else in the house. Encourage your family member to use the bathtub only if there is no potential for losing consciousness during the bath. To maximize bathing safety, follow these guidelines.

• Think through how you will help the older person into and out of the tub. To be sure of your moves, practice the procedure on a friend or family member. If you determine the task may be difficult alone, get someone to help you. Use good transfer technique, as follows:

To get the older person into the tub, hold his or her weak side, with your arm around the trunk. Have the older person step into the tub using the strong side. Have him grasp the grab bar. With your free hand, help him raise his weaker leg into the tub. While you support both sides, have him lower himself into the tub.
To get the older person out of the tub, let all the water run out, to prevent slipping and sliding from a standing position.
Dry the upper body and arms while he is still in the tub, for

a slippery, wet person is much more difficult to help move from the tub. Then have him draw his knees up close to the chest and, holding on to the grab bars, rise with your help. Have the older person turn toward you so that the strong side of the body leads out of the tub. As he steps out of the tub, provide support by placing your hands on each side of his body.

• Consider renting or buying a bath chair or bath bench, if sitting down in the tub will be difficult. Bath chairs in various designs and heights are placed at the middle of the tub with water all around. The bench is for showering with a handheld shower while sitting over the tub. With a transfer bench, one can easily swing the feet into the tub. Half of the bench stands outside the tub; the bather sits down and lifts the legs over the edge of the tub and then slides over on the bench to sit at the middle of the tub.

• An essential purchase is an *in-the-tub mat* with a suction base. Flower decals and adhesive strips do *not* prevent slipping and are not a substitute.

• Grab bars firmly mounted on the wall are also essential. The soap dish is not a substitute, because many are not firmly attached to the wall.

• A safe bath temperature is 100 to 101 degrees F (37.8 to 43.3 degrees C). Test the water on your wrist or with a cooking thermometer to be sure it will not burn the older person.

• Caution your family member not to adjust the temperature of the water, once in the tub. Very hot water, even when tolerable, can dilate the blood vessels and cause a drop in blood pressure as well as dizziness and fainting.

• Allow no more than twenty minutes in the tub. A prolonged soak will contribute to skin dryness and bring on fatigue.

• Allow privacy for the person in the bath if reasonable, but do be on standby — with the door ajar.

15

Help and Where to Find It

NO MATTER HOW well-informed you are about current medical
issues and about helping an older family member or friend lead a
comfortable and dignified life, you may eventually have to find help
beyond that which you or others can provide at home.

You may get this help from visiting nurses, home companions,
volunteers from church, or synagogue, Meals on Wheels, home health
aides, or even federally funded handymen who will do the necessary
carpentry around bathtubs and showers, toilets, and other places to
make the environment safe for the older person.

If the older person needs more around-the-clock care than you
and other caregivers can provide, you may face the daunting decision of looking for a nursing home or institution where your parent,
spouse, or older friend can receive full-time care by nursing professionals and social workers. By choosing a home wisely with help
from the suggestions we offer, you can stay completely involved with
your loved one.

In most cities and rural communities across the country, you'll
have to look for services among a patchwork of innovative programs that have sprung up in recent years to meet the needs of our
aging population. To make your job easier, we've sorted through
these services to find some designed to satisfy the almost universal
desire to keep frail, chronically ill older people in familiar surroundings and not in nursing homes. If a nursing home does seem the right
choice, however, you have a choice of ways to find good ones and
programs that help families come through the difficult decisions.

No question — for any of these services, you will probably have to pay. You may well discover that you can gain access to some free or pay-what-you-can services, but don't count on such good fortune. If you become efficient about networking in the local social-service system, you may succeed in arranging a combination of services, some free, some not.

The truth is hard: only a few services for long-term care of chronic illness are paid for out of community, state, or federal funds. Older people and their families end up paying for most help for long-term care problems out of their pockets. In the United States today, reimbursement is available from Medicare and most insurance policies, but only for those who succumb to critical illnesses and medical emergencies. Only the very poor and those who have exhausted their savings on long-term care are eligible for free, limited services for long-term care under Medicaid.

Like most who need help, you and others in your family probably have very little idea of what's available beyond the front door. This chapter should make it easier for you to reach intelligent decisions, with your parents or other older people, about how and where they will live. Don't get discouraged, because help is out there. You simply need to find out what it is and how to get it. Brace yourself — you have a big job ahead.

And good luck!

GETTING YOURSELF ORGANIZED

Files to Pull Together

Before we tell you about the wide array of services for the elderly, some careful organizing has to be done. The job of finding services and planning care will be much more wearing than it need be unless you pull together information about the older person's affairs, including health status, insurance coverage, financial status, and personal records.

As you network, seeking services and solutions to problems, you need to be armed with very specific information. In phoning around town and visiting agencies, strangers will ask you all kinds of questions. Being organized and having quick access to answers will save you time, frustration, and money. The people you procure to help will find their jobs easier if you have records and documents with which to plan care.

You may find it awkward getting access to your parents' more personal information. Older people commonly resist anyone's meddling in financial affairs, wills, and other important documents. They may come around to understanding your need for information if you explain that with it you can find out if they are eligible for the services they need, if they can collect insurance benefits, and what arrangements are needed for financial planning. You must also make it clear that documents need to be put in order so that you can have access to them if they become sick or incapacitated. Together you and your parents can make decisions early, before a crisis hits.

We suggest that you start "super files," which you can expand as time goes along. We call them "super" because each file category will be broken down into subfiles. If you don't organize papers in this way, soon piles of brochures, documents, bills, and more bills will grow insurmountable.

Buy a cardboard or metal filing cabinet specifically for long-term care planning, and keep it near a telephone. Also buy a looseleaf notebook for taking notes in telephone and person-to-person interviewing. Your notes can later be slipped into appropriate file categories.

We list here some basic super-file categories you should pull together at the start, with the essentials to go in them. Some of the legalese and government wordage may be new to you. If you need to define what terms mean, use the Index to look them up as they are described in the remainder of this chapter.

The Medical-Information File
- List all doctors.
    Doctor's specialty and the problem being treated
    Phone numbers and addresses
    State how you found each doctor
- List chronic health problems with dates of diagnoses.
- List surgeries, injuries, and acute illnesses, with dates.
    Doctors who treated each condition
    Hospital or clinic where treatment was provided
- List any tests beyond those done in routine checkups, with dates (such as x-rays, CAT scans, cardiac tests).
    Name of doctor who did the test

Where test was performed

Include copies of test findings

- List all medications.

  Name and phone number of your pharmacy, and the pharmacist

  Strength and frequency of dosage, who prescribed it, and date of first prescription

  Nonprescription items, such as vitamins, aspirin, and home remedies

  Allergies and past drug reactions

- Identify what to do in a medical emergency.

  Hospital to go to, including emergency-room phone number

  Ambulance service to call, including phone number

  Doctors to call

  Family members and friends to call

- Include all useful brochures, tip sheets, and newspaper articles on appropriate categories of disease.

The Financial-Resources File

- List all bank accounts.

  Checking, savings, money market

  Names and phone numbers of banking officers, stockbrokers, and so on

- List names and telephone numbers of all financial advisers, accountants, social-service workers.

- Put together a monthly income statement, with any of these that apply:

  Salaries, wages

  Social security for both husband and wife

  Pensions for both husband and wife

  Annuities for both husband and wife

  Stock dividends

  Rents

  Royalties, IRAs

  Bonds

  Mutual funds

- Estimate a monthly expenses statement, with any of these that apply:

  Mortgage or rent

> Utilities
> Telephone
> Maintenance, repairs
> Paid housekeeping services
> Legal
> Accounting
> Equipment rentals
> Insurance premiums
> Food
> Clothing
> Transportation
> Unreimbursed medical and dental
> Medicines
> Gifts
> Charitable contributions
> Miscellaneous

- Estimate a net-worth statement from the information above.

The Health-Insurance File

- Include Medicare card and any hospital or clinic cards.
- Put together all private insurance policies, including major medical and medigap policies.
- List names of insurance agents, with agent's phone number, address, and firm.
- Gather brochures about Medicare and Medicaid policies.

The Bills-and-Receipts File

- Organize all bills and receipts into categories, such as one operation and hospital stay, one chronic illness (not an acute illness).
- Include a bill-paying master flow sheet for filling in and quick review. To fit everything in, tape two sheets together. Headings across the top can include: date, service provided, provider, institution of provider, amount of bill, how bill was paid (including date), date Medicare reimbursement arrived, date private insurance arrived, notes, amount paid out of pocket, and date transaction completed.

The Documents File

- Gather legal documents.
  > The will
  > Power of attorney or durable power of attorney

- List names, phone numbers, and addresses of all lawyers, and their bills.

How Much Help Does the Older Person Need?

Most people make the mistake of seeking help for caregiving only when they're already in difficult straits, or when they're submerged under the hard work of it all, and the wrenching experience of watching an older relative or friend deteriorate physically and lose abilities. Under such stress it's not at all easy to take stock and sort out what the older person needs from you, as well as from outside helpers.

We next list questions like those a social worker or nurse would ask in a home visit, so that you can step back from the jumble of problems to identify the specific ones the older person may have. Once you have a clear list of "cans" and "can'ts," an objective assessment of the older person's limitations, you can start a plan of action to get you started seeking appropriate services.

Can the older person:

Take medications on time and in the correct dosage?
Go shopping for food and clothing?
Visit friends?
Drive a car?
Travel by bus or taxi?
Do light housekeeping?
Do heavy housekeeping chores?
Do the laundry?
Do yard work?
Afford to pay the bills?
Write checks and pay bills efficiently?
Take care of legal matters?
Maintain personal cleanliness?
Get dressed?
Use the toilet?
Sleep through the night?
Safely use the stairs and outdoor steps?
Look up telephone numbers and make calls without help?
Be left alone?

How to Network by Telephone

A few communities have well-organized eldercare programs set up to help older people and their families get along without excessive stress and strain. Your family may be lucky enough to live in such a community. Such programs may even be manned by polite, kind people who are willing and able to tell you all they know about available solutions to problems that you and your parents, and other relatives, may face. What's more, some programs may even be free or reasonably priced.

But as you will find out, if you haven't already, getting help can be a rocky road. The truth is that in most parts of the country the need for quick and easy solutions is far from met. Realistically, you're likely to call all over town, digging for answers to questions among an unconnected array of social workers, volunteers, and personnel at agencies and companies that have some link to long-term care of the elderly.

Prepare for the worst so that you won't get discouraged. Unsympathetic, annoying people may steer you in the wrong direction, give you the wrong information, talk down to you if you don't understand what they mean, fail to call you back, stay out to lunch interminably, and even put you on hold indefinitely. You may find yourself tempted to slam the phone down in frustration more than a few times.

To help you negotiate calls, we offer the telephone prompter on page 349. Copy it and put it by the phone. It should get you where you need to be, especially if the person on the line is not able to give you direct answers.

To be effective in getting the information, you need these few tips:

Make a call only after organizing in your mind exactly what you are after. Calling back with further questions can be awkward. And always ask about costs.

Be precise. The person on the other end of the line will appreciate your being very concise and specific about what you need.

Make morning calls whenever possible. Agency workers seem more willing to talk and be helpful fairly early in the workday. Many agencies take calls only in the morning.

If the person you need to talk to is out, *write down* the name and extension number, in case your call is not returned.

My name is —————————————————.
I'm caring for ——————————————————,
   who is my —————————————————.
I need ——————————————————.
The hours I need this help are ——————————————.
Can you help me? ——————————————.
   If no:
Can you give me another name or agency to call?
   If yes:
What services do you provide?
What are the costs? How are they paid?
What are the eligibility requirements?
How long must we wait?
Can you send a brochure or application?
To whom am I speaking?
Do I need to speak to anyone else?

Take notes in your looseleaf notebook on *every* call. Any information may be relevant later.

Be assertive if the person on the line seems to be withholding information and giving you a difficult time. Call back and ask to speak to a supervisor. If you get no resolution in this way, document the time, date, and content of your call and file a complaint with the Area Agency on Aging, the Better Business Bureau, or the Chamber Of Commerce.

Where to Start Networking

Now that you have some networking know-how and perhaps a dose of healthy pessimism, you need to make a beginning so that you can build up information for a total plan.

Your Area Agency on Aging. As we have described kinds of services, you may have noticed that we keep suggesting you first try to find out about them through the Area Agency on Aging. Most families have no idea that their community has an AAA.

A local AAA is a clearinghouse of information on programs for the elderly. Its purpose is to marshal and arrange services for older people from resources within a community. How good one is depends on the vagaries of budget and staffing constraints in any one place. Many AAAs across the country are quite good, a few are excellent, and some are hardly any good — those need a kick to shape up from federal regulators and their community's powers that be.

You can find the telephone number of the closest AAA in the yellow pages of the phone directory under "Social Service Organizations" or "Guide to Human Services" or "Aging Services." Although the title Area Agency on Aging is widely used across the country, some communities have come up with substitute titles, such as Administration on Aging, Mayor's Office on Aging, or County Senior Citizens' Office.

Across the country, about 660 agencies are in service, financed with federal funds under the Older American's Act that was set up by Congress in 1966. Sometimes the programs that an agency coordinates are run directly by its staff, but often the agency will contract services and assistance out to other organizations, such as churches and synagogues or the United Way and American Red Cross.

The AAAs are mandated by the federal government to administer and set up programs for nonmedical services within communities: home-delivered meals, illness prevention programs, adult daycare, free transportation to doctors' offices, shopping and housekeeping help, and social activities, among other functions. They also perform the important function of steering elderly people and their families to companies that manage and provide professional home-care services, including nurses, home-health aides, and physiotherapists. Some AAAs provide financial-planning assistance, or will advise where to find it.

More than a third of the agencies offer a service they call case management, or service coordination. A social worker comes to the older person's home to do an assessment and find what help is needed and how it can be organized. Usually this extremely valuable service is free of charge to everyone in a community. If case management is not an AAA service in your area, or if the service seems limited, the agency may have information about private case-management services.

As we have said, the quality of help provided by agencies varies from place to place. Nevertheless, any office should be able to provide at least something on these services, whether government-funded, for-profit, or volunteer-run.

Adult day care
Assistance with shopping

Case management
Employment opportunities
Friendly visiting
Home health aides
Homemaker and chores services
Housing services
Legal assistance
Meals programs
Mental-health services
Nursing-home and adult-home placement
Ombudsman services (investigating complaints)
Respite care (for caregivers)
Retirement planning
Senior-citizen centers
Telephone reassurance
Transportation
Visiting nurses

The Hospital Social-Work Department. Most hospitals have a social-work department, whose employees arrange for patients to leave the hospital with any necessary services ready to go. For this service, called discharge planning, they charge no extra fee.

Ask to speak with a social worker for information about community services, even if you are taking care of someone who is hospitalized for a minor reason that does not require professional aftercare at home. These hospital employees can provide you with a wealth of free information. Once your parent has left the hospital, though, you are no longer entitled to work with them.

The social-work department will help you make arrangements if your parent needs home care after the hospital, or to stay in a convalescence facility. Because finding properly supervised home health care can be time-consuming, make an appointment with the socialwork department as soon as it seems obvious that home care will be needed. Do the same if nursing-home placement is a definite prospect.

Other Sources of Help

• The local library — it may have all kinds of useful resources.

• Your doctor — often doctors are not familiar with nonmedical services, but you may get good leads and real help with arrangements.

• A local senior-citizen center — ask if staffers can refer you to services.

• A university department of gerontology — ask if it has community projects.

• Local hospitals — ask for a social-service department case manager or someone in the geriatrics department (if there is one).

• A clergyman — all the major denominations are involved in aspects of support for the elderly and their family caregivers; you may find one nearby.

• Your friends — usually those who have already arranged services — may be able to give you the first-hand story on good people to contact and their experience with long-term care.

Private Geriatric-Care Management

A new profession, geriatric-care management was spawned by growth in the older population. It is proving especially helpful for those who live far from their parents and for those who work at full-time jobs. These professionals have filled in where services provided by social workers on the government payroll leave off. Care managers, compared with caseworkers for government agencies, can be more available and more flexible in the service they can offer, for those who can afford their services. Caseworkers, often overwhelmed by large caseloads, can offer only limited assistance.

Care managers are social workers, nurses, psychologists, and those with degrees in nonmedical aspects of gerontology, who set themselves up for hire in private practice to counsel and assist families in planning for long-term care. They will help families at any level, with details or extensive responsibilities. Many work in group partnership with other care managers.

If requested — for hefty and continuing fees — a case manager will take on the entire job of planning and supervising an older person's long-term care, including financial arrangements. At this level the manager becomes a surrogate in the burdensome job that families have traditionally, and by necessity, taken on for elderly members.

Care managers function like other professionals, who do consulting as well as hands-on work. You can make an appointment with a practitioner and for an hourly fee learn from his or her experience. Or you can pay the practitioner to do the hard work you are unable or averse to doing. Depending on your geographic area, costs range from $50 to $120 an hour (in 1991 dollars). Some managers ask for an advance retainer, against which hourly rates are charged. A few specialized insurance policies will pay fees. Managers will also help families work out how to pay for management services out of the older person's funds or estate.

Case managers arrange for community-based services such as visiting nurses; occupational, physical, speech or other therapists; homemaker chore workers; and home-delivered meals. Often case managers work with families, bank trust officers, or attorneys, to ensure that an older person's government benefits are maintained and assets preserved. Others help complete insurance or government forms to pay for services, and provide advocacy when disputes arise over coverage. Some include financial and bookkeeping services that help clients organize their bills, write checks to creditors, resolve payment disputes, and prepare accounts and taxes.

Although the private-manager field is expanding rapidly and making inroads everywhere, usually they are found only in large cities. The National Association of Private Geriatric Care Managers (NAPGCM) was formed in 1986 to set standards for the profession and give prospective clients a national referral service. If you call or write to the association you will receive a packet of information about geriatric care management and names and credentials of managers in your area. Call (602) 881-8008 or write to NAPGCM, 655 North Alvernon Way, Suite 108, Tucson, AZ 85711.

Anyone can set up a practice as a care manager. More and more people are entering the field, some without proper credentials. If possible use a practitioner who has been approved for membership in the NAPGCM. Once you have found a care manager, determine if he or she is qualified by asking these questions:

What is your training and experience in gerontology?

How long have you been in private practice?

What state licenses do you hold permitting you to practice as an independent?

How do you provide backup when you are ill or on vacation?

What are your fees? How do they compare to those of other practitioners?

What services do you provide directly, and which do you arrange through outside providers?

Can you provide references from other clients?

Arranging and Checking Care from Afar

If you live many miles from your ailing parents, you face specific problems and the guilt and frustration of not being able to do enough to help with day-to-day difficulties, as well as crises when they arise. You may have tried in vain to get your parents to move closer to you, or even to live with you. But as you know, along with so many adult children in today's mobile society, the family home and the community they retired to are where most older people like to stay put, as long as they possibly can.

If you must manage the task of caring from afar, at least until your parents agree to move, here are suggestions to make it easier.

Before You Visit

• Obtain a telephone directory for your parents' community. Use it to network for community help programs, and to call friends and neighbors.

• Make appointments with personnel at agencies and with your parents' doctors, and with friends who can help. These contacts will save networking time while you are there and will also allow you to talk frankly with these people over the phone without having to worry about what you say in front of your parents. Calling ahead will also prevent the frustration of being unable to schedule appointments because personnel are booked up weeks in advance.

• Arrange for any needed services to start as soon as you arrive. You will have a chance to evaluate them, and, if necessary, hire and fire personnel while you are there.

While You Are There

• Be observant about health and safety issues. Is there a change in health status? Are they eating properly? Are friends coming around? Are finances being handled? Is the house clean? Is the house or apartment in good repair?

• Talk with your parents about their needs and how potential problems and crises will be resolved in your absence.

• Enlist their help whenever possible in arranging services. Be honest about their abilities and the supports that you foresee they will need.

• Talk to neighbors, friends, and helpers about how your parents cope when you are not there. You may uncover all kinds of problems needing resolution that your parents have kept from you.

• Arrange for and hire services well before you leave.

• Find out if any support system is formed by friends, neighbors, or club or congregation members. Make a list of these people and contact them to keep in touch and to thank them for any help they have given.

• Ask for specific help from people within the support system. You may be pleasantly surprised at people's willingness to run errands, drive for, and check up on your parents' safety.

• Make sure you have a back-up system for an emergency, and give key people within the support system the names of people to contact. Include your own name and work and home phone numbers, other family members, doctors, a social worker or care manager, nurses, and neighbors who can help locally.

• Leave a house key with a trusted neighbor, for use in emergencies, or to gain access to the house if your parent is hospitalized.

• Finally, consider hiring a private care manager to act as your representative and as an overseer for your parents' plan of care. Ask the manager to report to you regularly and as emergencies arise.

From Afar

• Establish a routine for telephone calls to your parents. Try to get other members of the family to help with the job of staying in touch. Assign days of the week to different family members.

• Encourage friends and relatives to send brief, newsy letters, photos, and clippings as much as possible. Make tape recordings as well.

• Encourage all grandchildren to make an effort to send letters, drawings, and copies of their work.

• Encourage other family members and friends to visit your parents.

• Keep in touch with all those who help your parents, including friends, volunteers, and paid help. Show your appreciation with letters, cards, and gifts for special occasions.

• Be alert to changes in your parents' mood and health. From their end, increased frequency of telephone calls, calls at odd times of the day or night, and calls for no apparent reason are tipoffs that things are not right. You need to find out what's wrong and take steps to settle anything that is bothering your parents. Frequent repeating of information, forgetfulness, and slurred speech over the telephone are signs of a medical problem and reason for the doctor to be consulted.

Help-Planning Guide

Look in the first column of the table on page 358 for many of the problems you may be up against. The second column lists ideas for solving these problems. In the third column are organizations to contact for help beyond any you can provide.

We have used the lingo that is used across the country for various kinds of long-term care programs. Many of these programs are described in the pages ahead, under home-based services and services in the community. (Note: All cost figures are in 1991 dollars.)

SERVICES PROVIDED AT HOME

All home-based services have one aim — to help older people keep living at home in safe, comfortable, clean surroundings with basic needs for food and health care provided. Care at home can consist of just a few hours a week of a service, ranging from friendly volunteer visitors to hot meals brought to the home, to housekeeping, to twenty-four-hour nurse's aide or skilled nursing care for a very ill older person who does not want to go to a hospital or nursing home.

Although in-home services are primarily designed to help older people who would not be able to live at home without such help, they are also a godsend for family caregivers who for any reason cannot be there to provide care themselves, or for hardworking caregivers who need to take a break from the job.

Home Repairs and Maintenance

After Mr. Jones's heart attack it was against the doctor's orders for him to go up ladders and to do any of the heavy yard work and house maintenance needed to keep his small house and quarter acre of ground livable and safe at all seasons. Their daughter made calls to find if a low-cost home-maintenance service was available in town. Through the Area Agency on Aging she found a work-study program at a nearby technical high school. Two well-trained and super-

vised twelfth-grade students came to the house for an afternoon, once a week, to do house chores at a minimum-wage charge. After graduation the students continued to work for the Joneses for a slightly higher fee.

What Is It?

Chore services are handyman programs, usually provided by local youth groups, retirees, and volunteers, for older people who can no longer do it themselves. The services do not include major improvements such as putting on a new roof, painting the house, or blacktopping the driveway. Tasks performed are for home and garden maintenance so that elderly people can live safely and comfortably in their house or apartment. Services include repairing steps, installing handrails and other safety features, putting in lightbulbs, fixing leaks, replacing windows, putting in or taking out storm windows, raking leaves, cutting down branches, and mowing lawns.

How Much Does It Cost?

Some communities have free services for senior citizens living on fixed incomes who are in clear need of assistance. If payment is involved, it is far less than it would be for professional handyman or gardening services. Costs range from the minimum wage up to $7 an hour.

Possible Resources

    Area Agency on Aging
    United Way
    Classified ads in the local paper
    Chamber of Commerce
    Yellow pages
    Local high schools
    Churches and synagogues

Friendly Visitors

After turning ninety-three, Mrs. Smith moved to Cincinnati to live with her daughter and family. Although the move made life easier for everyone, Mrs. Smith suffered loneliness and boredom during the day while the family was at work and school. Her poor eyesight prevented her from going out on her own, or reading, or doing the writing work she had enjoyed all her life. Never much of a joiner of

Your relative's problem	How you can help	Whom to contact in your community
Needs to get out and do something.	Include your relative in your social activities. Encourage friends, relatives, members of social organizations to include your relative in their plans. For a special occasion, pay for your relative and a friend to go out to dinner or a show.	Join a volunteer program: local church, hospital, synagogue, museum, zoo, library
		Federally funded action programs through the AAA:
		Foster Grandparents Program
		Retired Senior Volunteer Program (RSVP)
		The Senior Companion Program
		American Association of Retired Persons (AARP)
		Talent Bank
		Meals-on-Wheels
		Red Cross
		Big Brother/Big Sister
		Girl Scouts/Boy Scouts
		Become a member of an activist organization for seniors:
		American Association of Retired Persons
		Gray Panthers
		Older Women's League
		National Council of Senior Citizens
		National Caucus and Center on Black Aged
		Attend senior services:
		Nutrition sites
		Senior centers
		Mall walking clubs

Situation	Action	Resources
Needs company but cannot get out of the house.	Schedule visits with family and friends. Call local scout groups, civic and fraternal organizations, churches, and synagogues for volunteer visitors.	The Senior Companion Program (through the AAA) Telephone Reassurance Program Respite Volunteers Friendly Visitors Bright Moments Youth in Elderly Service (YES) Organizations specific to illnesses
Can do light housekeeping but needs help with heavy tasks.	You can do tasks. Hire a teenager to do tasks. Check yellow pages and contract help. Call senior-citizens center for retired worker who can do repairs. Arrange for swapping services with family and friends (for example, your relative can house-sit, babysit, feed pets in exchange for plumbing repairs, heavy garden maintenance).	Area Agency on Aging Churches and synagogues United Way Local youth groups Local high schools and community colleges
Cannot drive or use public transportation for appointments or shopping.	You can drive your relative to appointments, shopping. Call the function relative needs to attend and ask for a volunteer driver. Arrange car pooling and arrange for yourself or a substitute to drive. Call local church or synagogue for transportation volunteers.	Taxi transportation Handicapped transportation (services through Area Agency on Aging) American Red Cross transport programs Senior-citizens' centers
Cannot prepare nutritious meals.	You shop and prepare all meals. You drop off meals. You organize a schedule for family and friends to drop off meals. You arrange for a restaurant to deliver meals. Arrange for a certified dietitian to do a home visit for recommendations.	Area Agency on Aging Meals-on-Wheels Programs Senior centers, churches, and synagogues

Your relative's problem	How you can help	Whom to contact in your community
Needs assistance with personal care (bathing, grooming, dressing, toileting).	You can plan and provide care. Hire a certified home-health aide.	Local hospital-discharge planning office Visiting Nurse Association Home health aide agencies
Needs specialized equipment.	Call for catalogs. Compare prices. Arrange for an occupational therapist, physical therapist, or visiting nurse to do a home evaluation for specific recommendations.	Organizations specific to illness Volunteer ambulance corps Local churches and synagogues County office for the disabled
Is depressed.	Call or visit frequently. Encourage older person to participate in social activities. Be sure they sleep well. Watch for signs of overeating or undereating.	Geriatric Evaluation Unit Geropsychiatrist Psychologist Mental-health association
Has trouble managing money.	Add your name to the checking account. Have the bills sent to your address for you to pay and process. You do income tax or organize records for accountant. Obtain power of attorney.	Area Agency on Aging Bank officers Private accountants Case managers who do money management
Has unmanageable health-care costs.	Supplement your relative's income. See a lawyer about estate planning so that elder is eligible for publicly funded programs.	Private insurance companies Medigap insurance companies Medicaid or Medicare United Way Social Security Office Pharmacies with senior-citizen discounts Mail-order prescription services

Situation	Action	Resources
Has limited income; having problems with home-ownership-related bills.	Supplement income. Encourage relative to explore federal and local programs for savings for seniors who own their own home. Winterize the home. Have local utility company do a home energy evaluation.	Area Agency on Aging or State Energy Office for Information on Home Weatherization Assistance or Utility Assistance Program
Has legal matters that need attention.	Call local bar association for list of lawyers who work in geriatric law. Take time to discuss what to do in case of emergency or death. Encourage your relative to have will in order, have a living will, durable power of attorney. Know where legal papers are kept.	Area Agency on Aging Legal Councils for the Elderly Legal Aid Adult Protective Services Senior-citizen groups Association for specific illness Family-service organizations
Lives alone and worries about health emergencies and crime threats.	Call or visit on a schedule. Pay a neighbor to check on a schedule. Crime-proof home. Alert local police department that relative lives alone.	Emergency Response System Telephone Reassurance Systems Vial-of-Life Medi-Alert Program
Cannot be left alone during day.	Stay with relative. Schedule family and friends to eldersit. Hire home health aide. Hire companion.	Adult Day Care Visiting Nurse Association Home health aide agencies Friendly Visiting Service Companion Service United Way

clubs and groups, she refused to go to a local senior-citizen center to be with other older people.

Worried that her mother would become severely depressed without company and the stimulation of conversation, her daughter found out about a friendly-visitor program at their church. Mrs. Smith needed visiting five days a week, and so the church program arranged for a retired librarian to come to the house twice a week and a young housewife three times a week. Both arrangements worked out very well. Both visitors read to Mrs. Smith and enjoyed joining in her lively recounting of times gone by. Some days they took her on outings to lectures and concerts, or to sit outside in a local park.

What Is It?

The Friendly Visitor Service offers companionship to isolated older people. Volunteers visit them at home, usually for two hours once or twice a week. Often volunteers are older people interested in companionship with other older people. While visiting, the volunteer can offer ways to lighten the older person's day, including chatting, playing cards, reading out loud, or writing letters. The volunteers' main purpose is to provide company, and they do not perform personal, medical, or housecleaning tasks.

How Much Does It Cost?

The service is usually free, although from those who can afford it, a donation is always appreciated by the charity arranging the service.

Possible Resources

    Area Agency on Aging
    Local churches or synagogues
    Universities and colleges
    Retiree volunteer programs
    Junior League
    Local high schools
    Boy-scout and girl-scout troops

Senior Companions

Mrs. Levin became lonely after her husband died suddenly of a heart attack, and, being on a number of medications for painful arthritis, among other problems, she was subject to dizzy spells. Her son wor-

ried that she was heading for depression. He and other family members could easily manage visiting in the evenings, taking her to dinner and setting her up for bed, but they worked during the day and despaired at the idea of her being alone all day. On weekends they would work out ways for Mrs. Levin to visit the family or to receive visitors at home.

The family hired Mrs. Scharf through a social worker at the Area Agency on Aging. A retired waitress, she had been trained in a program set up by the American Association of Retired Persons (AARP). Mrs. Scharf came five days a week from noon to four o'clock to be a companion, helper, and safety watch for Mrs. Levin. The two women ate lunch together, which Mrs. Scharf picked up at a local restaurant. The rest of the afternoon they enjoyed each other's company by playing cards, cooking, reading, and watching television. When Mrs. Levin needed to get to appointments and to see friends, Mrs. Scharf drove her.

What Is It?

A companion provides company and services to older people unable to handle basic tasks of daily living. They are not trained to administer medical assistance, or to help with dressing, bathing, personal hygiene, or toileting. Their job description also includes no heavy-duty housecleaning. They are ideal for the older person who is isolated and unable to manage alone during the day.

How Much Does It Cost?

In some communities the service can be arranged through a social worker. Most programs are set up through the Area Agency on Aging or some other social-services department, and families pay the companion's wages out of pocket. Depending on the area, costs range from the minimum wage to $12 an hour.

Possible Resources

    Area Agency on Aging
    Visiting Nurse Association
    Private-home service employment agencies
    Department of Social Services
    American Association of Retired Persons
    Classified ads

Telephone Reassurance

Mary felt she needed to telephone her mother every morning and at night before bedtime, to make sure she had taken her pills and gone through the night and day without incidents. Mary's mother depended on the calls, and started to use them to talk on and on about a litany of woes. It was all getting to be too much for Mary, whose boss told her that long morning calls to her mother had to stop.

A friend told Mary to inquire about a volunteer telephone-reassurance program at a local senior-citizen center. Mary arranged for service, and every day a regular caller made a phone call at a prearranged time to inquire about her mother's health and safety and to remind her to take medications. Her mother was told that if she didn't answer, Mary would be contacted as well as the police. An added benefit from this new arrangement was that Mary's mother agreed to be picked up twice a week to join in the senior-citizen club's activity program.

How Does It Work?
Telephone reassurance programs go under different names, such as House Calls, Call-a-Day, and Care-Line. Most are staffed by volunteers working through organizations funded by grants from government or charity funds. Groups range from senior-citizen organizations, to the Visiting Nurse Association, to hospital social-work departments. In some areas where volunteer programs are sparse or nonexistent, private companies have filled the void for this valuable service. Usually a client is telephoned once a day and the caller keeps a chart including daily information about medication, meals, and appointments of which the older person needs to be reminded. Some for-profit services offer twenty-four-hour reassurance programs, which allow the older person to call a central office at any time.

How Much Does It Cost?
Usually the service is free. For-profit businesses charge a monthly fee, usually based on the time used up between the client and personnel working for the telephone service.

Where to Find It
Area Agency on Aging
A for-profit home health-care agency

A not-for-profit home health-care agency, such as the Visiting
   Nurse Association
Senior centers
Local hospitals

Medical-Alert Products

*After recovering from her broken-hip operation, Mrs. Gonzalez swore
she would never again be helpless, even for a minute, in a medical
emergency. The day she slipped and fell on the kitchen floor, the
telephone was inches away but impossible to grasp. She was discovered hours later, when her neighbor came by to borrow some milk.
Badly frightened by the experience, she kept thinking "I was found
this time, but what will happen next time?"*

*She shared her feelings with a social worker in the hospital, who
recommended she purchase a waterproof medical-alert button to wear
at home on a necklace and a medical identification card to carry in
her wallet, which included medical information and telephone numbers for emergency personnel.*

What Is It?
Medical-alert products allow older people at high risk for accidents
and medical emergencies to live independently — with peace of mind.
The three categories of products are personal-response systems,
medical-identification cards, and medical-identity jewelry tags.

Emergency Response Systems. The response systems link people to
twenty-four-hour assistance at the push of a button. A small device — the help button — is worn around the neck on a chain,
strapped to the wrist like a watch, or clipped to clothing. Help buttons can also be installed in convenient locations, such as next to the
bathtub or bed, in a wheelchair, or on a walker. Most people choose
to wear help buttons around the neck.

In an emergency, the wearer activates the help button, which initiates a call for help to an emergency-response center. As soon as the
call is received, someone at the center calls the person in distress and
talks over a speaker phone attached to the home telephone. If no
answer is heard, someone at the emergency-response center next calls
one of three "responders" who have agreed to enter the distressed
caller's home in an emergency. An ambulance can also be sent on its
way, depending on circumstances and prior agreements.

Your Area Agency on Aging or a nearby hospital can tell you who runs the medical-alert program in your parents' community. You can also look for programs listed in the yellow pages, under "medical alarms." In some communities, service is arranged through local hospitals or home-health agencies, such as the Visiting Nurse Association.

If no such programs are available where your parents live, or if waiting lists for service are long, you can get direct service from one of the national or regional companies, which supply emergency-response centers with equipment to lease to customers. These companies have set up their own emergency-response centers at company headquarters. Such companies may be listed in the yellow pages of the telephone directory.

Lifeline Emergency-Response Systems is the largest company in the business throughout the United States and Canada. Call the company at 800 451-0525, to make arrangements for service anywhere in North America that has telephone communications.

Some community-based centers offer free service to senior citizens, although they usually have a one-time installation charge and a monthly fee. Basic service ordered directly from Lifeline costs $35 a month, with a $50 installation fee. Be wary of unscrupulous companies offering similar services at exorbitant prices. If you're shopping for a service, comparison shop against what Lifeline has to offer, because they will forward literature on their products and quote all prices over the telephone.

Medical-Identification Cards. Wallet-size medical cards provide vital information for medical personnel to review in an emergency. They cost from $2 to $12 and are particularly helpful if the card owner loses consciousness or the ability to communicate.

Check with your primary physician about a suitable card arrangement, or contact:

STAT Medical ID Company, P.O. Box 9874, Alexandria, VA 22304-9874. The STAT Company offers a credit-card-size copy of a detailed application reduced onto microfilm but readable without magnification. Physicians' names and a medical history are included.

National Medic-Card Systems, P.O. Box 4307, Oceanside, CA 92054. This company's folded card includes medical history, insurance information, and treatment consent forms.

Medical Passport Foundation, P.O. Box 820, Deland, FL 32721.

The Foundation's card provides space for a variety of general health information.

Identification Tags. Emergency personnel are trained to look, in emergencies, for medical identification tags on bracelets or pendants or in clothing on incapacitated patients. Such tags are good for those with health problems who are out and about. Besides the wearer's name and a few basic items of medical information, the tag carries a call-collect telephone number of a central office at which vital patient information can be quickly obtained. Calls can be handled twenty-four hours a day, from anywhere in the world. The service is particularly valuable for those prone to confusion, angina, diabetes, and allergies to penicillin and other medications.

Medic-Alert is the leading medical signaling company; the basic service costs $20 as a one-time fee. The products, made of metal, look like jewelry. For information about these products call Medic-Alert: 800 ID-ALERT.

Lifesaver Charities offers a plastic tag free, but will welcome a small donation. Send a self-addressed, stamped envelope to Lifesaver Charities, P.O. Box 125-BH&G, Buena Park, CA 90621.

Meals on Wheels

Mrs. Jones's shingles flared on and on for weeks, leaving her weak from lack of sleep, depressed, and so exhausted that she was unable to prepare proper meals, let alone drive to the supermarket for food. Her neighbor gradually realized that she wasn't getting the nourishment needed to keep up her immune system, and he worried that Mrs. Jones would never conquer the disease.

The neighbor called a meals-on-wheels program organized by the local Kiwanis Club. He was able to arrange for the program's volunteers to drop off a cold lunch and a hot dinner for Mrs. Jones five days a week. Within a month, starting to feel like her old self, she discontinued the home-delivered meals. She was so grateful and so deeply impressed with the service that she signed up to do fund raising for it, and even arranged to be a volunteer deliverer of meals once a week.

What Is It?
Home-delivered meals, usually called Meals on Wheels, are a nutrition service provided by public and nonprofit organizations, or both.

Most programs are provided with some funds by the federal government under the Older Americans Act. According to government estimates, more than 375 million meals are served to senior citizens nationwide by federally funded services, either by Meals-on-Wheels programs or at sites such as senior centers and churches and synagogues. Meals-on-Wheels programs are for older people of all income levels who simply can't prepare nourishing meals for themselves, either for a short time or always. Meals must meet approval by state nutritional standards, and usually they are well prepared. Dinner usually has a soup course, bread and butter, full entrée with meat or a protein substitute, vegetables, and dessert.

In recent years nonprofit private programs have been started by churches and synagogues and civic organizations such as Kiwanis Clubs, Rotary International, and other social-service organizations.

How Much Does It Cost?
A donation for each meal is suggested, to pay for the food and its packaging. For lunch the charge is usually about $3; for dinner, $5. Programs receiving federal funds are not permitted to turn people away because of inability to pay. Private nonprofit programs generally charge a fee, but sometimes meals are provided to a limited number of nonpaying clients.

How to Find It
    Area Agency on Aging (especially for programs funded through
        them)
    Civic clubs
    Local churches and synagogues
    National Association of Meal Programs: 204 E Street N.E.,
        Washington, DC 20002, telephone (202) 547-6157. Call or
        write for names of local member programs.

Hospice

When Mrs. Morris was diagnosed as having terminal cancer, she told her daughter Cynthia that her biggest fear was not death itself, but dying in a hospital among strangers. Cynthia, an only child, wanted to do all she could to make her mother's last months as meaningful and comfortable as possible; however, she felt awed by the responsibility of providing for her mother's terminal care at home.

The doctor encouraged Mrs. Morris and Cynthia to meet with a representative of a hospice program run by the Visiting Nurse Association and supported by an interfaith group of volunteers, found through churches and synagogues. Cynthia and her mother signed up for hospice service, pleased to know that they would be supported by well-trained people who would help Cynthia care for her mother at home. A hospice nurse put in charge of Mrs. Morris's case worked out a plan for Cynthia and team members to follow. This nurse also taught Cynthia how to give pain medication and do basic bedside nursing tasks.

As the weeks went on, Mrs. Morris's condition deteriorated and she became bedridden. The nurse in charge recognized that Cynthia needed help and a break from the job. In response, a nurse came every day for an hour to help Cynthia do a bed bath, check on Mrs. Morris's comfort, her nutritional needs, and her skin condition, which was in danger of breaking down as she spent more and more time in bed. The hospice program arranged for a volunteer to sit with Mrs. Morris three hours every afternoon so that Cynthia could leave the house to take a break or a nap. Another volunteer was available to help Cynthia in any way she wanted for two evenings a week.

On the day when Mrs. Morris seemed near death, the afternoon volunteer and the nurse arranged to stay with Cynthia until the end. Friends dropped by all day, but the volunteer who had worked with her for so many weeks was her mainstay. After the funeral, Cynthia joined a bereavement group run by the hospice.

What Is It?

Hospice is a form of care that was developed by grass-roots organizations determined to find ways for people to die with dignity, without curative treatments for medical problems. Hospice care can be planned as home care, in a hospital setting, or in a free-standing facility. Most of the 1,600 hospice programs around the country help a family member or friend to care for a dying person at home. Programs in hospitals usually assign dying patients to their own ward and concentrate on palliating pain and giving psychological support.

Typically, hospice programs are staffed by several nurses, a few physicians, clergy, social workers, and volunteer coordinators. The bulwark of all hospice programs, though, are volunteers, many of them people who once cared for terminally ill relatives and saw how important other volunteers were to them.

How Much Does It Cost?

Most people using hospice services receive reimbursement for it out of Medicare funds. In some states, Medicaid pays. Many private insurance companies also provide coverage. Since 1982, when the Medicare Hospice Benefit Act was passed, the federal government has provided more and more funds for hospice care. The reason is obvious: hospice can save Medicare from the far greater expenses of hospital or nursing-home care. Medicare-certified hospice programs can receive Medicare reimbursement only if a primary doctor and the patient sign a statement saying that the patient has less than six months to live, and if care is palliative rather than curative. A few nonprofit, community-based programs have preferred to stay independent of the federal government and private insurance companies, and usually operate on a pay-what-you-can arrangement.

How to Find It

Write to the National Hospice Organization, Suite 901, 1901 North Moore Street, Arlington, VA 22209, or call (800) 658-8898. They will send a printout of hospices in your area and answer questions about specific programs. The organization represents most hospice programs, whether Medicare-certified or independent. Hospice has strict guidelines: programs must be volunteer-based and offer only palliative care and one year's bereavement counseling for the primary caregiver.

Licensed Home Health-Care Agency

Elana called a health-care personnel registry she found from an advertisement in the yellow pages and asked if the agency could send a woman — experienced in helping older people — to work for her parents. Elana's parents were in their late eighties and needed help with taking medications, cooking, tidying the apartment, and some personal care, including bathing and grooming. The agency staff sent a seemingly pleasant woman, who had been trained, they claimed, to work with the elderly.

After a few days, Elana and her parents recognized that the woman from the agency was inexperienced, inefficient, and dishonest. She refused to help Elana's parents with personal care, neglected to cook meals, and forgot to remind the mother to take medications. She spent most of her time in front of the television set smoking ciga-

rettes. What's more, the grocery money Elana had left was used up in two days, with only a few groceries in sight.

After calling the agency, which refused to pay back the finder's fee or replace its worker, Elana complained to the Better Business Bureau. They recommended she find a home-health aide through a bona fide home-care agency licensed by the state health department and certified by Medicare. Such programs meet strict standards.

Tips for Hiring Home-Care Personnel Through an Agency

The home health-care services industry is not well regulated. Anyone can open a mom-and-pop agency, advertise, and send workers classified as health aides into people's homes. Generally, you should stay away from such agencies because their owners have not subjected themselves to the scrutiny of state licensure and Medicare certification.

You can find well-run agencies that meet the industry's high standards, established by its membership body, the National Association of Home Care. Here are questions to ask yourself when hiring someone to work in your parents' home, so that you can set up a satisfactory arrangement without being taken advantage of by an unscrupulous home-care agency:

1. Is the agency licensed by the state department of health? This is a reliable criterion. Don't be taken in by glossy advertising, the largest ad in the yellow pages, or a sales pitch from an unlicensed agency.
2. Is it Medicare certified? Certification is not an absolute criterion for choosing an agency, but it is a good indicator of high standards. Some licensed agencies operate only on private payments and so have not needed to go through the complicated procedure leading to Medicare certification. Using such an agency does not necessarily mean that services can be reimbursed through Medicare. If you pay for services out of pocket, find out if your parent is eligible for insurance.
2. Are employees insured and bonded? If they are, the agency is responsible for any lawsuits against you, and damage inflicted on your parents' property by their employees.
3. Does the agency provide worker's compensation to employees? If it does, your parents will not be liable for a worker's job-related injuries.

4. Is the aide supervised by a registered nurse, to whom you and he or she can report? A good agency will provide case management by a registered nurse supervisor at least once a month. The nurse and other professional personnel should have malpractice insurance.
5. Is the supervisor or a substitute available around the clock, seven days a week? You need to know if you will have access to case management if the home-care situation changes.
6. Will a replacement be ready if a permanent worker gets sick or leaves? or if the worker provides unsatisfactory service? The agency should be able to send you a replacement, on the usual work schedule.

What Is It?

A health-care agency is set up to send personnel into the homes of people who are incapacitated, ill, or recuperating from illness. The personnel can be homemakers, home-health aides, registered nurses, physiotherapists, or speech therapists. Some agencies, such as the Visiting Nurse Association, are classified as not-for-profit organizations because they are primarily funded by fees paid either by insurance or by clients out of pocket, but also by community-raised funds and state and federal grants. Others are private companies that are funded solely by reimbursement from clients' insurance or payments.

How Much Does It Cost?

A bona fide agency supplying home health-care services will be able to determine whether or not your parent is eligible for insurance coverage, and for how long. Under specific, limited circumstances a primary doctor can "order" a home health aide (personal care aide), homemaker, or skilled professionals such as nurses and physiotherapists, so that fees are paid by Medicare and private insurance. Usually such short-term payment applies if restorative care is needed after a hospital stay. In most states Medicaid pays for limited long-term home health-care services.

Insurance reimbursement should always be attempted when someone with medical problems needs paid help. If the patient is not eligible for reimbursement, or if reimbursement ends, the patient is left to decide whether or not to pay for home-care services out of pocket.

If a homemaker or a home health aide is needed and your parents can't afford the cost, do investigate pay-as-you-can homemaker health-aide programs. Available in some communities, such programs are run by the Visiting Nurse Association or other nonprofit groups, for those who can prove from IRS forms and other documents that their income is below a specific limit.

How to Find It
The hospital discharge-planning office
Your primary doctor
The Visiting Nurse Association, or another nonprofit home
    health-care agency
A local branch of a private home health-care chain. Listed in order of numbers of nationwide branch offices, these are
    among the chains known for holding to good standards:
    Kimberly Quality Care
    Medical Personnel Pool
    Upjohn Health Care Services
    Norrell Health Care
    Olsten Health Care
A locally controlled, licensed agency giving home health care

In the following three sections, we supply costs of homemakers, home health aides, and skilled professionals. We describe jobs according to their strictest definitions. Job descriptions vary from state to state and agency to agency. For example, some agencies send out paraprofessionals who provide personal care as well as homemaking.

Homemakers
Mr. Martinez lived at his daughter Marianne's house after his wife died. After two months he announced that he wanted to go back to his apartment to try living alone. Marianne knew her eighty-six-year-old father was ready, but wondered how on earth he would cook for himself and take care of the house. He was slow on his feet and suffered from mild emphysema, and Marianne knew that he also had no experience with housekeeping.

Marianne contacted a home health-care agency and asked if she and her father could interview several people for the job of taking care of his household needs. They hired a homemaker who came in five days a week to do the shopping, cooking, and housecleaning for Mr. Martinez.

What Is It? Homemakers are trained to take care of the household needs of elderly people who cannot manage them. A homemaker usually has no training in personal care and nursing principles.

How Much Does It Cost? In some circumstances after an older person has been discharged from a hospital, homemaker fees are paid for by insurance. The cost varies greatly from location to location, but averages around $8 an hour.

How to Find It. A bona fide home health-care agency is the source (see section above).

Home Health Aides
Eighty-one-year-old Jack DeMille was still not strong enough to go home unattended after his operation for cancer of the colon. Before his discharge a social worker at the hospital arranged for a home health aide to help him for a couple of weeks. She came from nine to six, five days a week, and a substitute supplied by the agency took her place on weekends. She helped Mr. DeMille with his morning bath, cooked his meals according to a diet ordered by the doctor, and reminded him to take his medications on time. She also changed his bed every day and kept his apartment in order so that he could comfortably and safely move around. The nurse came in at the beginning of each week to supervise a care plan.

What Is It? Home health aides are trained to provide personal care for people who have health problems. They function much like nurse's aides do in the hospital, only they work alone in the patient's home, supervised by a registered nurse. Sometimes hospitals train and provide such aides for their discharged patients, but more often they are employed by community-based, not-for-profit home health agencies, or private for-profit agencies. Although home health aides are usually ordered by a doctor as part of the hospital discharge, families can secure health aides on their own through agencies.

How Much Does It Cost? Under specific, limited circumstances, a primary doctor can "order" a home health aide so that fees are paid by Medicare and private insurance. Usually such payment applies if the patient needs rehabilitation after, say, a stroke or a broken-hip operation, or for restorative care after hospitalization for a debilitating illness. Costs vary from location to location, and are around $10 to $20 an hour.

Skilled Home Care

Mrs. Spencer spent three weeks in the hospital recovering from a fractured hip. While there she contracted pneumonia, which slowed her recovery and left her very weak. Her doctor recommended she recuperate in a convalescence home, where she could be rehabilitated over several weeks. Mrs. Spencer balked at this idea and asked if professionals could rehabilitate her at home, where she lived with her daughter and son-in-law; they were willing to be involved with her care.

The hospital discharge planner arranged for a case manager from a private home health-care agency to meet with the family and primary doctor at Mrs. Spencer's hospital bedside. The nurse case manager worked out a plan of care with the doctor and the Spencer family so that Mrs. Spencer could be home in two days, under the care of several professionals employed by the agency. It turned out that Medicare and private insurance would pay the full costs of restorative care for up to five weeks.

On the day of discharge a home health aide came to the house, supervised by a registered nurse. The aide worked five hours a day, five days a week, and a substitute took her place on weekends. The nurse came to the house twice a week to supervise the aide and to perform skilled nursing tasks for Mrs. Spencer, checking her lungs and blood pressure. She also worked with Mrs. Spencer on a program of walking exercises. A physiotherapist came for one hour, three days a week, to work on restoring Mrs. Spencer's muscle strength, gait, and balance.

After a week, with everything running smoothly, the nurse determined that Mrs. Spencer probably had a urinary-tract infection. She consulted with the doctor, who asked her to send a urine sample to a laboratory for testing. When the test came back positive the next day, he prescribed antibiotic therapy, which was overseen by the nurse.

The skilled home-care team provided by the agency kept Mrs. Spencer out of a convalescence home or hospital, at lower cost than in such institutions. She was able to regain much of her lost ability in the security of home, and with her family around.

What Is It? Skilled home care is provided by licensed health-care professionals, such as nurses, practical nurses, physical or occupational therapists, respiratory therapists, and nutritionists. These professionals work in collaboration with the patient's primary physician, and perform many of the functions they were trained to carry out in a hospital setting.

All across the country, more and more insurance programs — the more expensive ones at least — are paying for a limited period of skilled home care, so that patients can leave the hospital system and receive care at home. The arrangement meets the needs of those who prefer to be home as soon as they can, and it is also cheaper for the insurance programs, which now give hospitals incentives for releasing patients as soon as possible.

How Much Does It Cost? If a doctor "orders" skilled care according to guidelines set by Medicare or a private insurance company, costs are usually paid in full. The rates for skilled care vary according to the profession involved. A reputable home health-care agency will quote prices over the telephone.

COMMUNITY-BASED SERVICES

Services that older people go to from their homes are called community-based. They may be social programs, for older people who are well and want to get out to meet and be with others of their generation. Or they may be for older people who are chronically ill and need a place to go to for minimal medical care and supervised therapy, as well as socializing.

Some community programs are designed especially for families who need a break from taking care of their aging relatives. These services allow a primary caregiver — the family member in charge — to work outside the home, take breaks, and even go on vacations from the job of taking care of an incapacitated relative who cannot be left alone.

Senior Centers

Edith James's eighty-year-old mother seemed lost after her husband died. Most of her friends had moved to a warmer climate when they were in their seventies, and her very best friend was in a nursing home.

Edith kept telling her mother she should join the senior-citizen's center downtown so that she could be with people close to her age. It had all kinds of social, exercise, and health-screening programs; a library; films; and a lecture series. But try as Edith would, her mother resisted. She even told Edith, "I don't want to be around all those decrepit old people learning how to dance and make potholders. The whole idea depresses me."

Then Edith's mother read in the paper that the senior-citizen center was having a Greta Garbo film festival, open free to people over sixty-five. Without telling Edith, she attended the first movie showing. She was thrilled to be there: the room was packed with interesting-looking people and the center had a spirited, stimulating atmosphere. After the film she signed up to meet with a social worker to discuss joining the club's lunch program.

What Is It?

A senior center is a place at which older people can gather and make friends. In some communities, the name "club" seems to be replacing "center," because it better describes the social aspect of such places. The centers can be a vital part of the continuum of services for older people, forming access points for other programs, disseminating information and benefits for older people. They are primarily for the well elderly who can get themselves to the center on their own. A limited number have transportation services for special events.

Styles of centers vary greatly from community to community and within communities. Some clubs are specifically for private interest groups, and others are run for the whole community and paid for out of community-chest and government funds.

How Much Does It Cost?

Most services and programs at senior centers are free, except that they usually charge for meals.

How to Find It

Area Agency on Aging Directory of Senior Clubs and Centers
Nationality associations such as Italian-Americans, Polish-
    Americans, and German-Americans
Civic organizations: Kiwanis, Elks, Rotary
Churches and synagogues
Union clubs
Company retirement clubs

Community Meals Programs

Rebecca and Peter Parson were obviously not eating correctly to maintain good health. Cooking full meals and shopping several times a week for fresh food seemed difficult. They turned increasingly to canned food, frozen dinners, and butter and toast.

Their daughter lived across the country and so was able to visit only once or twice a year. When she showed up to help celebrate her parents' sixtieth wedding anniversary, she was glad to find them still well able to manage for themselves, with only housecleaning help once a week. But she was shocked at how much thinner and frailer they were than just six months before.

Now at their daughter's recommendation, and after some friendly scare tactics by their doctor, Rebecca and Peter go every day to a local senior center, where nutritious meals are served to people over sixty-five. On days when they choose not to drive, the center's van picks them up and returns them home after each meal and visit.

What Is It?
Community-based meal programs operate in all cities and some small towns. Many are funded with federal money through the Older American's Act, and others are paid for out of community funds. Federally funded programs offer one square meal a day, usually lunch, in a group setting. Most meal programs operate five days a week, although in some communities they are offered seven days a week, and in others just three days. Meal programs are provided in local churches and synagogues, schools, senior centers, and other places.

The purpose behind these programs is to keep people healthy. Often health screening and lectures on health-related topics are offered at the meal site. Most programs provide transportation for those who cannot drive or otherwise get to the site on their own.

How Much Does It Cost?
When programs are federally funded, a donation for meals is suggested, usually $5 or less.

How to Find It
    Area Agency on Aging
    Local senior centers
    Churches and synagogues

Adult Day Care

After Alzheimer's disease was diagnosed, Patricia invited her mother to live at her house. At first her mother was able to manage alone during the day, with Patricia coming home at midday to prepare lunch. As her mother grew increasingly confused it became obvious that this arrangement was no longer safe and sensible.

Not wanting to put her mother in a nursing home, Patricia called the local chapter of the Alzheimer's Disease Association to ask about community services that could help take care of her mother. She learned about an adult day-care center on the other side of town, which had a special program for people suffering from permanent dementing illnesses. Even though Patricia had to get up an hour early every day to get her mother ready and drive her to the program, the effort was well worth it. Her mother seemed happier and Patricia was able to keep her job without worrying about her mother's safety and well-being during the day.

What Is It?
Adult day-care centers take frail or demented older people who can no longer remain at home alone but who do not need skilled nursing care. Although centers are a growing form of care, they are a fairly new idea and are not available in all communities. Centers within a community vary in specifying whom they will take. Some centers will *not* take demented people, those who use wheelchairs and walkers, or those who are incontinent. Others are set up to take people suffering from specific diseases, such as Alzheimer's or stroke damage. Besides providing a safe, structured environment, such centers give the frail elderly contact with other adults and medical and rehabilitative services. Lunch is provided and most centers have a space where clients can nap. Some centers provide transportation, although most don't.

How Much Does It Cost?
Fees at most adult day-care centers are not covered by Medicare or private insurance. Some states have Medicaid-funded centers for qualified older adults with less than a specified income. Some facilities are not-for-profit, and get federal and community assistance. Others are privately owned and operated for profit. Usually for-profit

centers cost more than not-for-profit centers. Fees generally range from $20 to $80 a day.

How to Find It

Area Agency on Aging

Disease societies, such as the Alzheimer's Association, American Heart Association, American Lung Association

Local hospitals

Write to the National Institute of Adult Day Care at the National Council on the Aging (see Appendix).

Respite

Mary and James Meldago care for James's mother in their home. Because she requires attention around the clock, Mary and James had not been able to take a vacation in three years. After their son announced he was getting married in California they decided they had to find a way to go to the wedding. They were able to leave without worries because a local nursing home took James's mother into an overnight respite program for two weeks. As their plane took off, Mary said, "Thank goodness for respite. Why didn't we do this sooner."

What Is It?

Respite programs are for overburdened caregivers, who without it are in danger of buckling under the strain of it all. The word derives from the Latin *respirare*, "to breathe." As a form of care, the program gives family caregivers breathing time before they must again get into the taxing job of caregiving. Respite can mean someone comes to the home to give a family caregiver a break; a program at a hospital or nursing home, where a disabled older person is dropped off; or a short stay in a nursing home, as for Mrs. Meldago.

Although the practice of care outside the home for short periods is controversial, it is slowly growing. Those in opposition say that changing an older person's living habits back and forth in a short time is traumatic and cruel. Supporters say that caregivers need such a service to survive, and ultimately to keep their relatives out of the nursing home.

How Much Does It Cost?
The daily rate for overnight respite care averages about $100. Such care is not usually reimbursable through Medicare, Medicaid, or private insurance. Volunteer-provided services in the home are free, and drop-off respite programs are either free or handled by a pay-as-you-can arrangement.

How to Find It
Finding a place to provide overnight respite care is not easy in many communities. Only 30 percent of the members of the American Association of Homes for the Aging offer residential respite care, according to an 1989 survey. Write for an updated list of such homes to American Association of Homes for the Aging, 1129 20th Street, N.W., Washington, DC 20036. Try calling local licensed nursing homes.

Some communities have in-home and drop-off respite services, which are found through:

Area Agency on Aging
Civic groups
Churches and synagogues
Home health agencies, such as the Visiting Nurse Association

HOUSING ARRANGEMENTS FOR OLDER PEOPLE

Like adult children everywhere who look after aging parents, you may be doing all you can to help your parents stay in the familiar surroundings of their house or apartment, with its comforts, time-worn possessions, and links to the past.

When it becomes all too obvious that living at home is no longer a good idea, the painful realization dawns that another living arrangement has to be worked out. The reasons for your parents having to move may be entirely practical. Maintaining a home, paying people to take over housekeeping and caregiving tasks may become too expensive. Or perhaps your parents have had enough, of muddling through, constantly coping with loneliness with the danger of accidents looming over them. In this section we cover housing arrangements for older people so that you can investigate options that might work for your parents and for everyone's peace of mind.

A Wrenching Decision

A change in living arrangements is always difficult for older people. Home holds special meaning for all of us, but for older people it represents identity, freedom, a familiar way of life, security, stability, and above all independence. A move from home to a more limited living arrangement means not just loss of a house but separation from ties to the past and giving up the feeling of being in full control.

If your parents deny the need to make a change, you will find this stage of caregiving particularly difficult. The classic scenario has the worried-sick adult children on one side of the fence, and on the other parents stubbornly hanging on to living alone. You may know what's best, that they can no longer live alone. And yet they will say, "We will go on living as we are, at our own risk." It's a seesaw conflict, in which you are bound to feel guilty and upset regardless of the decisions you make. You may wonder, "Should I force the issue, or should I yield and bear the worry of knowing that if something happens, the decision to live alone was theirs and not mine?"

We have no hard-and-fast answers to this prickly question; no one does. If your parents are mentally competent it is their civil right to do as they please, as long as their decisions do not endanger others. All you can do — when you believe they should move for their own good — is prepare for a breakthrough as best you can. Meanwhile, be ready to present a well-thought-out alternative living plan for the day you finally hear: "All right, but where do we go next?" Here are a few general suggestions that may help you get through to your parents so that they can be involved in making the decision and will accept an unwelcome but necessary change.

• Plan with, not for, your family members. No adults like to have decisions made for them. Even if they resist talking about change, it is usually best to inform your parents about any inquiries and serious discussions having to do with them.

• Try to find any hidden reasons for your parents' resistance. You may be able to resolve especially bothersome issues. Ask yourself: Do they think a nursing home is the only alternative? Are costs a worry? Do they fear abandonment? Do they worry about being under the care of strangers? Do they fear being sent where they must live by strict rules? Do they worry about having to give up cherished possessions?

- Deal with your parents' perceptions and feelings. If your father feels he is perfectly safe living alone, be specific and objective in explaining why you think he is not.

- Talk with your parents about their desires and priorities. Determine what is important to them in a living arrangement.

- Be positive about what a move will enable them to do. A move can represent a turnaround toward increased independence and a better life.

- Try not to focus on their limitations as a reason for moving. Avoid such statements as, "You can't cook for yourself any more," and instead say, "You will eat well-prepared meals at . . . ," or, "You can no longer drive to the store"; instead say, "You need to live where shopping is within the building or close by."

- Try enlisting the help of a social worker, a visiting nurse, a doctor, or a friend from outside the family. This person may meet less resistance in presenting problems and solutions.

- If your parents persist in saying, "Things are fine the way they are," try focusing on your own needs. Start with "Will you consider doing this for me so that I will worry less," or, "I can't worry about you any more, without losing my health," or, "I am exhausted. Unless we change your living situation, I will have no more energy left to take care of anyone."

Moving In with You

Too often, adult children harbor in the back of their minds the notion that "Dad or Mom can always come and live with us." Such a solution to the problem of where they will live when the time comes seems comforting to everyone — until the time comes to follow through on the idea. Often families don't have relationships or space to make a happy living arrangement. Many older people also don't want to live under their children's roofs, no matter how good and companionable everyone feels about one another.

Sharing a home with an aging relative always introduces stress into a household, and if the relative is in poor health or demented the stress can become unbearable. Moving in with family works well for some people, if major adjustments are anticipated and weathered.

This arrangement can mean an enriched life for everyone, from the top generation to the bottom. For the older generation it can mean sharing expenses and chores, feeling secure and useful, and for the younger generation it can mean someone will be there to watch over grandchildren.

If the grandparent is severely debilitated, providing hands-on care or supervising paid home-care personnel can be done as part of running the household. No more constant worry about what's going on when you're not there, difficulty in making arrangements from afar, and time taken away from your own family while you travel back and forth between locations.

The decision to permanently join households should not be made hastily. Thoughtful decisions will save everyone later resentment and guilt. Taking your time, you should carefully weigh the disadvantages and advantages in having all of you live together. Ask yourself, "Is this something I truly want to do?" or, "Am I thinking I should do this out of obligation, guilt for past behavior, sentimentality, or because this is what others want me to do? Above all, weigh whether or not your parent really wants to live with you.

Before making a commitment in words or in action, go over the questions listed here. These ideas should be considered by everyone in the family. They will help you come to a decision about whether or not living together is a sensible option. And if you do decide to live together, your answers may identify potential trouble spots so that you can work them through before they blow up into problems and hard feelings.

1. Can you get along day after day? Look at unresolved conflicts, pleasant and unpleasant aspects of earlier relationships, habits and all the little things that irritate, which could be magnified if you live together. Consider all areas of incompatibility: food preferences, use of alcohol and cigarettes, standards of cleanliness and order, choice of friendships, and religious practices.

2. How will the older person's presence complicate or relieve pressures within the household?

3. How does everyone in the household feel about a joint living arrangement? Involve your spouse and children in decisions. How good are the in-law relationships?

4. Who will be in charge if the older person becomes dependent and needs care? Who will provide the care? How will tasks be delegated and divided among the household? If help is secured, how will it be paid for? How will long-term caregiving affect the whole family? Is everyone well aware of the sacrifices required in giving selfless care to an ill, dependent person?

5. Does the home have enough space for another person? Is an extra room available? Is a bathroom near the room designated for the older person? Is closet space adequate? Are living areas sufficient to accommodate everyone, with space enough for privacy? For visiting? What changes need to be made to provide the elder with a room, and the family with the space it needs?

6. How will you work out financial arrangements? Consider how to plan specifically who will pay for what. Will someone in the family eventually have to give up working to be home for the older person?

7. How will joint living areas be set up? What about noise limitations? How will the temperature of the house be handled, if the elder needs more warmth and air-conditioning?

Group Housing Options

When a change obviously needs to be considered and acted upon, older people and their families often spin themselves into a state of high anxiety because of the erroneous notion that the only choice they have left, besides living together, is to find a place for mother or father in a nursing home. As they see it, this is the dreaded end of it all, for older people who can no longer live alone or with their family.

Less anguish can darken discussions and thoughts of your parents' making a move if everyone takes time to understand that the city or town where your parents want to live probably has a variety of intermediate housing. The choices bridge the gap between struggling to live at home and moving to a nursing home. These are groups of older people living together in such a way that their individual and collective needs can be met. A group can consist of three or four older people in shared housing, or thousands living together in a township.

Start networking now to find out what's available. Do it right away, because waiting lists are long for just about every kind of housing. Ask questions over the phone and send for written information and brochures. Once you have determined which places to consider, do some footwork, going from place to place. Look with your eyes, follow your instinct about the "feel" of a place, and talk to the staff and residents. Do some sleuthing about the general reputation of a place.

Besides your parents, let others help you in your quest for a resolution to the housing problem. Two or more heads are better in any decision about so great a change in lifestyle, particularly because it affects the whole family. Call a family meeting so that the final decision is shared and agreed upon. Consult your parents' doctor. Involve professionals in the planning as much as possible.

Together you can all look for a pleasant haven for your parent — a better place to be than home, as it now shapes up. They need a place where they can feel independent but can get assistance when they need it. Here are categories of housing arrangements for you to investigate according to your parent's state of health, needs, and finances. Use the same standard names as we do and you will save yourself time and aggravation while you gather information from housing providers.

Retirement Communities
Self-contained complexes for older people who want to live with others of their generation, away from the noise and bustle of the workaday world and activities that have to do with raising children: these are retirement communities. Usually minimal services are provided, such as security, recreation, and a communal dining room. Sometimes shops and health-service providers are in the community. Retirement communities may consist of a multiple-unit building, a townhouse or single-family housing development, mobile or modular homes, or even a small town. Living units may be for rent or for sale. Prices vary tremendously in different regions and according to the quality of housing and services.

Continuous-Care Retirement Communities
Retirement communities with continuous care are set up to supply their residents' needs for their lifetime. A community offers housing for independent living and personal and home nursing care if needed. A skilled nursing-home facility is run within the grounds. The beauty of this arrangement is that the elder's support system can remain uninterrupted as time goes on and needs change. Another advantage is that couples can stay in the same community, even when one partner needs nursing-home care.

Many of these communities are like miniature towns, including a medical clinic, shops, banks, libraries, transportation, and recreational and educational facilities. Because of the numerous services, living in a continuing-care community can be costly. They usually require a substantial entrance fee (called a founder's fee) plus monthly charges. Requirements for admission are usually restrictive, covering age, health, and finances. Most communities have long waiting lists. Communities are not all run by honest owners. Before signing any contracts, applicants should call the Better Business Bureau to find if any complaints have been lodged against the community. Also, seek legal and financial advice from someone not connected to the community.

Congregate Housing or Senior Housing

Housing designed specifically for older people and built with federal, state, or local government financing is called congregate or senior housing; if services are included it is also called "assisted living" or "enriched housing." This is not low-income housing, but rather a middle-income housing program. It is designed for assisted living, especially for the elderly on fixed retirement income, who are capable of living independently. Most congregate housing is rented and prices are kept affordable, with some rent subsidies available. Usually housing is in an apartment in a high-rise building or garden complex. Residents have their own private apartments, including a kitchenette for light meals and snacks. Limited services usually are given, ranging from meals in a common dining area to housekeeping, transportation, recreation, and security.

Board-and-Care Homes

In a well-run home, board and care is a small, friendly arrangement for people who need help with personal care. Usually fewer than ten people live in a house, which is run by someone licensed by the state health or social-service department. Levels of care within this housing option vary from state to state. Generally most homes provide assistance with bathing, grooming, dressing, getting in and out of bed or bathtub, and supervision of medication. Meals, housekeeping, and laundry services are also provided. Not all facilities accept people using walkers or wheelchairs, and prospective residents must be fairly alert mentally and able to take themselves to the toilet.

If you consider it for someone you love, investigate the home carefully before making a commitment. Reports of abuse are many and supervision by state agencies is said to be minimal.

Adult Foster Care
Families caring for a dependent adult in their home often own a large house and offer foster-care service to bring in needed income. For a monthly fee, meals, housekeeping, and help with dressing, eating, bathing, and other personal care are provided by trained personnel. If the arrangement is listed with a social-service organization, a case manager is required to monitor the care. This arrangement is available for older people who are mentally alert, continent, and able to move about.

ECHO Housing
Called "granny flats" in Australia, where the idea originated, Elder Cottage Housing Opportunity (ECHO) housing consists of small living units that can be ordered and set up through a city agency to be placed on the same lot as a family member's house. The units are not mobile homes, but are designed to fit in with local housing styles. A few towns offer this service through local zoning boards. Costs vary from community to community.

Home Sharing
Many community social-service agencies offer home sharing, a roommate-matching service for senior citizens. Programs match up individuals of any age, including students, who want to live in the home of an older person who needs some services and companionship. Home sharing between healthy, independent elderly people can also be arranged.

THE NURSING-HOME DECISION

"Father's dying wish was that mother would never have to go to a nursing home."

"My husband and children want me to place father in a nursing home. They say his illness is going to wear me out before him."

"We can't afford $60,000 a year for around-the-clock nursing care at home. And if one of us quits work to help provide it, we won't be able to pay our mortgage and bills."

The decision to place a relative in a nursing home is never an easy one. Like most family caregivers, you may have put off the decision as long as you possibly could. The necessity of nursing-home care may be thrust upon you suddenly, after a debilitating turn in your parent's state of health; or gradually, when you start to buckle under the strain of twenty-four-hour caregiving, even with the help of the kinds of services we have discussed in this chapter. Finances necessarily enter into your decision, for around-the-clock nursing care and services at home usually are prohibitively expensive, compared to similar care provided in an institution.

Any anguish and guilt you may feel about placing your parent in a nursing home partly reflects our pitiless stereotype of nursing homes as warehouses for the sick and the old, where they are "put away" in their hour of greatest need, left in the care of strangers. Mere mention of the name "nursing home" brings up terrible images of abuse, regimentation, neglect, abandonment, and at best, dingy and dreary surroundings.

Plenty of nursing homes in fact are truly awful places, where you would never want someone you love to live, but this ugly stereotype isn't necessarily valid everywhere. In most communities some nursing homes are well run and hospitable to chronically ill older people, places where the elderly are treated with dignity and respect. If you as a family have come to the decision that you cannot properly provide care to your parent at home, your job is to go out and find such a home. It is our hope that you will succeed.

Your role as loving adult child and caregiver need not stop once your parent is placed in a suitable nursing home. If you secure a place for your parent in a "better" home, your family will be encouraged to visit as often as you like and to participate in your parent's plan of care. The move can be positive for you and your parent, allowing you to be together and enjoy each other during visits, without having to devote all your time to strenuous caregiving tasks.

Even if your parent or an older friend goes to a nursing home that you believe is well run and pleasant, you still should stay involved. Your job is not just to show that you care for the older person, but to make yourself his or her advocate. Even in the "best" nursing homes, problems arise, and residents are never completely safe from subtle or frank abuses to their sense of worth and their health.

What Is a Nursing Home?

Before launching an investigation of local nursing homes, be sure you understand what such an institution should be. Your parent may not be eligible for a nursing home, but may be a candidate for the custodial housing arrangements described in the preceding section.

Admission to a nursing home has to be arranged through a doctor, who signs papers stating that the candidate has a medical need to be in the home. A nursing home is for people who require twenty-four-hour access to skilled medical care, or intermediate custodial care.

Skilled nursing care is provided around the clock by registered nurses, licensed practical nurses, and nursing assistants. This care includes such intensive services as oxygen therapy, feeding tubes, dressing changes, drainage of body fluids, and administration of intravenous fluids. A physician who is an official staff member is ultimately responsible for the patient's condition and for prescribing medication, therapy, diet, and other treatments. Only around 5 percent of nursing-home residents receive this kind of care at any one time, and often such patients are recuperating from a devastating illness that was previously treated in a hospital, or from a serious operation.

Intermediate custodial care is for people who can't live independently because of one or more severe, disabling, chronic illnesses. In such a "health-related" facility, people can participate in their own care, but in a limited way. This type is typically for the Alzheimer's patient, the badly stricken stroke victim, the patient with severe rheumatoid arthritis, or the patient who has severe trouble with balance and mobility. This kind of care is rarely paid for by Medicare and private insurance, except in limited circumstances for a few weeks. Once the patient's assets have been depleted by the nursing-home costs to a minimum, Medicaid can sometimes pick up the tab. Most private homes require two or three years of residence before payment through Medicaid is allowed. The for-profit nursing-home industry is where the better homes predominate, but because they are in business for profit they often shun patients on Medicaid, because that program provides limited reimbursement.

From Hospital to Nursing Home

Moving from hospital care, you have the advantage of being able to use the services of the hospital social-work department. But you can't therefore relax and let the hospital-discharge worker make decisions for you. No matter how much you yearn for freedom from the responsibility, you need to be in charge, and you are ultimately responsible for the nursing home your parent goes to.

Let the discharge planner work for you, and follow the suggested directives. This person will make inquiries about availability
of space in homes known to the planner or you. But let no final decisions be made without your approval. Go out and look at any homes
suggested, and if one does not appear suitable, insist on an alternative. Be highly involved too in arrangements for payment for a home.
You don't want the hospital-discharge planner to procure a place in
a private home that is not eligible for Medicare, during this period
when your parent may well be covered for Medicare reimbursement
for several weeks, or perhaps longer.

Discharge planners work for the hospital, and it is their job to
get patients out of the hospital by the designated discharge date, in
order to save the hospital penalties for keeping the patient longer
than the time allotted by Medicare. The discharge planner is more
likely to come up with a quick and easy solution rather than a careful, negotiated solution. The planner may be interested in procuring
just any place, rather than the most suitable place, in a good, Medi-
care-eligible home.

Selecting a Nursing Home

Most nursing homes with praiseworthy reputations have long waiting lists. Families who wait until the breaking point, or for a medical
catastrophe to strike, are often shocked and distraught to hear that
no places will be open for months, sometimes years, in the "best"
homes. Our advice is that you look around at nursing homes and get
yourself in line for those which look acceptable, as soon as you begin to determine that your parent's health is rapidly deteriorating.

Signing up before the need is obvious may feel like a betrayal of
your best intentions and your parent's expressed wishes, but it is a
step that you must take. Being on waiting lists and in contact with
homes you like may allow your parent to easily gain access after a
sudden hospitalization for a debilitating condition, or when the time
comes for you to relinquish your job of caring for your parent at
home. You and your parent can always say "no" to a place, if the
time is not right, and ask to keep your parent's name active on the
waiting list. You may have to pay a deposit to get on the list. Do find
out whether you forfeit the deposit in the event you do not want a
place when one opens.

Find out about nearby nursing homes from your doctor, a social worker, or nurses and friends who have placed older people in local nursing homes. You can get a list of homes from the Area Agency on Aging, a senior-citizen's center, and possibly from other local service organizations. Once you have compiled a list of compatible-sounding homes, make calls to arrange visits. If the personnel welcome your visit and answer questions respectfully, you know — at least initially — that the home may be a good one. Make at least one and preferably several visits to any home you are seriously considering. Take someone along with you. Two pairs of eyes are better than one, and you will be able to share opinions and together come to conclusions.

You should expect to meet the director of the home, several staff members, and some residents. A tour of the home should of course be part of your first visit and any subsequent visits you feel are needed. Excellent times to request an observation tour are during mealtime in the dining room and on weekends. Mealtimes are a challenge for the staff, for everyone has to be gathered together and fed in a reasonable time. You can sense the atmosphere in the dining room and whether or not residents are eating properly, are interacting with each other, and are being treated respectfully by the staff. Usually nursing homes have a smaller staff around on weekends and by observing then you can gauge how the home is run with limited staff.

The staff are the most important component of a home, more than beautiful surroundings and plentiful services. You need to observe how the staff talk to the patients. Do they look at them eye to eye and communicate with patience and respect? Do they care for patients gently and kindly, being considerate of their need for privacy? Do the staff answer your questions with reassuring and complete responses? In a "good" home the staff will encourage you to be involved in your parent's care plan, and the activities of the home as a community of patients and families.

Besides staffers, talk to residents and their families. Many homes have residents' councils and family councils. Members of these councils are excellent people to contact, so that you can get the inside story on the home from the consumer's point of view.

Selection Checklist
The following points are the most important for you to investigate carefully. Use these lists as you go from home to home, so that you know what to look for.

License and Certification

Is the home licensed by the state? (a must)
Does the chief administrator have an up-to-date license?
Is the facility Medicare and Medicaid licensed?
Is the facility a member of the American Health Care Association or the American Association of Homes for the Aged?
Will the director provide you with the latest annual survey prepared by Medicare and Medicaid?
Is the resident's Bill of Rights prominently displayed? Many states require homes to post it. In many better homes a complaint-referral procedure is also prominently displayed.

Costs

What is the basic monthly fee?
Does the home charge for doctor's fees, dental fees, medications, laundry, special feedings, frequent changes of linen, or special supplies such as wheelchairs and walkers?
Are therapies included in the basic charge?
Is there an extra charge for incontinent patients?
Is there a written statement listing all charges above the basic rate?
Is insurance counseling provided?
How long does someone have to live in the home to be eligible for Medicaid?
What is the involuntary transfer policy? What happens if a patient can't pay full rates, or is deemed "too difficult"?
Does the home hire an accountant to manage its financial arrangements?

Staff

Does the full-time staff include an administrator, director of nursing, social worker, and activities director?
What is the ratio of registered nurses to patients on any shift? (A minimal standard, effective October 1, 1990, is that all nursing facilities must have a licensed nurse RN or LPN or LVN on duty in each nursing home twenty-four hours a

day; an RN must be on duty for at least eight hours a day. An RN Director of Nursing is required.)

What is the ratio of licensed practical nurses to patients on any shift?

What is the ratio of nurses' aides on any shift?

What is the training of nurses aides? Do they receive continuing education?

Is a physician on call twenty-four hours a day, as required by law? Is a physician on permanent duty within the facility?

When would a medical situation be considered beyond the staff's capabilities? What is the hospital-transfer policy?

Is psychiatric or psychological counseling available?

Policies

What are the standard visiting hours?

In times of crisis can the family visit during the night?

Are children allowed to visit the home?

What is the checkout policy for the patient to travel outside the home?

Can residents bring their own furniture and mementos?

Can residents bring their own television set, radio, and books?

Is there a restraint policy?

Will the family be notified about changes in the medical regimen?

Can the patient's private physicians be involved in care?

Are families promptly notified about changes in the patient's medical and psychological condition?

How often do patients go outdoors?

The Environment

Do rooms provide space and privacy? If residents share rooms, find out if a screen or curtain is available for privacy.

Are rooms pleasant, light, and clean?

Are the bathrooms easily accessible?

Is the home well ventilated, warm or cool enough, and free from noxious odors?

Are smoke detectors and sprinkling systems visible? Is an emergency evacuation plan clearly posted?

Are hand rails and grab bars installed in hallways, staircases, and bathrooms?

Is the home accessible throughout to those in wheelchairs?

Are the grounds well kept?

Is the neighborhood quiet?

Does the facility have comfortable, spacious lounges and activity rooms?

Services and Activities

What are the daily activity programs for mobile patients and for bedridden patients?

Are religious services offered?

Does the home plan outside activities?

Is a hairdressing service available?

Is there a resident's council?

Is there a family council?

Are family support groups active?

Do volunteers come to the home from community-based programs?

Meals

Is there a dietician on the staff?

Are meals nutritious and well balanced, including fresh dairy products, fruits, and vegetables?

Are snacks provided?

Are special diets available for specific health problems? For religious dictates?

Will meals be delivered to rooms if patients don't come to the dining room?

Are patients weighed routinely?

Are aides available at mealtimes for patients who need help eating?

PLANNING LEGAL ISSUES

Margaret and Bill Johnson's mother was hospitalized with a stroke. On the second day of her hospitalization, the doctor told them that their mother would probably die within a few days. This was the first time they had considered their mother's death.

Grief-stricken and desperately wanting their mother to live, Margaret and Bill wondered how far to push the doctors to save their mother's life. They asked themselves if she would want to be put on life-support systems, including a respirator and feeding tube. They also agonized over issues they had never discussed with her. Where did she want to be buried? Did she have a will? How would they take care of her medical bills? Were her bills left at home?

Mrs. Johnson pulled through the critical stage. The stroke left her paralyzed on one side and unable to read or write properly. The doctors told her she might partially recover most lost functions, but only after months of rehabilitation therapy.

Now Margaret and Bill were left wondering how they could get to her bank accounts to pay for her care and daily living expenses at home.

They decided to call a lawyer. After meeting with a lawyer experienced in long-term care, they wished they had done so sooner, while their mother was still in full command of her mental and physical capacities.

Why Plans Are Important

Lifetime planning is the label that the legal profession applies to the kind of planning families need for worst-case scenarios involving death and incapacity. The planning involves setting up wills, joint bank accounts, and powers of attorney, which arrange financial affairs; and living wills, which enable someone to specify whether or not heroic medical treatments are to be provided.

Be sure that your parents have well-thought-out life-planning arrangements. If such arrangements are not set up when your parent is incapacitated, you may face untold anguish, and the expense and inconvenience of lengthy court proceedings.

When the family has no sensible life planning, it can take months of visits to lawyers' offices and court proceedings for adult children to get access to their parents' bank accounts and business arrangements. In the interim, the parents' bills are put on hold (with creditors banging at the door), unless they are paid out of the adult children's pockets. Also, unless a living will has been written and signed, medical decisions fall to the older person's doctors rather than the family, which will have no immediate power to ensure that the older person's philosophy and wishes will be respected.

Such issues usually are extremely difficult for adult children to bring up with their parents. Discussion of worst-case scenarios having to do with illness force into the open deep-seated fears: death itself, pain, mental incapacity, losing independence, and being a burden on one's family. Nevertheless, discussing how to plan for critical illness and incapacity is essential, as is taking legal measures to set up a plan.

Do Use a Lawyer Who Knows Elderlaw

The key to putting affairs in proper order is a lawyer who knows about planning for incapacity and lifetime planning. Choose this lawyer carefully, because lawyers are not all familiar with the complexities of such planning and how it ties in with reimbursement by Medicare and Medicaid and private insurance. Even lawyers in top firms who routinely write out wills and estates may not be well versed in elder-law issues. Plenty of families find out too late that arrangements were not complete.

To find a lawyer befitting the job, you may want to contact your local bar association, state bar association, or the Academy for Elderlaw Attorneys (see Appendix), and ask for names of lawyers who specialize in elderlaw. Another place to inquire is a local or national disease organization, such as the Alzheimer's Disease and Related Disorders Association (ADRDA), which may have a roster of attorneys familiar with incapacity planning for the specific disease. If a private attorney seems too expensive, your Area Agency on Aging will recommend Legal Services Offices funded by the Older Americans Act, which provide free legal assistance to people over sixty who are unable to pay private fees. Ask these questions of any attorney you consider using:

1. Are you familiar with Medicaid issues in estate planning?
2. Are you familiar with Medicare?
3. Are you familiar with property-management alternatives?
4. Are you familiar with the use of trusts in planning for incapacity?
5. Are you familiar with the legal aspects of planning for medical care of the critically ill?

Basic Legal Arrangements

Everyone's case is different, depending on the relationships within a family and the financial assets of those who seek life-plan arrangements. Nevertheless, there are basic legal instruments or directives that your parents need to arrange. If these are planned, you can avoid the woeful scenario of having to go to court on their behalf.

Power of Attorney for Financial Arrangements

The power-of-attorney arrangement works very well for temporary or terminal illness, or if the older person is unable to pay bills easily and properly for any reason. If an older person signs over power of attorney to an adult child or to another specified person, this person can act as a surrogate in paying bills and in buying and selling property, including real estate. The older person can sign over limited powers, such as the right to write checks from a simple checking account; or broad powers, such as selling stocks, bonds, or real estate, and running a business. A power of attorney can be revoked at any time.

A durable power of attorney is the preferred form, because it allows stated powers to continue if the older person can no longer make clear, well-thought-out decisions. If someone wants power of attorney to go into effect only after complete incapacitation, as determined by a doctor, then a document called a springing power of attorney should be arranged. This arrangement springs into action as soon as the person granting the power over his or her affairs becomes incapacitated.

Joint Checking Accounts

Arranging a joint checking account, on which both parent and adult child can write checks, can make things easier for paying bills on the parent's behalf. The arrangement works well when the parent fully trusts the child, and if the child is trustworthy. If a joint account is created, it is extremely important that only the parent's funds enter the account. A joint bank account with commingled funds can create serious obstacles for the parent if the time comes to apply for public benefits. A joint account can be arranged at the bank.

Representative Payeeship

The payeeship option has to do with a family member or friend's gaining access to the benefits of an incapacitated person in order to pay bills on his or her behalf. The option is a provision of the Social Security Administration, the Veteran's Administration, and the Railroad Retirement Administration. To apply for access, the family member or friend must make an appointment with the administration governing the pension. Once access has been granted, the family member or friend can deposit the check in the incapacitated person's checking account.

A Will

Those who die without a will have the fate of their full estate determined by a court, according to state laws. Without a will, a surviving spouse faces possible financial hardships, and children as well as the surviving spouse have to pay considerably higher estate taxes than they would with a will.

A will provides explicit instructions for distribution of property and designates a person or persons who will be responsible for distribution of the property. The will can also specify funeral arrangements.

A Durable Power of Attorney for Health Care

This document allows someone to make medical decisions on behalf of a relative or friend if this person becomes incapacitated. The appointee acts as a surrogate for the incapacitated individual. Specific directives can be set down in the document. Not all, but most states allow such documents.

Living Will

The living will is a legal document stating an individual's expressed wishes about treatment decisions if he or she becomes terminally ill, or is in a vegetative state with no hope of being able to regain the ability to make decisions.

Living wills are a relatively new phenomenon. The first living-will law took effect in California in 1976. At the time of writing, only about 9 percent of Americans had set up living wills, most people not wanting to plan specific directives for their dying days. Although the American Medical Association and most doctors endorse the idea, probably more wills are not signed because many doctors are reluctant for some reason to talk with patients about death and what a living will can reasonably cover. On the other hand, more and more doctors are taking the time to gently urge their terminally ill patients — while still mentally alert — to sign a written directive about how much technology they want to sustain them.

The move toward living-will laws, which now apply in most states, came about as doctors became able to keep people alive with artificial measures long after life-sustaining body functions have ceased to function on their own. Few deaths in a hospital these days are peaceful and natural, unencumbered by medical machinery. With laws as they stand today, doctors are legally obliged to do all they can to keep patients living, even if they are very old and are in pain with a terminal illness. Families often find themselves in the anguish of watching an older dying relative put on life supports that no one wants — the dying relative, the doctor, or themselves.

The Society for the Right to Die has made up forms for living wills to comply with state laws in every state. These forms are available without charge from the Society for the Right to Die, 250 57th Street, New York, NY 10107. Living wills must be signed, dated, and countersigned by two witnesses (ideally not the heirs). Copies of the will should be given to the primary doctor and the attorney who has arranged lifetime planning. Your attorney will be able to advise you about the wording of the will and if it is valid in your state.

Appendix
Index

Appendix: Resources for Caregivers

Organizations Dedicated to the Concerns of Older People

ACTION
1100 Vermont Avenue N.W.
Washington, D.C. 20525
(202) 634-9108

This agency is also known as the Federal Domestic Volunteer Agency. It is the umbrella organization for all federally sponsored volunteer programs, including three for older adults: Foster Grandparent Program, Retired Senior Volunteer Program, and Senior Companion Program. ACTION offers information, including free publications about its programs directed to seniors.

American Association of Retired Persons
1909 K Street N.W.
Washington, D.C. 20049
(202) 872-4700

A membership organization dedicated to improving the lives of people who are fifty and over. Local volunteer groups provide a variety of services, including a widowed persons' service, driver improvement programs, and health information. Members may participate in group health insurance, travel services, auto and home insurance, and investment programs. The mail-order pharmacy service offers excellent discounts on prescription and over-the-counter medications. AARP publishes many free pamphlets on aging, housing, retirement planning, travel, and the whole range of support services for caregiving, hospitalization, and health and exercise, plus a bimonthly magazine and monthly newspaper. Information about the organization and its publications is available upon request. Annual membership is $5.

American Society on Aging
Suite 512
833 Market Street
San Francisco, CA 94103
(415) 543-2617

The largest nonprofit membership organization for professionals, practitioners, researchers, and advocates in the field of aging. The society publishes a quarterly magazine and a bimonthly newsletter for members.

Gray Panthers Project Fund
1424 16th Street N.W.
Suite 602
Washington, D.C. 20036
(202) 387-3111

An activist group that works to change laws and attitudes that discriminate against people on the basis of their age. Local chapters sponsor public education seminars and provide information about resources for older adults. Membership ($15) allows participation in local networks and their advocacy efforts.

National Association of Area Agencies on Aging (NAAAA)
1112 16th Street N.W.
Suite 100
Washington, D.C. 20036
(202) 296-8130

This umbrella organization represents more than 650 area agencies that have been mandated by Congress to help older people gain from social and medical services across the country. The names of local agencies vary from community to community, making it difficult to find telephone numbers, especially for caregivers at a distance. Call the NAAAA to find the telephone number of your local agency for information and referrals to services.

National Council on the Aging, Inc. (NCA)
409 Third Street S.W.
Washington, D.C. 20024
(202) 479-1200

A national nonprofit organization, primarily directed to professionals and volunteers in aging and related fields, which provides information and training and supports research related to this field. Within the NCA are many subgroups, including the National Institute of Adult Daycare, the National Institute of Senior Centers, and the National Institute of Senior Housing. A number of NCA publications that are of direct help to caregivers are available upon request.

National Council of Senior Citizens
1331 F Street N.W.
Washington, D.C. 20004
(202) 347-8800

Founded in 1961 during the struggle to create Medicare legislation, NCSC is a national social activist association of councils, clubs, and community groups that work toward a better life for older people, as well as people of all ages. Call or write to join ($12 a year), so you can use the information and referral service, which provides information about federal housing programs, job programs under the Older American Act, Medicare, and long-term-care insurance.

National Institute on Aging (NIA)
Public Information Office
Federal Building, Room 6C12
Bethesda, MD 20892
(301) 496-1752

The NIA is part of the National Institutes of Health and is the principal agency for conducting and supporting research related to aging. It offers a variety of free publications for older people, including Age Pages, which are fact sheets on a wide range of topics related to aging and health promotion. A list of free materials is available upon request, and calls for information are answered by specialists.

National Interfaith Coalition of Aging (NICA)
c/o NCA
409 Third Street S.W.
Washington, D.C. 20024
(202) 479-6689

NICA is a division of the National Council on the Aging. Its members include representatives of Catholic, Jewish, and Protestant religious bodies as well as individuals of all faiths. Members work together to support research and plan assistance to religious groups that serve older adults. They have been instrumental in setting up caregiver support groups.

Older Women's League (OWL)
Suite 300
730 11th Street N.W.
Washington, D.C. 20001
(202) 783-6686

OWL seeks to educate the public about the problems and issues of middle-aged and older women, including caring for spouses and parents. Local OWL chapters offer mutual aid and supportive services, especially to women who are alone.

United Way of America
701 North Fairfax Street
Alexandria, VA 22314-2034
(703) 836-7100

This is the national association office of the 2,300 independent local United Way agencies across the country. Local offices raise money within the community for social services, including those to help older people, such as Meals on Wheels, respite programs, senior centers, and volunteer programs. You can contact the national office to find out about local offices nationwide; however, the best first approach is to look in the white pages of the local telephone book.

Arthritis

Arthritis Foundation
P.O. Box 1900
Atlanta, GA 30326
(800) 283-7800 (information line)

This voluntary organization supports research to find a cure for arthritis and provides services to improve the quality of life for people who have arthritis and other rheumatic diseases. There are 150 offices nationwide. Contact a local office, or call the information line for answers to questions, free brochures, and locations of chapters, which provide physician referrals, exercise programs, support groups, and courses in arthritis management.

National Arthritis and Musculoskeletal and Skin Disease Information Clearinghouse
Box AMS
Bethesda, MD 20892
(301) 495-4484

Contact this National Institutes of Health Resource Center for information about federal programs related to rheumatic and musculoskeletal diseases and skin diseases, such as psoriasis, vitiligo, and eczema. A number of free publications are available upon request.

Bones and Feet

American Academy of Orthopaedic Surgeons
P.O. Box 618
Park Ridge, IL 60068
(708) 832-7186

This is a professional organization of doctors who specialize in treating diseases and injuries of the musculoskeletal system. Free brochures are available upon request on subjects including total joint replacement; arthroscopy; common foot problems; neck, low back, and shoulder pain; and sprains and strains. Send a self-addressed envelope and a request for particular topics.

American Podiatric Medical Association
9312 Old Georgetown Road
Bethesda, MD 20814
(301) 571-9200
(800) FOOT CARE

The APMA is a professional organization of doctors of podiatric medicine, who specialize in the diagnosis and treatment of foot injuries and disease by medical or surgical means. Call their 800 number to obtain free brochures on a wide range of subjects, including diabetes, arthritis, bunions, heel pain, Medicare benefits, and finding a local podiatrist.

Cancer

American Cancer Society (ACS)
1599 Clifton Road N.E.
Atlanta, GA 30329
(404) 320-3333
(800) ACS-2345

This voluntary organization funds cancer research and offers programs to educate the public and health care professionals about cancer prevention, detection, and treatment. Around 50 ACS division offices and 3,000 divisions offer a variety of services, including self-help groups, support groups for families, transportation programs, and home care items. The ACS sponsors Reach to Recovery, which helps breast cancer patients cope with the physical, emotional, and cosmetic needs related to their cancer and its treatment. I Can Cope and CanSurmount are support groups for patients and their families to learn about cancer, locate local resources, and cope with the disease. Laryngectomy Rehabilitation and Ostomy Rehabilitation offer pre- and post-operative support.

Make Today Count, Inc.
101½ South Union Street
Alexandria, VA 22314-3323
(703) 548-9674

This nonprofit organization provides information and emotional support to people with life-threatening illnesses and their caregivers.

It publishes a bimonthly newsletter that offers tips on caregiving and inspirational reading and sponsors workshops and seminars. Through local chapters it offers volunteer-based services such as group meetings, a telephone "buddy" system, home and hospital visits, and emergency transportation. There are approximately 150 local chapters. To contact the one nearest you, call the national office or send $1 for a national registry of local chapters.

National Cancer Institute
Cancer Information Service (CIS)
Building 31, Room 10A24
Bethesda, MD 20892
(800) 4-CANCER

The NCI, a section of the National Institutes of Health, is the government's principal agency for funding cancer research and distributing information about cancer to health care professionals and the public. Through the Cancer Information Service, the institute provides, toll free, the latest information about cancer treatment and where to get it. The NCI distributes a variety of excellent detailed, free publications about different forms of cancer. To obtain a list of its publications, call the 800 number.

National Coalition for Cancer Survivorship
328 8th Street S.W.
Albuquerque, NM 87102
(505) 764-9956

The mission of the coalition is to communicate that there can be vibrant, productive life following the diagnosis of cancer. It operates an information clearinghouse and referral service on all aspects of problems related to cancer treatment, costs, insurance, employment, and support groups. Free publications and resources are available upon request. *Practical Resources For Cancer Survivors* is available for $12 to members.

Caregiving Support and Information

Brookdale Center on Aging
425 East 25th Street
New York, NY 10010
(212) 481-4426

The Brookdale Center is an academic gerontology center funded by Hunter College, City University of New York. It offers professional training and advice to those who provide social services to older people. The center compiles information on aging research and provides assistance to communities planning Alzheimer's respite services for caregivers. Information is available upon request on respite services and legal services for older adults.

Children of Aging Parents
2761 Trenton Road
Levittown, PA 19056
(215) 945-6900

CAPS is a nonprofit self-help organization that provides information and emotional support to those caring for older adults. It publishes a bimonthly newsletter that addresses areas of concern to caregivers, a directory of national support groups, and many helpful pamphlets. Information about the organization and a list of publications is available upon request.

National Federation of Interfaith Volunteer Caregivers, Inc.
105 Mary's Avenue
P.O. Box 1939
Kingston, NY 12401
(914) 331-1358

The federation helps congregations of all faiths minister to frail, disabled older people and their families. More than 200 interfaith caregiving programs in 45 states have been started through the federation. Contact the national office for the name of a local program or for assistance in setting one up.

Shepherd's Centers of America
6700 Troost, Suite 616
Kansas City, MO 64131
(816) 523-1080

This is the national association office of the 95 Shepherd's Centers, which are primarily in the midwestern and southeastern states. A Shepherd's Center is an organization of community-based interfaith volunteers who provide programs to improve the quality of life for older adults and their family caregivers. Each center develops services, which may include support groups for those who have Alzheimer's, Parkinson's, or other disabling diseases, respite programs for caregivers, and senior companion programs. Contact the national office for information about the Shepherd's Center movement and the name of a center near you.

Diabetes

American Association of Diabetes Educators
500 North Michigan Avenue
Suite 1400
Chicago, IL 60611
(312) 661-1700

A professional organization of certified diabetes educators, who counsel those who have diabetes about managing the disease. Call or write to find an educator in your area.

American Diabetes Association (ADA)
1660 Duke Street
Alexandria, VA 22314
(800) 232-3472

The ADA is a national voluntary organization that supports diabetes research and seeks to improve the lives of people with diabetes and their caregivers. The ADA reaches over 800 communities through local affiliates and chapters, which offer educational seminars for those with Type II diabetes, support groups for older adults and their families, and health screenings. Call the toll-free number for a list of excellent free publications and a quarterly newsletter, *Diabetes,* which includes self-help and caregiving tips, recipes, and exercise information.

National Diabetes Information Clearinghouse
Box NDIC
9000 Rockville Pike
Bethesda, MD 20892
(301) 468-2162

The National Institutes of Health sponsors this clearinghouse as a resource and local referral service for those who have diabetes, their caregivers, and medical professionals. A list of free publications is available upon request. *Diabetes Dateline* is a helpful newsletter containing news about research, self-care techniques, relevant publications, and new products. Numerous patient guides to diet, exercise, medications, and diabetes monitoring are available, as is a bibliography of diabetes-related literature.

Digestion

> National Digestive Diseases Information Clearinghouse
>   (NDDIC)
> Box NDDIC
> Bethesda, MD 20892
> (301) 468-6344

The National Institutes of Health sponsors this clearinghouse as an information and local referral service for those who have disorders of the digestive tract, including constipation, hemorrhoids, ulcers, diverticulosis, dry mouth, and swallowing difficulties. A list of its publications is available upon request. *DDNotes* is a helpful newsletter about new research and literature, common signs and symptoms that merit medical attention, treatment options, and new products. Numerous patient guides are available, as are extensive lists of literature pertaining to various digestive disorders.

Financial Planning

> Institute of Certified Financial Planners
> 7600 East Eastman Avenue
> Suite 301
> Denver, CO 80231
> (800) 282-PLAN

This is a national organization of licensed professionals who provide financial planning for long-term care, medical insurance, life insurance, and taxes. Call the toll-free number to obtain up to five names of financial planners anywhere in the country and a brochure about how to select a licensed planner.

International Association for Financial Planning (IAFP)
2 Concourse Parkway
Suite 800
Atlanta, GA 30328
(404) 395-1605

A national organization of those who work in various financial services fields, including planning services for older people and their support network. Contact IAFP for a free copy of the *Registry of Financial Planning Practitioners Directory,* which lists names and addresses of the organization's members in each state. Also free to the public are helpful brochures, including *The Financial Planning Consumer Bill of Rights* and the *Consumer Guide To Financial Independence.*

Hearing

American Hearing Research Foundation
55 East Washington Street
Chicago, IL 60602
(312) 726-9670

A nonprofit organization of otolaryngologists (ear, nose, and throat specialists). Contact the organization for names of local otolaryngologists and information about hearing disorders.

American Speech-Language-Hearing Association (ASHA)
10801 Rockville Pike
Rockville, MD 20852
(800) 638-8255 (except Maryland)
(301) 897-8682 (Maryland)

A membership association of more than 6,400 audiologists (licensed professionals who diagnose hearing problems and fit hearing aids) and speech language pathologists (licensed professionals who diagnose and treat speech disorders). By calling their toll-free helpline you can get answers to questions, referrals to professionals in their registry, and free publications. Their publications include pamphlets on communication disorders and aging, hearing aids, assistive listening devices, and tinnitus.

American Tinnitus Association (ATA)
P.O. Box 5
Portland, OR 97207
(503) 248-9985

A voluntary organization that supports research to find a cure for tinnitus. They also distribute information about the disorder and sponsor self-help groups nationwide. Contact ATA for referral to medical specialists in tinnitus and support groups in your area. A list of their publications is available upon request, including a helpful magazine containing current information and self-help tips.

Better Hearing Institute
P.O. Box 1840
Washington, D.C. 20013
(800) 327-9355

The institute educates the public about the issue of uncorrected hearing problems and available medical, surgical, hearing aid, and rehabilitation assistance. Call the toll-free number to request free pamphlets about various topics, including hearing aids, nerve deafness, and cochleal implants, and information about financial assistance for treatment and a list of local hearing professionals, including audiologists and doctors.

Hearing Aid Helpline
20361 Middlebelt Road
Livonia, MI 48152
(800) 521-5247 (U.S. and Canada)

A call to this helpline sponsored by the hearing aid industry will give you specific responses to questions about all aspects of hearing loss and its treatment. You can send for free written materials on a wide range of topics, from hearing aids to dogs trained to assist the hard of hearing. Also available are names of licensed hearing aid specialists (in states that offer licensure), who have passed the test standards of the National Hearing Aid Society.

National Institute on Deafness and Other Communication Disorders Clearinghouse
Information Office

9000 Rockville Pike
Bethesda, MD 20892
(301) 496-7243

This clearinghouse is a division of the National Institutes of Health. Call the toll-free number to ask for free written information about hearing, balance, smell, taste, voice, speech, and language.

Self Help for Hard of Hearing People, Inc.
7800 Wisconsin Avenue
Bethesda, MD 20814
(301) 657-2248 voice
(301) 657-2249 TDD (Telecommunications Display Device)

This volunteer-based organization is designed to help those who are hard of hearing help themselves through 280 chapters nationwide. A $15 membership includes an informative bimonthly magazine, *SHH Journal,* and information about conventions for the hard of hearing, local self-help groups, and publications.

Heart Disease and Stroke

American Academy of Physical Medicine and Rehabilitation
Suite 1300
122 South Michigan Avenue
Chicago, IL 60603-6107
(312) 922-9366

A professional organization of physiatrists, who are doctors specializing in physical rehabilitation. You can contact the academy to locate board-certified physiatrists in your area.

American Heart Association
7320 Greenville Avenue
Dallas, TX 75231
(214) 373-6300

This is the nation's largest voluntary health organization that funds research and sponsors public education programs about the prevention and treatment of heart disease and stroke. The 56 affiliate offices and numerous local divisions offer programs, such as stroke clubs and exercise, diet, and smoking cessation programs, and excellent pamphlets about heart disease and stroke. Look in the white pages of your telephone directory for a local chapter, or contact the national office.

National Heart, Lung, and Blood Institute
Information Center
4733 Bethesda Avenue
Suite 530
Bethesda, MD 20814
(301) 951-3260

NHLBI, a section of the National Institutes of Health, is the government's principal agency for research on diseases of the heart, blood, and lungs; it distributes information to health care professionals and the general public. A list of materials is available upon request.

National Institute of Neurological Disorders and Stroke
    (NINDS)
Office of Scientific and Health Reports
Building 31, Room 8A06
9000 Rockville Pike
Bethesda, MD 20892
(301) 496-5751

NINDS, a division of the National Institutes of Health, is the government's principal agency for research and dissemination of up-to-date information about neurological diseases, including stroke, Parkinson's disease, multiple sclerosis, epilepsy, and Alzheimer's disease. Contact it for fact sheets, brochures, and current reports.

National Rehabilitation Information Center
8455 Colesville Road
Suite 935
Silver Spring, MD 20910-3319
(800) 346-2742

This organization was set up by the U.S. Department of Education to provide information about disabilities and rehabilitation. A call to the toll-free number will introduce you to its resource, research, and referral services. The free quarterly, *NARIC Newsletter,* is available upon request.

> National Stroke Association (NSA)
> Suite 240
> 300 East Hampden Avenue
> Englewood, CO 80110
> (800) 367-1990

This is the only national organization that focuses solely on stroke prevention, treatment, and rehabilitation. It has an information and referral center for stroke survivors and their caregivers, including information about the 800 Stroke Clubs nationwide, rehabilitation facilities, and professional services. The center will provide publications, including a quarterly newsletter and a widely used book, *The Road Ahead: A Stroke Recovery Guide.*

Home Care

> American Red Cross
> 17th and D Streets N.W.
> Washington, D.C. 20006
> (202) 737-8300

The American Red Cross offers safety and health programs through nearly 2,700 local chapters nationwide. These include courses in first aid, CPR, aquatics, back injury prevention, stress management, and health for people over fifty. Many chapters train nurse assistants who work in long-term-care facilities. Not all courses and programs are available from all chapters. Contact your local chapter for more information.

> Foundation for Hospice and Home Care
> 519 C Street N.E.
> Washington, D.C. 20002
> (202) 547-7424

This foundation is dedicated to helping people set up quality home care, including hospice, as an alternative to institutional care. It sets up certification programs and workshops for home health aides and publishes educational materials. Two free pamphlets, *All About Home Care* and *Consumer's Guide to Hospice Care,* as well as names of home health care agencies, are available upon request.

National Association of Home Care
519 C Street N.E.
Washington, D.C. 20002
(202) 547-7424

The NAHC is a professional association representing a variety of agencies that provide home health services, including home health agencies, hospice programs, and homemaker/home health aide agencies. *How To Select A Home Health Agency* and *The Patient's Bill of Rights* are available upon request.

National Association of Meal Programs
204 E Street N.E.
Washington, D.C. 20002
(202) 547-6157

An association of professionals and volunteers who provide congregate and home-delivered meals to elder individuals. It can refer you to local meal programs.

Hospice

National Hospice Organization
1901 North Moore Street, Suite 901
Arlington, VA 22209
(703) 243-5900
(800) 658-8898

The NHO promotes quality care for terminally ill patients and provides information about hospice and about local hospice services. A list of publications is available upon request.

Housing and Nursing Homes

American Association of Homes for the Aging (AAHA)
901 E Street N.W.
Suite 500

Washington, D.C. 20004-2837
(202) 783-2242

The AAHA is a national nonprofit organization representing not-for-profit nursing homes, housing, health-related facilities, and community services for the elderly. It publishes free consumer brochures on health and housing options for older adults. For a publications catalogue, including a directory of the association's member facilities, write to Publications at the above address.

Concerned Relatives of Nursing Home Patients
P.O. Box 18820
Cleveland Heights, OH 44118
(216) 321-0403

This nonprofit organization, which is not connected with the nursing home industry, monitors the quality and costs of care in nursing homes and is an advocate group for patients' rights. It publishes a newsletter that includes updates of legislation affecting nursing home patients and changes in Medicare and Medicaid. A list of publications is available upon request, including one on selecting a nursing home and one on the Patient's Bill of Rights.

National Citizens Coalition for Nursing Home Reform
1224 M Street N.W.
Suite 301
Washington, D.C. 20005
(202) 393-2018

The coalition initiates and watches over nursing home reform laws and regulations, with a primary mission of improving the quality of care and life for nursing and boarding home residents. Call or write for a free consumer packet containing brochures about nursing homes and a list of officials to contact in your state if you have questions about a particular problem. A list of their excellent publications is also available upon request.

Nursing Home Information Service
National Council of Senior Citizens
1331 F Street N.W.

Washington, D.C. 20004
(202) 347-8800

Contact this information and referral service for information about all aspects of long-term care, including nursing homes, retirement communities, board and care homes, and home health care agencies. Written materials are available upon request, including listings of local licensed residential facilities and home services.

Insurance

National Consumers League
815 15th Street N.W.
Washington, D.C. 20005
(202) 639-8140

This is the oldest consumer advocacy group in the U.S. It advocates to protect consumers from fraud in all industries, including health services and health insurance. Contact the league for brochures and information about medigap insurance and long-term care services, including hospice, home health care, and ambulatory services.

National Insurance Consumer Helpline
Suite 1200
1025 Connecticut Avenue N.W.
Washington, D.C. 20036
(202) 223-7780
(800) 942-4242

This helpline, sponsored by the Health Insurance Association of America, will put you in touch with experts able to answer questions about health insurance, including supplementary Medicare insurance and long-term care. Specific questions about policies cannot be answered. Consumer guides and other printed materials are available upon request.

Legal Services

Concern for Dying — Society for the Right to Die
250 West 57th Street
New York, NY 10107
(212) 246-6962

This national organization provides information about the complex issues of terminal care and the right of patients to control treatment decisions. It will send living wills for all of the states. A list of publications is available upon request.

National Academy of Elder Law Attorneys
655 N. Alvernon Way
Alvernon Place, Suite 108
Tucson, AZ 85711

The members of this rapidly growing professional organization are attorneys who specialize in the legal needs of older people. You can send a self-addressed envelope for a free booklet, *Questions and Answers When Looking for an Elder Law Attorney.*

Lung Diseases

American Lung Association
1740 Broadway
New York, NY 10019
(212) 315-8700

This voluntary organization funds research and conducts educational programs on lung diseases. Local chapters in all major cities and towns offer smoking cessation programs as well as educational programs about lung diseases, including influenza, pneumonia, emphysema, chronic bronchitis, and lung cancer. The association offers a variety of excellent free publications, and a list is available upon request.

National Jewish Center for Immunology and Respiratory
   Medicine
1400 Jackson Street
Denver, CO 80266
(800) 222-LUNG

This teaching and research center provides clinical care for patients with respiratory diseases. By calling the toll-free number you can get information about respiratory diseases and their treatment, and the names of physicians who have completed their training program at the center.

Mental Health

American Psychiatric Association
1400 K Street N.W.
Washington, D.C. 20005
(202) 682-6000

This society of doctors of psychiatric medicine supports research, sets standards for care, and offers educational programs for its members. Write to the above address for the free packet *Let's Talk Facts About Mental Illnesses,* which includes a brochure about mental health of the elderly, and for names of local psychiatric associations that will refer you to geriatric psychiatrists.

American Psychological Association
1200 17th Street N.W.
Washington, D.C. 20036
(202) 955-7600

This is a national society of psychologists who counsel people with mental, emotional, or behavioral problems. Contact the society for the addresses of local societies, which have the names of psychologists who work with the elderly. Numerous free publications on various mental health topics are available upon request to the national office.

National Institute of Mental Health
Public Inquiries Office
Room 15C-05
5600 Fishers Lane
Rockville, MD 20857
(301) 443-4513

The NIMH, a section of the Alcohol, Drug Abuse, and Mental Health Administration, conducts and supports research on the causes, prevention, and treatment of mental illness. An extensive list of free publications is available upon request.

Neurological Diseases

Alzheimer's Association
919 North Michigan Avenue
Suite 1000
Chicago, IL 60611-1676
(800) 272-3900

This national voluntary organization funds research on the prevention, cause, and treatment of Alzheimer's disease. The toll-free information and referral line directs caregiving families to local chapters for support and respite services information. You can also request written information on a wide range of topics, including financial arrangements, medications, and caregiving.

National Institute of Neurological Disorders and Stroke
    (NINDS)
Office of Scientific and Health Reports
Building 31, Room 8A06
9000 Rockville Pike
Bethesda, MD 20892
(301) 496-5751

NINDS, a division of the National Institutes of Health, is the government's principal agency for research and dissemination of up-to-date information about neurological diseases, including stroke, Parkinson's disease, multiple sclerosis, epilepsy, and Alzheimer's disease. Contact the institute for fact sheets, brochures, and current reports.

Osteoporosis

National Osteoporosis Foundation (NOF)
2100 M Street N.W.
Suite 602
Washington, D.C. 20037
(202) 223-2226

A voluntary health agency dedicated to reducing the widespread prevalence of osteoporosis. A list of free publications is available upon request. An NOF membership entitles you to the quarterly newsletter *The Osteoporosis Report,* which contains updated information on diagnosis, prevention, treatment, and support groups, among other topics.

Parkinson's Disease

American Parkinson's Disease Association
60 Bay Street
Suite 401
Staten Island, NY 10301
(800) 223-2732

This national nonprofit organization promotes research and supports patient care for those who have Parkinson's disease and their families. A call to the toll-free number will put you in touch with one of the 43 information and referral centers in hospitals throughout the country. A nurse coordinator can refer you to medical specialists, local chapters, and support groups, as well as answer questions about any aspect of Parkinson's disease. *The Parkinson's Disease Handbook,* which includes frequently updated information about medications, is an essential resource available free upon request. Also available free is *Be Active* and other manuals.

United Parkinson Foundation
360 West Superior Street
Chicago, IL 60610
(312) 664-2344

This nonprofit organization funds research and educates patients, health care professionals, and the public about all aspects of Parkinson's disease. Its referral service can help you locate a physician who specializes in Parkinson's as well as a support group for patients and their families. Personal questions will be answered by the staff. Various helpful, up-to-date, free publications are available upon request, covering topics such as medications, caregiver tips, day care, nursing homes, and legal issues. Also free is a quarterly newsletter.

Professionals Who Work with the Elderly and Their Families

American Dietetic Association
216 West Jackson Boulevard
Suite 800
Chicago, IL 60606
(312) 899-0040

The professional society for registered dietitians. An information specialist will answer questions about health, food, and nutrition and will provide you with a list of registered dietitians in your area. Free publications are available upon request, including several about chronic conditions such as heart disease and diabetes, and the brochure *Guide for Elder Americans*.

American Nurses Association
2420 Pershing Road
Kansas City, MO 64108
(816) 474-5720

A professional society that represents the nation's registered nurses. The ANA sets standards for nurses and educates the public and Congress about the nursing profession. A publications catalogue is available upon request, as well as a list of state associations.

American Occupational Therapy Association, Inc.
P.O. Box 1725
1383 Piccard Drive
Rockville, MD 20849-1725
(301) 948-9626

The national professional organization for therapists who help disabled patients restore their ability to perform daily living skills such as cooking, eating, bathing, dressing, employment, and other activities. Brochures about occupational therapy and a list of state associations are available upon request.

American Physical Therapy Association
1111 North Fairfax Street

Alexandria, VA 22314
(703) 684-2782

A professional organization of physical therapists, who help patients recover from injury, stroke, or other illness by strengthening muscles and improving coordination. A free list of stroke rehabilitation facilities nationwide is available upon request, as well as brochures on the role of physical therapy.

National Association of Private Geriatric Care Managers
655 N. Alvernon Way
Suite 108
Tucson, AZ 85711
(602) 881-8008

An organization of social workers, nurses, and psychologists in private practice who counsel and assist families at any level of caregiving. Call or write for a packet of information and names of managers in your area.

National Association of Social Workers
7981 Eastern Avenue
Silver Spring, MD 20910
(301) 565-0333

A national organization of social workers, who help individuals and their families obtain housing, transportation, meals, health care, counseling, family support, and other social services. They can also provide counseling and case management services to older adults and their families.

National League for Nursing (NLN)
10 Columbus Circle
New York, NY 10019-1350
(212) 989-9393
(800) 669-1656

The NLN works to improve standards of health care. It accredits home health care agencies, nursing homes, and community health programs to ensure that patients receive quality care. Contact the NLN for a list of accredited home health care agencies.

Urinary Tract and Incontinence Problems

American Urological Association
1120 North Charles Street
Baltimore, MD 21201
(301) 727-1100

An association to encourage research on treatment of conditions of the urinary tract. Contact it for names of local board certified urologists.

Continence Restored, Inc.
407 Strawberry Hill
Stamford, CT 06905

This nonprofit organization was set up to establish a network of support groups throughout the country and to disseminate information on incontinence. Upon written request it will provide information on local support groups and direct you to sources of care. A telephone number is included in the mailings they send out.

Help for Incontinent People (HIP)
P.O. Box 544
Union, SC 29379
(803) 579-7900
(800) BLADDER

HIP is a nonprofit advocacy organization for people with urinary incontinence. Its mission is to educate the public and health care professionals about causes, diagnosis, treatment, and management of this problem. Call for information and referral services. Personal questions about incontinence will be answered by mail when accompanied by a long, stamped, self-addressed envelope. A list of publications is available upon request, including the quarterly newsletter *The HIP Report* and a comprehensive guide to continence products and services.

International Association for Enterostomal Therapy
2081 Business Center Drive
Suite 290
Irvine, CA 92715
(714) 476-0268

The IAET is an organization of nurses who specialize in the prevention and treatment of pressure ulcers and the management of incontinence, wounds, and ostomies. You may call for the name of a nurse in your area.

The Simon Foundation for Continence
Box 835
Wilmette, IL 60091
(800) 237-4666

This nonprofit membership organization educates the public and professionals about incontinence and its management. The toll-free number provides information about basic membership ($15 annually). You can also order a free information kit about incontinence issues as well as a copy of *The Informer,* a quarterly magazine for those interested in incontinence control.

Vision

American Academy of Ophthalmology
P.O. Box 7424
San Francisco, CA 94120-7424
(415) 561-8500
(800) 222-EYES (3937) (8 A.M. to 5 P.M. Pacific time)

A professional organization of physicians who specialize in the diagnosis and treatment of eye diseases. The National Eye Care Project has a toll-free information line that will give you names of ophthalmologists nationwide who provide free or low-cost eye care to financially disadvantaged older adults. Publications about common eye diseases affecting those over sixty-five are available upon written request.

American Council of the Blind
1155 15th Street N.W.
Suite 720
Washington, D.C. 20005
(800) 424-8666

The council seeks to improve the lifestyles of those who are blind or visually impaired. The toll-free referral service provides up-to-date information on low-vision devices, treatment, and services. It publishes a variety of free educational materials in large print or audiocassette, including a free bimonthly newsletter *The Braille Forum*. A list of publications is available upon request.

American Foundation for the Blind
15 West 16th Street
New York, NY 10011
(212) 620-2000
(800) 232-5463 (New York State residents call 212-620-2147)

This nonprofit foundation offers services to those who are blind or visually impaired and their families, as well as educational and training programs to educators, health care workers, and other professionals and volunteers who work with them. The toll-free number provides information about blindness and low vision, informative publications and videos, local community services, and low-vision products sold through the foundation. A catalogue of free publications and products is available upon request.

American Optometric Association
243 North Lindbergh Boulevard
St. Louis, MO 63141
(314) 991-4100

The professional organization of optometrists, primary eye care providers who diagnose and treat conditions of the eyes and vision system. Contact them for information about finding a local low-vision specialist. Free written materials are available upon request, including brochures on the low-vision specialty and appropriate eye care in nursing homes.

Lighthouse National Center For Vision and Aging (NCVA)
800 2nd Avenue (temporary location until early 1994)
New York, NY 10017
(800) 334-5497
(212) 808-5544 (TDD)

The NCVA hotline provides information and resources on vision and aging, as well as on the dual loss of vision and hearing. Also provided are referrals to low-vision clinics, rehabilitation services, and support groups nationwide.

National Association for Visually Handicapped (NAVH)
22 West 21st Street
New York, NY 10010
(212) 889-3141

The only nonprofit national organization devoted to those who are not totally blind but who do not have adequate vision, even with the best corrective lenses. NAVH distributes more than 1,600 free titles in large-print book form as well as a large-print newspaper and provides counseling in the use of low-vision aids. Contact NAVH for a kit, including a visual aids catalogue, large-print library catalogue, and listings of low-vision clinics and services in your state.

National Eye Institute
Information Office
Building 31, Room 6A32
Bethesda, MD 20892
(301) 496-5248

The NEI, a section of the National Institutes of Health, is the government's principal agency for funding research and distributing information to health care professionals and the general public about the prevention, detection, treatment, and rehabilitation of eye disorders. A list of brochures is available upon request.

National Society to Prevent Blindness
500 East Remington Road
Schaumburg, IL 60173
(800) 221-3004

The primary mission of this national nonprofit society is to educate the public about preserving sight and preventing blindness. The toll-free information line provides answers to questions, and you can request free written materials on eye diseases, including cataracts, macular degeneration, and glaucoma. An excellent free publication is the family home eye test, which includes a grid test for macular degeneration.

Opticians Association of America
10341 Democracy Lane
P.O. Box 10110
Fairfax, VA 22030
(703) 691-8355

The OAA is a professional association of opticians, who fit, supply, and adjust glasses and contact lenses that have been prescribed by an ophthalmologist or optometrist. It can help you locate a local licensed optician.

Acknowledgments

RESEARCHING AND WRITING A book of the depth and magnitude of *The Caregiver's Guide* has certainly been an arduous, although most gratifying task. I would not have been able to do the job without the help of many kind and dedicated people who work exceedingly hard to dignify the lives of older people.

Janet Reynolds has been a mainstay of the project, and numerous physicians, nurses, social workers, and specialists in the field of aging have shared their knowledge on various topics. Many people whom I did not have the opportunity to contact directly have helped through their contributions to the literature of gerontology and social work. Many family caregivers and older people, especially Katharine Divine, herself in the ninety-five-plus age group, gave me insights into the issues of older people's health concerns and particular needs. It is not possible to name all of those who have contributed to this project; however, certain people have been very generous, and to them I am exceedingly grateful.

First I would like to thank those who gave a great deal of time in extensive interviews and in review of chapters. These people have made sure that all relevant topics are included according to current standards of geriatric and social service practice. Special gratitude goes to Carolyn Robertson, R.N., M.S.N., C.S., clinical specialist in diabetes, New York University Medical Center; Mace Rothenberg, M.D., special assistant for clinical science, Division of Cancer Treatment, National Cancer Institute; Frederic L. Sax, M.D., F.A.C.P., F.A.C.C., assistant professor of medicine, Cornell University Medical College; Anne Smith Young, C.U.T., president of Continence Restored, Inc.; Cynthia Stuen, D.S.W., director of the Lighthouse —

National Center for Vision and Aging; E. Douglas Whitehead, M.D., P.C., assistant clinical professor of urology, Mount Sinai School of Medicine, and director of the Association for Urinary Continence Control, New York City.

Special gratitude also goes to Susanne Fields, M.D., chief of Geriatrics Section, St. Vincent's Hospital and Medical Center, New York City; and Newton Gresser, M.D., chief of the Department of Geriatrics, Hackensack Medical Center in New Jersey.

In addition I want to thank Anne Belcher, R.N., Ph.D., associate professor, University of Maryland School of Nursing; Edna Dunnery, R.N., M.S., orthopedic nurse clinical specialist, St. Vincent's Hospital and Medical Center; Edward Farkas, M.D., geriatric psychiatrist, New York City; Theresa Galsworthy, R.N., coordinator of the Osteoporosis Center, Hospital for Special Surgery, New York City; Margot Harris, program associate in lung disease care and education, American Lung Association; Kathryn Haslanger, senior program adviser, United Hospital Fund; Martha Hill, R.N., Ph.D., associate professor, Johns Hopkins University School of Nursing, and the American Nurses Association representative to the National High Blood Pressure Education Program; David Isralowitz, M.D., geriatrician, Department of Geriatrics, Hackensack Medical Center; Mary Lakaszawski, R.N., clinical enterostomal therapist, St. Vincent's Hospital and Medical Center; Sheree Loftus, M.S.N., C.R.R.N., R.N.C., rehabilitation specialist and coordinator of the Information and Referral Center, American Parkinson's Disease Association; Nancy J. Olins, director of program development, Retired Persons Services, Inc., the AARP Pharmacy Service; Joan Petrlik, R.N., C.R.N.P., nurse specialist in pacemakers, Department of Cardiology, Johns Hopkins Hospital, Baltimore; Peter Podore, M.D., chief of the Division of Vascular Surgery, Jewish Hospital of Cincinnati; Emmanuel Rudd, M.D., emeritus associate professor of clinical medicine, Cornell University Medical College, and rheumatologist, Hospital for Special Surgery, New York City; Vicki Schmall, Ph.D., gerontology specialist, Oregon State University Extension Service, Corvallis; Martin F. Schulman, Ph.D., M.D., ophthalmologist, Hackensack Medical Center and Pascack Valley Hospital, New Jersey; Andrew L. Siegel, M.D., attending physician in urology, Hackensack Medical Center; Joel Zonszein, M.D., F.A.C.P., associate professor of medicine, Albert Einstein College of Medicine, New York City.

Appreciation and thank yous go to Sia Arnason, C.S.W., co-director of the Institute on Law and Rights of Older Adults, Brookdale Center on Aging, Hunter College, New York City; Wendy Avery-Smith, M.S., O.T.R., coordinator of the Swallowing Team, New York Hospital–Cornell Medical Center; Elizabeth Barret Connor, M.D., professor of community family medicine, University of California, San Diego; Rona Bartlestone, A.G.S.W., L.G.S.W., president, Rona Bartlestone Associates, Inc.; Amanda Barusch, D.S.W., chair of Gerontology Emphasis, University of Utah; Morton Bogdonoff, M.D., director of clinical geriatrics, New York Hospital–Cornell Medical Center; Barbara Bohny, D.N.S., R.N.C.S., gerontological clinical specialist, assistant director of nursing for long-term care, Bergen Pines Hospital; Michele Brandenberg, R.N., hospice nurse, Hackensack Medical Center; Lawrence Brandt, M.D., professor of medicine, Albert Einstein College of Medicine, and director of the Division of Gastroenterology, Montefiore Medical Center, New York City; Sarah Greene Burger, R.N., M.P.H., gerontological nurse consultant, National Citizens Coalition for Nursing Home Reform; Diane Burnett, R.N., M.S.N., cardiovascular surgery clinical specialist, Johns Hopkins Hospital; Dorothy Colvani, R.N., G.N.P., geriatric nurse clinician, Department of Geriatrics, Mount Sinai Medical Center; Rita Considine, R.N., M.S.N., cardiovascular clinical nurse specialist, Lenox Hill Hospital, New York City; John Coppola, M.D., head of the Department of Cardiology, St. Vincent's Hospital and Medical Center; John Cornwall, M.D., assistant attending in medicine, St. Luke's Roosevelt Hospital Center, New York City; Cathy Custer, R.N., M.S.N., clinical nurse specialist, Department of Surgery, Johns Hopkins Hospital; Noreen Daly, R.N., B.S.N., oncology public health nurse, St. Luke's Roosevelt Hospital Center; Barbara Dashow, M.S., C.D.E., board of directors of the New York Diabetes Association; Dennis Desilvey, M.D., assistant clinical professor of medicine, University of Vermont School of Medicine; Denise DeSylvia, O.D., director of clinical services, Optometric Institute and Clinic of Detroit; Gregory Disanto, O.D., assistant clinical professor, State University of New York College of Optometry; Andrew Drexler, M.D., clinical assistant professor of medicine, New York University Diabetes Complications Center; Rose Dubroff, D.S.W., director, Brookdale Center on Aging, Hunter College; Lawrence Fishberg, Ph.D., geriatric consultant, New York City; Jerry Flegg, M.D., cardiovascular and senior investigator, National Institute of Aging; Hal Freiman, M.D., attending gastroenterologist,

St. Vincent's Hospital and Medical Center; Rose Gerber, R.N., Ph.D., associate professor, University of Arizona College of Nursing; Gary Gerstenblith, M.D., associate professor of medicine, Johns Hopkins University School of Medicine; Marylyn Gilbreath, O.D., chief, Low Vision Rehabilitation Services, Optometric Center of Fullerton; Lou Glasse, president, Older Women's League; Dorothy Goldstein, M.S., director of medical affairs, New York chapter of the Arthritis Foundation; Andrew Guccione, Ph.D., P.T., assistant professor, Department of Physical Therapy, Boston University; Sol Gussberg, M.D., past president emeritus, American Cancer Society; Rebecca Hahn, M.D., instructor in medicine, Cornell University Medical College; Cathy Handy, R.N., M.A., oncology nurse clinical specialist, St. Vincent's Hospital and Medical Center; Ada Sue Hinshaw, R.N., Ph.D., director, National Center for Nursing Research; Andrew Hoffer, National Association of Families Caring for Their Elders; Ira Jacobsen, M.D., assistant professor of medicine, Cornell University Medical College; Katharine Jeter, Ed.D., E.T., director, Help for Incontinent People; Adrienne Karp, M.A., consulting audiologist, the Lighthouse and Helen Keller Services for the Blind; Sharon Keigher, Ph.D., assistant professor, University of Michigan School of Social Work; Christen Kerr, M.D., assistant professor of psychiatry, Psychiatric Day Treatment Center, Georgetown University Medical Center; Paul Kleyman, editor, *Aging Today;* Rita LaMell, A.C.S.W., Geriatric Assessment Program, Hackensack Medical Center; Barry D. Lebowitz, Ph.D., chief, Mental Disorders of Aging, National Institute of Mental Health; Helen Sloss Luey, L.C.S.W., communication specialist, University of California, San Francisco; Michele LeNoir Palamountain, R.N., M.A., clinical liaison nurse, Pain Management Program, St. Luke's Roosevelt Hospital Center; Jackie Luke, Pharm.D., critical care specialist, Pharmacy Department, Hackensack Medical Center; Susan Massatelli, R.N., director of patient services, New York Hospital–Cornell Medical Center; Mary Ellen McCann, R.N., M.A., coronary health and stress counselor, New York City; Mary McDonald, R.N., M.S., National Heart, Blood, and Lung Institute Support Contract; Cindy K. Merkel, R.N., M.A., C.N.R.N., clinical neurology and neurosurgery nurse specialist, St. Vincent's Hospital and Medical Center; Sheila Merolla, M.S.W., A.C.S.W., director of Self-Help Program, Morningside Health and Retirement Services; Paul Miskovitz, M.D., associate professor of clinical medicine, Cornell University Medical College; Charles

Nechemias, M.D., assistant clinical professor of medicine and assistant attending physician for diabetes, Mount Sinai School of Medicine; Jeffrey Nichols, M.D., director, Frances Schervier Home, Riverdale, New York; Leonie Nowitz, M.S.W., A.C.S.W., director, Center for Lifelong Growth, New York City; Guy Renvoize, M.D., attending physician in gastroenterology, St. Luke's Roosevelt Hospital Center; John Richardson, D.P.M., attending podiatrist, St. Vincent's Hospital and Medical Center; Richard Rosenbluth, M.D., chief of oncology, Hackensack Medical Center; Joseph T. Ruggiero, M.D., professor of medicine in Hematology-Oncology, Cornell University Medical College; Virginia Schiaffino, executive director, National Federation of Interfaith Caregivers; Craig Smith, M.D., assistant professor of surgery, Columbia University Medical School; Carole Smyth, R.N.C., A.N.P., nurse practitioner and clinical associate in the Division of Geriatrics, Montefiore Medical Center; Alan G. Snart, M.D., chief of the Medical Vascular Department, New York Hospital, and assistant professor, Cornell University Medical College; Thomas Spicuzza, A.C.S.W., Geriatric Consultation Program, St. Vincent's Hospital and Medical Center; Joseph Stillman, M.C.P., partner, the Conservation Company; Sunny Sutton, R.N., senior vice president of Medicare Services, Kimberly Quality Care; Sharon Tennfredt, R.N., Ph.D., project director, Massachusetts Elder Health Project, and senior research scientist, New England Research Institute; Margaret Tietz, R.N.C., M.S.N., nursing home educator, Center for Nursing Care, Jamaica, New York; David Turner, M.Ed., program manager, Salt Lake County Aging Services; Judith Tyler, M.A., R.N., assistant director of educational resources, *American Journal of Nursing;* Jeanette Vaughan, R.N., president, Age View, Inc.; Barbara Ventura, R.N., administrative clinical assistant in cardiology, Montefiore Medical Center; Annette Warpheha, R.D., nutrition consultant, New York City; Barbara Weinstein, Ph.D., associate professor, Lehman College, City University of New York; Myron Weisfeld, M.D., president and director, American Heart Association; Ann Williams, health and science editor, American Heart Association; Mark Williams, M.D., director, Program on Aging, University of North Carolina at Chapel Hill; T. Franklin Williams, M.D., director, National Institute on Aging, National Institutes Of Health; Judy Wingate, R.N., nurse clinician, Osteoporosis Center, Hospital for Special Surgery; Catherine Wondolowski, R.N., M.Ed., project director, Gerontological Nurse Practitioner Program, Hunter Bellevue School of Nursing, City University of New York; Anna Zimmer, A.C.S.W., director of the Institute on Mental Aid and Self-Help, Brookdale Center on Aging; Michael A. Zullo, M.D., associate professor of clinical medicine, Cornell University Medical College.

I am especially indebted to three friends who helped with the production of the book: Francis Greenburger, Bill Friedman, and Kittsie Watterson. Also to Ruth Nivola, a grandmother and a great friend of my husband's parents, who contributed most of all her wisdom and encouragement, as well as the beautiful workroom in her garden during my summers in Easthampton.

This book would never have come to be without Ruth Hapgood, senior editor at Houghton Mifflin Company. Her enthusiasm to publish the project kept it going, and she has shepherded it through all its various stages, showing me kindness and respect for the time and care it needed. Jane Dystel, of Acton Dystel Literary and Dramatic Management, must be thanked for believing in the project from its very beginning.

Acknowledgments are not complete without a particular thank you to Tom Reynolds, Janet's husband, and their daughter, Sarah, who gave support to the project, and to Janet, over its long haul.

Caroline Rob
New York City

Index

Note: Page numbers in *italic* indicate resource addresses.